Finalist, Gay Memoir/Biography
Lambda Literary Award

"A remarkable collection of hard-earned, melancholic wisdom. Currier is a masterful essayist, adept at lingering over a meaningful detail or capturing a complex emotion in a simple phrase."
—*Kirkus Reviews*

"A wealth of wisdom about our collective past can be found within our personal stories when they are told with such humility, humor, and profound introspection."
—*Chelsea Station*

"Achingly poignant and full of humor. Currier addresses topics familiar to gay men—sex and the search thereof, love and relationships, AIDS and loss—all rendered in vivid details that ring with the clarity of Truth."
—*Art & Understanding*

Until My Heart Stops

intimate writings by Jameson Currier

Until My Heart Stops assembles more than fifty works of nonfiction written by the author over four decades, including many published during the height of the AIDS epidemic. The result is a searing and poignant memoir of an artist finding his voice during difficult times. Once again Currier doesn't shy away from revealing personal moments and emotions, this time his own, including his love and retreat from the theater, his grappling with boyfriends and long-term relationships, and the details into his own medical diagnosis of HCM—hypertrophic cardiomyopathy, a condition of excessive thickening of the heart muscle for which there is no apparent cause or cure.

"Currier is adept at drawing a fine line between the erotic and the tragic, and at telling stories that 'although personal, are also the stories of our community.'"
—*The New York Times Book Review*

"A writer who consistently surprises and delights, Currier's dynamism will surely carry his literary career to higher heights."
—*Bay Area Reporter*

"The breadth of Currier's personal experience is evident in his writing, which is moving without resorting to melodrama, familiar without feeling clichéd."
—*Windy City Times*

Also by Jameson Currier

A Gathering Storm

Based on a True Story

Dancing on the Moon: Short Stories about AIDS

Desire, Lust, Passion, Sex

Still Dancing: New and Selected Stories

The Forever Marathon

The Haunted Heart and Other Tales

The Third Buddha

The Wolf at the Door

What Comes Around

Where the Rainbow Ends

Until My Heart Stops

intimate writings

Jameson Currier

Chelsea Station Editions
New York

Until My Heart Stops
by Jameson Currier

Copyright © 2015 by Jameson Currier.

All rights reserved.

No part of this book may be reproduced in any form without written permission from the publisher, except by a reviewer, who may quote brief passages in a review where appropriate credit is given; nor may any part of this book be reproduced, stored in a retrieval system, or transmitted in any form or by any means—electronic, photocopying, recording, or other—without specific written permission from the publisher.

In some cases factual names and details have been altered or fictionally created as composites in order to shadow a specific person. In other cases, the author has relied on artistic license for thematic or narrative intent.

Book design by Peachboy Distillery & Designs
Cover art by Patrick Bremer

Published by Chelsea Station Editions:
362 West 36th Street, Suite 2R
New York, NY 10018
www.chelseastationeditions.com
info@chelseastationeditions.com

Limited edition hardcover: 978-1-937627-14-0
Paperback ISBN: 978-1-937627-17-1
Ebook ISBN: 978-1-937627-64-5
Library of Congress Control Number: 2015951908

Contents

Until My Heart Stops	9
What She Gave Me	12
Stages	25
Hometown Sweethearts	36
On A Day I Am Not Myself	66
Actors	68
July	73
Passing Grades	84
Invitation to Dance	89
The Last Minute Friend	93
Rock Hudson's Vacation	107
Isn't It Romantic?	120
Threads	124
Why I Live Where I Do	134
Haircuts	139
Desperado	143
Caution	146
Something from the Rain	152
Between the Lines	154
How Does My Garden Grow?	156
Dates	160
The Child in Me	164
The Right Man	168
One Way or Another	172
Just Looking	175
Friends	182
That Summer	187
Finding New Hope	190
Behind the Screen	196

Where You'll Find Me	199
Strength	202
Old Things	205
What Comes Around	208
Still Dancing	215
Excerpts from a Stonewall Diary	220
Funny Guy	240
It	248
Treats	251
Art History 101	254
Dicks	263
Lessons	266
Glasses	279
The Pot	282
Writers	290
A Personal History of the Epidemic	295
Magic Carpet Ride	299
Buddies	303
Remnants	317
A Few Minutes with Liberace	321
Twilight on the Esplanade	327
What Did Not Change	354
Do I Know You?	359
Lovers	363
My Haunted History	371
A Bookstore Tourist	384
A Gathering Storm	387
Hearts	391
The House of Ten Thousand Temperatures	394
Fifteen Minutes More	414

Until My Heart Stops

UNTIL MY HEART STOPS

By the time you read this introduction I will have reached the age of sixty. As long as I have been writing I have wanted to publish a collection of my nonfiction, but throughout my writing career I have tread a thin line between what is fact and what is fiction in my work, often using details from my own life to flesh out those of my fictional characters and sometimes using narrative creativity to embellish the point of my own life in an essay. In some cases I have published a story as both fiction and nonfiction. What you have here is no different, though this collection of stories leans as close as I may come to publishing a memoir. As is stated on the copyright page in some cases factual names and details have been altered or fictionally created as composites in order to shadow a specific person. In other cases, I have relied on artistic license for thematic or narrative intent. But the truth remains behind why I write and what I write: I write to understand my own life better and to comprehend my place in the world.

The earliest written work included in this collection was created in the early 1980s as I was experimenting with subjects and expressions. I'm not a graduate of an academic writing program; I found my voice one word at a time, often by trial and error, and often as self-therapy. Much of the tone of this collection owes birth to the short essays I created for a column for a men's magazine in the late 1980s, and since then, this collection has expanded as my career and relationships evolved. I've organized the order of these selections by a chronology that mirrors the main events they cover. One obstacle of being both the author and publisher of a collection of writing whose contents were created over the course of four decades is the ability to self-edit. Because many of these works were created during different parts of my writing career, influenced by certain individuals and events, and sometimes tailored for specific outlets, you may notice some repetitiveness in these tales, though my hope is that you will appreciate the impact the detail has had on the storyteller's life. This is not an exhaustive collection of my nonfiction, nor is it the only collection of nonfiction that I hope to write, assemble, or publish. It is neither a comprehensive depiction of my life nor an all-inclusive examination of my writing career.

I've subtitled this collection as intimate writings, relying on the definition of the word "intimate" as revealing something that is private and personal. The main topics of these intimacies revolve around being both a gay man and a writer, among them sex, dating, romance, relationships, love, friendships, family, health, AIDS, loss, self-acceptance, coming out, and change, not necessarily in that order.

I do not maintain an ongoing daily diary, and as I assembled material for this collection I realized that I had not written about many key moments in my life. I've published little work that relates to my boyhood, what it was like to grow up in the mid-twentieth century suburbia in the South with unexpected detours to Los Angeles, London, and upstate New York. I've left out the amusing failures at my first jobs in Georgia as a zookeeper at an amusement park and as a paint salesman in the hardware section of a large department store. I have not included details of many of the remarkable places I have been fortunate to visit: Italy, Japan, and a summer behind the Iron Curtain. I have not included any of the numerous reviews I have published on gay literature, or the interviews I have conducted with other gay writers or members of the HIV community. And I have not written of many family issues, including the long illness my mother suffered before her passing last year.

Sometime after the attacks on the World Trade Center on September 11, 2001, the trajectory of my writing career changed. The opportunities to contribute book reviews on gay and AIDS literature to many newspapers and magazines disappeared. The market for writings about the impact of AIDS and HIV shrank. Gay literature became a niche market. But I also stopped examining myself and my life so thoroughly and began to examine the place of gay men in the world, with a particular focus on the crimes and injustices committed against us as individuals or as a community. As I also settled into a full-time job during these years, a job that was not devoted to my career as a writer, my time to write became more limited. But my day job allowed me to pay down the years of debt I had amassed trying to become a writer, provided me with health insurance, and offered me the opportunity to travel.

And I am keenly aware of how change has occurred since I began writing and publishing in the 1980s. It's easy to chart that in the progress of technology with the mere availability of an e-book edition of one's work, but gratefully, it is also as easy to recognize it today in the growing cultural acceptance of gay lives, thanks to the many efforts of activists and, most recently, the decision of the Supreme Court to legalize same-sex marriages.

But what hasn't changed is how important writing is to me, how important reading is to the shape and direction of one's life, how important it is to find yourself in the pages of your own writing or within someone else's work. I know I've certainly become more sentimental about this as I have aged. Perhaps that is the root of why this particular collection has been so hard for me to release out into the world. I am convinced my heart is on every page.

Jameson Currier
October 2015

WHAT SHE GAVE ME

On my twenty-fifth birthday my mother explained to me how I was born. We were sitting in the kitchen of the house where she had lived for seventeen years, the house I had grown up in, a two-story suburban ranch kind with a half-acre of land in the back yard and the swing set still standing but now dented and rusty. I had come to visit her in Atlanta for the weekend, a stopover on my way home to New York City from a vacation in Fort Lauderdale. My mother, once a slender, breezy Southern woman, now reminded me more of my grandmother: round and pudgy with curly, cottony white hair and silver wire rim eyeglasses. She had finished her morning cup of coffee and was now opening cabinets and the refrigerator, withdrawing flour, eggs, measuring spoons, milk—all the ingredients she needed to bake a cake from scratch. "Your favorite," she said in that light drawl of hers which could stretch the syllables of any word into a sentence. "Pineapple upside-down," she announced proudly, as though it were a secret. "Because it's your birthday."

She stopped and retrieved a large mixing bowl from the cabinet beneath the kitchen counter and as she straightened herself up, her face flushed and she let out a tiny giggle. "I never told you this," she began, "but one weekend when I was about seven, no, I guess seven-and-a-half months pregnant with you, your father took me along with his scout troop to Red Top Mountain. They were all camping out by the creek, but your daddy had made me stay in one of the cabins by the Information Center. Well, they all got up early to hike to the top of Red Top and help the forestry service put markers on a new path, and I was to meet them later that night back at their campsite. I woke up early and got so bored sitting around and walking back and forth to the stream that I decided I would walk up the main road and meet them at the observation point at the top. Red Top really isn't a big mountain, you know.

"Well, it started getting hot. It turned real fast into one of those awful hazy, humid Indian summer days when you just can't breathe, and here I was walking up this windy road that was just all dirt and sand and gravel and, you know, it just wasn't fun. I hadn't brought anything along to eat or drink and by the time I got just half way up I was exhausted. So I sat down and right then a pickup truck comes down from the top of the mountain and the driver stopped when he saw me by the side of the road. This old farmer opened the door and asked me if I was okay and I said yeah, but just a little hot, and then he asked me if I wanted a ride back down to the Information Center. I said sure, because I thought at least I was tired enough now to take a nap. Well, down we went on that bumpy road and that truck—which must have been made before they invented shock absorbers—just kept going bump-de-bump-de-bump all the way down. That road seemed endless. By the time we reached the Center I had gone into labor. Thank God that old man had sense enough to stick around and take me to the hospital.

"You were less than five pounds when you were born," she smiled. "Four pounds, eleven and three-quarters ounces to be exact," she said, opening the top of the package of flour and placing the measuring cup on the counter space in front of her. "You were a preemie," she added. "We were really worried about you."

As I walked out of the kitchen and up the stairs to my old bedroom I realized I found my mother's story humorous, part of some Southern Gothic charm I had always invented about her and my family, and for a while I retold the story of how I was born to my friends in Manhattan, at a party or at a bar or when I was out on a date. I tried to use it to explain a lot about me—why I never wanted to live in the South, how the mere smell of dirt sent me rushing toward civilization. I used it to rationalize why I always wanted to get out of suburbia, moving away from quirky, middle-class-All-American-too-Christian parents. I joked that it accounted for my determination to provide myself with a college education, and how I used that education to find employment in New York City. I felt it answered why I sometimes became compulsively neat: cleaning, washing, filing, sorting. And I thought it explained why I preferred to read a book instead of going camping or hiking or anywhere that meant following a dusty, rocky path. My mother had, after all these years, given me the reason for my own quirkiness.

* * *

Not long after I heard my mother's story, I had an operation to repair an inguinal hernia. I'd spent a few years working out, trying to put my body in better shape, only to wake one hot July morning with a swelling in my groin so severe I could not bear to even wear cotton briefs. I'd never been an athletic child—a season on a little league baseball team as an outfielder (where the ball seldom appeared) and an attempt at intramural basketball in high school (where I never saw the ball, either, due to being shorter than the other players)—and my attempt to transform my physique into something other than its scrawny frame had clearly backfired in a way I hadn't expected. My doctor wasn't at all convinced that it was entirely due to straining too hard with heavy weights at the gym, and offered another possibility, that the hernia could have been present since birth. Whatever its cause, I lived through the operation and a painful six-week recuperation period just as I had such childhood illnesses and accidents such as tonsillitis, chicken pox, measles, and a broken arm. To assuage my mother's concern over the operation—which involved spinal anesthesia—and to amend her fear that my hernia could be hereditary—I flew down South to have the operation, staying a few days at her home before flying back to Manhattan.

It wasn't long after that that I began feeling my vision changing. I had been working long hours as a theatrical publicist, reading small print newspapers for tearsheets for clients, and fighting off severe headaches which I had attributed, at first, to on-the-job stress. One evening as I made my way through Times Square to deliver some tickets and press releases, I noticed that my long range vision was blurring. Through a friend, I found the name of an ophthalmologist in the West Village near my apartment.

I'd worn eyeglasses for reading since a child, been diagnosed with astigmatism, and had spent a year of adolescence doing a series of exercises of looking through hand-held prisms to strengthen the muscles of my left eye. (I had been diagnosed with a "wandering eye" as a boy—something which sounds now as an adult as so unnecessary to want to correct.) At the back of my mind was the idea that because of technological advances in the making of contact lenses, I could get soft lenses which might change my green eyes to blue.

The doctor, a stocky, handsome man in his late thirties with deep brown eyes, gave me a stronger reading prescription and then said it was impossible for me to wear contact lenses because I had unusually large cataracts for my age growing in my eyes. I wasn't alarmed by the news, but found it strange that this had never been detected before, and I agreed to return in six weeks in order for the doctor to measure the growth of the cataracts. In the interim I discussed my diagnosis with friends and coworkers who urged me to seek a second opinion. Instead, I decided to return to the doctor for a second measurement and I would decide on a second opinion after that appointment— once I had learned exactly how severely these cataracts were growing. When I arrived to see the ophthalmologist for the second appointment, the doorman of the building where his office was located told me that the doctor had moved and had not left a forwarding address.

This news took me by surprise and I walked to the corner and then walked back to the building, wondering if I had made a mistake about the location. I asked the doorman again about the doctor—I had only been there a few weeks before—and told him that there had been no contact with me about the office closing. Then came his response, "He wasn't well, you know." As I left, thinking I could locate his office via the phone book, I remembered there had been some fumbling during my first appointment about whether or not I had shown up on the right date.

And then I heard through my friend who had recommended the ophthalmologist that the doctor had died. I went to another ophthalmologist—this one recommended through a coworker—who said I had not a single cataract and I ordered tinted contacts. But the story doesn't end there. Not long after that first eye doctor died, I also went to visit my general physician to take an HIV test for the first time. This was a period in the mid-1980s when every little skin blemish and bug bite and unexplained bruise was causing me considerable worry. As my doctor listened to my heightened panic over sexual partners who were ill and the story of a coworker who had died, before withdrawing my blood, he tested my blood pressure, my reflexes, my breathing, and my heart beat and determined that I had a heart murmur.

"It's not a cause for alarm at this point," he said. "But I'd like you to go for some tests so that we can measure it against future readings." He explained that a murmur is usually the result of an irregular flow of blood through the heart and it rarely affects the overall health. I answered a few questions about my general health and the health of my family members, and somewhere in the doctor's explanation, there was a hint of a possibility that my heart murmur could have underlying hereditary causes.

A few days later I arrived at a cardiology clinic on Madison Avenue and, at the age of twenty-nine, was subjected to a series of pulmonary function and exercise tolerance tests that were also being administered that day to a seventy-three year-old man—walking on a treadmill strapped with wires and plugs and bands attached to different points of my body. After the exams were over—(and I was told nothing of their diagnosis;

the reports were to be sent to my doctor)—as I was waiting for the elevator to leave the clinic, I had a premonition of my own death, that if I was lucky enough to survive the AIDS epidemic, then I most likely would die of a heart attack. I never went back to that facility for other measurements. Instead, life intruded: My job consumed my energy, and my murmur receded into the subconscious of my mind, and I began to find myself among a growing number of friends and coworkers who were testing HIV-positive and growing ill, while learning that I, myself, had thus far escaped the virus.

Months later, fighting off a bout of stress which landed in a spot beneath my right shoulder blade, I went to a chiropractor who had been recommended by an actor I was dating. Like the optometrist, the chiropractor was a darkly attractive fellow. I undressed and he went through his inspection of my body, answering his questions as he manipulated muscle groups around my back, neck, and legs. At the end of the examination, he told me that my spine was crooked and that I would need several follow-up appointments to begin to correct it. Instead of returning to him, I went back to my general physician and asked for anti-depressants.

Over the years as I have moved from apartment to apartment and changed physicians with different jobs and different health insurance plans, I have learned to tell my doctors about my heart murmur. Every single one has become alarmed by it; over the last two decades I have ended up in clinics from Beth Israel Hospital to Cornell Medical Center to be measured and monitored, testing the strength of my heart through noninvasive cardiology exams such as electrocardiograms, MRIs, and ultrasound echocardiographs, only to be thanked for my time and sent on my way. I sense that some day down the road that I will be presented with bad news: a decision between surgery or death. But as for now at the age that I am writing this, forty-four, other than recommendations for antibiotics when I had some dental work done, my heart has not interfered with my day-to-day life. I have used it and abused it as well as ringing it emotionally dry, from living in a fifth-floor walk-up that always left me panting for breath to breaking up with a boyfriend and dropping to an alarmingly thin shell of myself after subsiding for weeks on nothing but anti-depressants and booze.

* * *

I was raised as a Southern Methodist and though my parents were not strict, certain things were simply not discussed. Even though it was the era of free love, inside our home sexual matters were hidden, suppressed, or not talked about at all. We were made to go to church every Sunday—Sunday school and worship services following, and brought back again in the evenings, for choir practices and youth fellowship groups. My parents set out to raise their children via an accepted standard version of morals, a belief in honesty, freedom, and trust, instilling their offspring with equal portions of politeness and guilt. But by the age of thirteen I knew I was different from my parents, detached by some other schism than the separation of generations. I became aware that I was attracted to men; I began studying them carefully, the way the sweat formed on my father as he mowed the yard bare-chested, the way dark hair wrapped around my band instructor's wrists, the way the older boys at school touched themselves as they showered in the locker room. I started locking myself in my bedroom, staring at the pictures of athletes in magazines, memorizing the firmness and energy of their bodies, fantasizing they were next to me, touching me, wanting me, needing me. I read every book I could find on sex, even the ones my parents kept hidden in my father's workroom in the basement, alarmed and even more confused by the descriptions of homosexuality as a deviation and a perversion.

Almost every gay man can list certain pinpoints of recognition on their trajectory toward gay self-identification, even if he hadn't admitted the possibility to himself at that period in his life; in retrospect, it's clear that it was a moment of gay awareness. The signs are obvious to me now that this happened to me long before I left the South for Manhattan. I remember at the age of fourteen comparing definitions of homosexuality in the different dictionaries of my library. Even earlier I recall a boyish fascination for comic book superheroes morphing into a sweating discomfort while watching Hercules movies.

Growing up in the South I felt only my difference from my family and others. I wanted to change the way I talked, the way I thought, and the people around me into different persons. Yet one thing a gay Southern boy learns early on is to keep his difference to himself or face ridicule. I flattened my accent, hid my desire to be campy, and set about constructing my life into two camps: those who might be gay or sympathetic, and those who most definitely were not. Because of their narrow religious view, my parents were part of the latter group in my mind, and I began to withdraw from them in regards to my life.

There were many years as an adult when I disregarded my parents, presuming geographical distance would keep us out of each other's thoughts, believing any discussion of my life would make them embarrassed, ashamed, or unable to accept and understand. Parents, of course, do not want their children to be different from themselves. But the truth is I could not shake the imprints that they had left on me, both mental and physical. Even now, every day in front of the bathroom mirror, I notice my father's face and hairline, and the skin of my body, the translucent color of my mother's complexion, has become a patchwork of blue veins so close to the surface they resemble the tattoo of a roadmap.

Even though she had been there for visits to see her sister—my aunt—my mother hated and feared New York City; she had gathered enough suspicion of the city simply from watching the nightly news. When I settled there the year after I graduated college, she was worried I would starve, that the building where I lived would burn down, or that I would be mugged late at night while waiting for the subway. Early on, right after I had moved to Manhattan, we spoke every Sunday on the phone and after quizzing me about my job, my furniture, my friends, what I had eaten for dinner the night before, her voice would take on the petite, Southern belle quality that I knew was the end of our conversation. "Why don't you come home and live?" she would ask. I would answer with something like "Not yet," or "I can't," or "I'm not ready," never what I was really thinking, what I really felt was the truth but was too impolite for a Southern man to express, that where she was, where she lived, was not my home anymore.

I never told my mother many things about my life in New York; many details I knew would upset her. I told her about the jobs I had, what the city looked like, how the weather was, and how I wanted to furnish the apartment where I lived. I remember telling her about the apartment I shared on Bleecker Street, a top story walk-up with a floor so lopsided in the kitchen that we had to wedge a piece of wood underneath the refrigerator to keep it from rolling against the front door. But I never told her that one night, after a heavy rain, as I brushed my teeth before going to sleep, the plaster ceiling collapsed on top of my bed and had I been there, in the bed asleep, I would now be dead.

But I did tell her about the new friends I was making and a few of the things we did together. I told her about going to the movies and plays, and trips to the beach or Atlantic City or Boston or the Hamptons. At first she used to ask me if I had met any nice girls, then one Sunday I noticed the question had stopped, maybe she realized something in the fact that most of my friends were male. My decision at that point in my life not to tell her I preferred to sleep with men was not because I was ashamed of my life, it was that there was nothing in the stating of the fact which would serve any purpose to either one of us; it would not change our relationship, she was my mother and I was her son, we loved each other, and she was there and I was here. I didn't tell her that the true reason why I left home was not so much to pursue a graduate degree at New York University but to openly explore gay life in the West Village without any parental intrusion. Such things were not really necessary for a parent to know about their child.

And I never told my mother about the incident after a party at a restaurant near Times Square. As I exited the building a man tried to rob the woman I was with of her purse. I yelled to distract both the victim and her assailant, and as I reached out to prevent him from grabbing my friend's purse, his arm changed direction and his fist socked me in the eye. The next time I saw my mother, six months later, she noticed the scar above my left eyebrow. I said I had fallen in my apartment, tripped over the phone cord and hit my head against the side of my bedroom bureau. I told her it was nothing; it only looked worse than it really was.

And as the years went by I held more and more things back from my mother. I didn't tell her about the friends who were dying, or the ones I was taking care of, hoping that they would survive. I never told her about the married man I dated who took me on an expensive trip to Palm Springs, never told her, either, of the time I was threatened with losing a theatrical job when it was discovered I was having an affair with a member of the cast. I never told my mother about the time I returned to Atlanta on business because I wanted to spend my evenings checking out the gay club scene I had heard about for so many years but had never fully experienced; never told her about the trip to Chicago I made to see a musical I had written performed because I was sleeping with the composer. I never told her, either, that I, like her father, have, as the years progressed, developed a "tendency to imbibe too much." Once, when I returned home to attend my niece's wedding, I brought with me my own bottle of wine, hiding it in my suitcase and drinking in my bedroom after the rest of the household was asleep. Another time, during a period when I was a cigarette smoker, I excused myself to do errands in the car in order to smoke and not be seen by my mother. My parents never approved of these habits in my older brother and younger sisters, and even before I had come out as gay to them, I had enough facts on my side to weigh in their disapproval of the way I was living my life.

And I never told her about the cataracts, my back problem, and certainly nothing about my heart murmur. Once, when she visited me in Pennsylvania where I was living at the time, she mentioned that I looked unhappy and distracted. It would be another year before I would summon up the courage to let her know I was gay and what she didn't know then was that I had just ended an unhappy affair with a man. She twisted her hands together and said, "You know, honey, you can tell me anything you want." And I sensed then that perhaps she understood more about my life than I wished her to know. For in the next breath she asked me about my health; mothers possess instincts their children spend years trying to comprehend. At the time I was only suffering from depression and trying to stop smoking, in order to give my life some sense of a different direction. But I opted not to discuss this with her. I had learned from my father that there are things a Southern gentleman simply does not talk about with a Southern woman, particularly his mother. (At the time my father was battling prostate cancer—and even between father and son, the discussion of its progress was limited to simple phrases, "Doin' fine" and "Doc says there's hope.")

This never prevented my mother from telling me stories about her own illnesses—her arthritis, her hiatus hernia, and her trips to the dermatologist at age seventy-one to remove deposits which had blemished her forehead—or the illnesses my grandmother suffered—my mother's mother—the memory loss of Alzheimer's, the hip replacement while in the nursing home, a second stroke which left her immobile. My mother felt that by telling her stories—filling up the empty spaces between us with sound—that she was re-connecting us as we had been years before as mother and infant son, and, in a way, she did. The last time I saw her—a weekend in the Poconos while my father searched for his genealogical roots in the area—she talked incessantly about the irritation her metal jewelry was causing to her skin. A watch she had worn on the drive north had made the area of her wrist break out into red welts which had crusted over after she had applied a cortisone crème. I had arrived at the lodge where they were staying with a cold which had progressively gotten worse during my stay with them, so bad, in fact, that I had become worried about it transforming into something more serious. It was a beautiful fall weekend—sunny and cool, and the maples, oaks, and hickory trees were full of orange, yellow, and red leaves which had transformed the mountainside into tufts of color. But this was the second serious cold I had suffered in the space of two months and I had admitted that fact to my mother upon my arrival. All I wanted was to stay inside, lie on the couch, sleep or watch TV, and get better. My mother twisted her hands nervously and urged me to eat or drink something every few minutes. "I hope none of this is my fault," she said, when I had drained another glass of orange juice.

"Why? What do you mean?" I asked.

"You being so sickly," she said.

"I'm not sickly," I answered defensively. "I'm just sick."

"You were such a sickly baby," she said. "You got all the stuff babies get right on cue."

"So that hardly makes it unusual," I said.

"I never told you this," she added. "But we didn't expect you to live when you were born. You were so tiny—we were all so worried." Her eyes had taken on a wet, ashamed look and she tilted her heavy body forward in the chair as she spoke in a soft tone so that my father, napping in the other room, could not possibly hear.

"You had to stay at the hospital for something like two weeks in an incubator," she said. "Your daddy went to visit you every day, but I had your brother at home to take care of and I couldn't always make it there, and I was so worried about you. I was so just worried about you not making it and my not being there for you. So we convinced the hospital to install an incubator at the house. It was the first time they had ever done it. They set it up in the living room. We had to rearrange everything. A nurse came out and stayed over at the house to make sure it went okay." She leaned back, pleased with herself, and she lifted the corner of her lip into a crooked smile that I clearly recognized as one I have also inherited.

"You were so, so tiny," she added. "All I wanted to do was to hold you but the doctors wouldn't let me. So when no one was around I would lift you up out of that stupid glass box and hold you in my arms. I think it made you want to live. I didn't care what any of those silly doctors said; it didn't hurt you, did it? I didn't I hurt you, did I, honey? You're not damaged goods."

Of course I didn't respond to this. It's impossible to say if my mother did any damage. As far as I am concerned, in comparison with other gay men of my generation, my own health travails—my heart murmur included—play simply like minor skin irritations. And as for affairs of the heart, most have been of my own doing and undoing. But the older I become the clearer it is to me that my parents provided me with a basic education in survival and faith, passing along a few genetic traits in the mix as well. I now understand how my mother felt standing over that glass incubator looking at her child struggling to live in a small, enclosed glass box. She not only gave me life, but she also passed along a will to help and hold someone in their arms, something I've been hoping to find since the day I left home.

STAGES

I must confess now that I was a rather serious child. I was serious about minding my parents, serious about looking both ways before crossing the street, serious about mittens and mufflers and galoshes and raincoats in inclement weather. I was serious about keeping my hair combed, my fingernails cleaned, my clothes off the floor, and my bed made every morning. I was also a serious student, my head stuck in an encyclopedia or locked in my room reading *Dr. Doolittle* or *Treasure Island*, turning in perfect penmanship papers and math homework without eraser smudges.

From the moment I learned about Broadway musicals, however, my world changed. The summer I was eight years old my father took our family to see *The Unsinkable Molly Brown* at the outdoor amphitheater in Atlanta. The production was one of those rickety semi-professional touring summer stock let's-throw-together-a-moneymaker shows which starred an actress whose biggest credits to date included cameo appearances on *Gunsmoke*, *The Flying Nun*, and *Gilligan's Island*. Still, it was the most inspirational thing I had ever seen; it was as if I had personally discovered the face of Jesus on the side of a potato. There it was, right in front of me, the miracle of the live theater experience for the first time: rich, glorious sounds of an orchestra spilling out of a hole in the ground, grown men and women dressed in strange costumes with raccoon-lined eyes and clown-red cheeks acting out a story communicated by overly enunciated words and dramatic hand gestures, so effervescently that it prompted applause from everyone watching. *Applause*. Imagine that!

When I got home that night it was like I had been infused with a silliness drug, as if someone had slipped LSD into my glass of vitamin-enriched chocolate milk. I couldn't shake the images and sounds off of me for days—I pranced around the house, goose-stepping down the stairs and slapping my knees with the palm of my hand singing, "Belly up to the bar, boys! Belly up!" Show tunes were *ringing* inside my ears. *Molly Brown* was only a start, of course. That season they were also doing *The Music Man, My Fair Lady,* and *How to Succeed in Business Without Really Trying.* I never imagined that, well, people could go through life singing and dancing (and get paid for doing it, too).

By the end of the summer the musical comedy desire had welled up in me so much that I was practicing choreography as I brushed my teeth. "I believe in *yooooooouuuuu*," I sang to the skinny little image of myself in the mirror. "*Eeeeeyyyyeeee beee-leeve innnnn yoooooouuuuu.*" It wasn't that music had never moved me before—I had been cognizant even by then of the power of Judy Garland to realign my DNA structure even though I couldn't give a name to what it was that was happening. Whenever I heard "Over the Rainbow" I was frozen into place, unable to do anything but listen, and, well, *worship*. But suddenly, with *Molly Brown*, I had been bequeathed with the knowledge that there was a whole new live medium I had never known existed before—one with a heritage and a structure and an endless supply of Original Cast Albums, as if some pious pilgrim had said to his boyfriend while stepping off the Mayflower, "Let's invent a new art form that will drive little sissy boys crazy."

The image of those early days of becoming, well, *serious* about Broadway musicals and show tunes was so vivid and gratifying to me that several times a day I imagined myself sweeping onto a Broadway stage and throwing kisses to a grateful and admiring audience. "Thank you," I'd say, as though nothing were out of the ordinary about an eight year-old having just performed every role of *Camelot* by himself to himself in the privacy of his bedroom mirror. "Thank you *sooooooo* much." In retrospect, however, I can't help but see this new-found obsession as a product of my remoteness. My life growing up in suburbia had been normal and serious and, well, just a bit too solitary. My mother was busy with her house chores, cooking and cleaning for four children in a too-small-but-with-more-stairs-than-you-can-want split level home; my father was off-site making an income designing airplanes that could drop atomic bombs; my brother and sisters were either too old or too young or wanted nothing to do with me. I had been a too serious sibling, really, and then, well, I became a silly one. And most of the neighborhood kids were on little league baseball teams or mini-football squads or out riding bikes and playing Frisbee with their dogs, all of which I had no talent for—especially trying to learn to catch a Frisbee with my teeth. Left to my own devices, it's only reasonable that I emerged as Mr. Wanna-Make-It-Big-In-Show-Biz.

On one of the shelves of my bedroom bookshelf, I kept all of the programs and playbills and ticket stubs of the shows that I had seen, that my father or mother had, at first, willingly, and then later, suspiciously, taken me to thus far, from the church production of *Annie Get Your Gun* to the junior college presentation of *You're a Good Man, Charlie Brown*. I treated these souvenirs like reference tools. Didn't the composer who wrote *Hello, Dolly!* also write *Mame*? Wasn't the woman who did *Once Upon A Mattress* related to the man who did *Carousel*? Didn't Ethel Merman have a loud voice? Why did I know the lyrics of "People" before I ever heard the song? And why did I listen to that cast album over and over and over again? On my bottom bookshelf I stored the cast albums I had acquired, shows like *Sweet Charity* and *Bye, Bye Birdie* and the television version of Mary Martin's *Peter Pan*; a few I had appropriated from the back of my mother's closet, those standard mainstream all-stars such as the soundtracks to the movie versions of *West Side Story, Gypsy,* and *The King and I*. They were all neatly alphabetized and stacked upright so that the records inside wouldn't warp.

Many of the albums were soon scratchy from overuse,

however; I spent hours and hours memorizing the lyrics of every new album I got, moving the needle back across the record in search of a previous groove. There was one album, a musical called *Wish You Were Here*, which I always kept out of order, however, the album cover sitting on top of my record player. The cover featured a black and white picture of a shirtless man carrying a yellow bathing-suit clad woman in his arms. I spent more hours studying that picture than I ever did trying to learn those inane Harold Rome lyrics, trying to imagine the width and bulk of the man's arms and shoulders or how much hair was growing on his chest—that chest above that silly woman who dangled where I wanted to be dangling. The man wasn't exactly a title holder in the brawn department, though to a young boy what he did exhibit was a wide berth of photographed skin. Something moved inside me when I saw that man in the photograph, the same sort of feeling, really, that I had felt when I had watched, mesmerized, the old Steve Reeves *Hercules* movies on television.

This obsession with bodybuilders didn't really begin to haunt me till years later, however, somewhere around that inexplicable age of thirteen, the same year I kept lifting my arms up over my head wondering when I was going to begin sprouting hair beneath my underarms. Everyone I knew was going through puberty before I was. *Girls* were even going through puberty before I was. My dog was going through puberty before I was. Every day I would run home and lock myself in my bedroom and examine my armpit for hair follicles. In the gym class that I had been forced to take that year there were boys who already had dark, coarse hair on their chest and arms and legs and underneath their arms. I had nothing but the fine silky brushings I had always had on my forearms. When I stood in the mirror and flexed my biceps nothing in my arm moved or hardened. I had neither muscle tone nor bulky fat nor even *shape* in those days—only the skin and bones of a worried what's-to-become-of-me youth.

On the days when I wasn't so eager to examine my armpits I would ride my bike to the twenty-four hour convenience store which had opened about two miles away and order one of those icy fruit-flavored slurpy drinks. When I had finished and my lips were framed by an orange- or red-colored mustache, I would stand in front of the magazine counter and look through the racks. There were copies of those general interest Apple Pie Americana periodicals such as *Look* and *Life* and *Time* and *Saturday Evening Post* on the racks, ladies monthlies like *McCall's* and *Glamour* and *Woman's Day* and *Vogue* were given a whole shelf, and the sports and hobby magazines like *Car and Driver*, *Motor Trend*, and *Popular Electronics* had a whole case on the other side of the aisle. But my gaze was always searching with burning-eyed neck jerks to where two specific magazines were located within that last rack—*Muscle Builder* and *After Dark*. I pretended, with all my stagey rehearsed nonchalance, not to want to look at them by feigning interest in a whole slew of other magazines. I would stand there and flip through *Sports Illustrated*, for instance, unable to read the articles or even look at the pictures because all I wanted to do was to look at one of those two other magazines instead. When I had spent enough diversionary time not to be studied by the salesclerk, I picked up a copy of *Muscle Builder* first, holding the spine gingerly between my palms as if I were Superboy and the pages were to ignite from my overheated stare.

    Muscle Builder was full of workout routines photographed with bodybuilders such as Lou Ferrigno, Franco Columbo, Larry Scott, Dave Draper, and pre-Hollywood Arnold Schwarzenegger—huge, thick-shouldered men with ridges of abdominals and striations across their chests and massive sets of muscles called deltoids and triceps—all of whom looked like they would be the winner of a national tractor pull contest. They made the guy in *Wish You Were Here* look like a leprechaun who had wandered out from behind a four-leaf clover by mistake. I would stand there and look aghast at the sizes of these powerfully-built men, many photographed in skimpy swimsuits in poses where their muscles popped obscenely to the surface of their skin. The pictures never failed to arouse me—me, a tiny, scrawny thirteen year-old yearning for hair under his arms—and I would stand there, shifting back and forth on the heels of my feet, feeling myself growing erect, a sensation I had not yet adapted to, furtively looking about to see if anyone understood what was happening to me but not wanting them to know about it, of course, my throat drying out and my heart beating in my ears, frustrated because I didn't understand anything except that I shouldn't tell anyone what I was feeling. I could seldom muster up the courage to buy a *Muscle Builder*, especially if a guy was working the check-out counter, but, oddly, I never had a problem taking the newest issue of *After Dark* to the register. To me, *After Dark* was just like one of those hobby magazines, except, of course, it was all about *my* hobby.

The true irony about *After Dark*, however, was that it tried to pass itself off as a legitimate entertainment monthly magazine, something like *People* before *People* was invented. Only there were no stories about aging soap stars recovering from alcohol abuse or movie stars supporting charity causes; instead, there were articles about Broadway revivals and choreographers and ballet dancers all throughout *After Dark*, all accompanied by glossy studio photos of young male dancers without their shirts on, or young sports jocks breaking into show business without their shirts on, or up-and-coming male models without their shirts on, or recently unemployed television actors looking for stage work without their shirts on. These young men were not nearly as beefy as those in *Muscle Builder*, of course, those older men were *professionals*, but these guys were just as fit. And *After Dark* treated their subjects more like gods who had landed on earth than those sweaty gym idols. Those men in those photographs were styled and posed and airbrushed and lighted with every kind of gel and make-up and super hair-dryer and micro-strobe technique imaginable. I have no idea how this magazine ever found its way to my small hometown in north Georgia, but *After Dark*, I believe, even to this day, awakened my sexual desire for other men with its soft core erotica. I didn't want to be a skimpily clad dancer in those pages. I wanted to be the big, beefy bodybuilder *with* that skimpily clad dancer. It's as if those two magazines were the culminations of my fantasy world come true.

Not a day went by without my fretting over these magazines once they had found their way into my consciousness. I soon had such a collection of magazines to compliment my musical theater library (including a few discreetly-hidden-in-my-closet muscle magazines that I had found the courage to buy). About that time my older brother abandoned his basement lair and I took to working out with the set of weights he had left behind. I borrowed my sister's portable Swinger phonograph with the flip-down turntable and took it downstairs, exercising to show tunes in the chilly, damp space of our basement, a room that smelled like carpet which had been flooded on too many times. I huffed and puffed and tried to blow the walls of that basement apart with my new super-exercised strength, but more than once I would abandon those dumbbells in favor of, well, just dancing and lip-synching to my favorite songs, always trying to end my routine by stretching my legs into an impossible split. The door to the basement stairs was always opening and closing, and I suspected my mother and father and siblings were peering down from their worried perches, wondering what all that noise was about—what could I possibly be doing that could make the foundation of the house literally, well, vibrate in that kind of manner?

About that time, too, I discovered in my father's workroom of tools and hardware—the dusty, sunless location-of-the-power-drill closet that was adjacent to my new personal-and-very-own-private rehearsal studio and gym—a flimsy, dark yellow paperback book on one of his shelves wedged between old copies of *National Geographic*, titled *The Parents' Guide to Sex*. It was the scariest book I had ever seen up to then, and just the kind of book for parents to leave in a well-hidden-but-not-too-well-hidden spot so that the child-in-question will discover it on his own. It had been written decades before, but inside were sketches of male and female genitalia and reproductive systems. In the back of the book were horrid black and white pictures of men and women with swollen lips and running sores and scabs and rashes on their bodies—all illustrating a chapter entitled Venereal Diseases. The pictures were both repugnant and magnetizing, but what worried me more was a chapter in the middle of the book on homosexuality. The book was specific on the distinguishing characteristics of homosexuality in young boys, describing the potential he-will-grow-up-to-be-a-nasty-man-and-a-pervert as exhibiting a "desire to dress up like little girls" and "moving around in a way identified as feminine." Homosexual boys, the author informed the reader, had sloped, rounded shoulders (Okay, whew, not me), hairless chests (Uh, oh, maybe me), soft, delicate skin (Uh, oh, maybe me again), and a peculiar swinging motion of the hips when he walks (Whew! Not me at all; I only swing my hips when I *dance*). What I needed was someone to tell me what to do with those *feelings* for other men, which were, needless to say, crowding out everything in my brain except the lyrics for all those show tunes.

It shouldn't come as a surprise, then, when I admit that I wasn't much of a jock in high school, even with all the playing (and dancing) I did with dumbbells. In tenth grade, I mustered enough courage to audition for the school production of *Oliver!*, believing, well, just *knowing*, really, that I was perfect for the title role of Dickens's orphan circa nineteenth century London. I wasn't cast in the lead, of course, even though I knew every note and lyric and word of dialogue by heart and had demonstrated so at my boisterous and too-cocky audition for Mrs. Prentice, the elderly drama club sponsor-cum-choral teacher who always smelled of alcohol and rose-infused perfume. Mrs. Prentice didn't much care for my over-the-top rendition and when it came right down to it, I couldn't sing the boy-soprano part, either; I had developed underarm hair by then (thank goodness for something) and my voice had changed an octave lower. No boy in my school could sing the part, or so Mrs. Prentice announced one afternoon, and she cast an eleventh grade *girl* as Oliver—a *girl*, mind you, creating a wave of raised eyebrows throughout the drama club and the first time I ever heard the word *lesssz-beee-innnnsss* whispered in public. It wasn't like we were doing *Peter Pan* and *expected* to cast a girl as a boy.

Mrs. Prentice did cast me as Mr. Brownlow, Oliver's *grandfather*, a grand faux pas if you ask me, since the fake gray that had been sprayed in my hair for the part failed to age my pageboy coiffure—it had turned it silver and I still looked *younger* than the *girl* playing Oliver. My stage debut was nonetheless memorable, however. I knew nothing about vocal projection and breathing from the diaphragm and all that stage-actory stuff, nor was Mrs. Prentice smart or sober enough to impart that sort of wisdom to her assemblage of wanna-be theatricals. By the day of the first performance I was so nervous and sore from shouting my grand total of three lines that I had developed laryngitis. I spent my off-stage time coating my throat with a cold spray. Mrs. Prentice, helping me into the jacket of the costume my mother had sewn which looked more like a revised Confederate soldier's uniform rather than an English gentleman's topcoat, and which Mrs. Prentice had complimented me on only days before when I had shown it to her, said, just before pushing me on to the stage, "No one will ever believe you are supposed to be in *this* play. But, hell, at least, you *sound* old."

The next year I didn't fare much better as Pontius Pilate in *Jesus Christ, Superstar,* though I had studied voice in the year since my stage debacle and I could carry a tune, even project it across the footlights. *Superstar* was Mrs. Prentice's concession to the students that the drama club should be more *au courant,* though there was a backlash against the production from a group of Baptist parents about a singing and dancing Son of Our Lord during His Last Days on Earth. I had wanted to be Jesus Christ, but when they made the student who was cast in that role wear a fake beard, I was relieved to have been overlooked. My costume was a white dress shirt and white bell-bottom pants and since our version was an abbreviated one, I was only onstage once, to sing "Pilate's Dream."

By my senior year I had gained some weight and some muscle tone from my on-going basement exercises when I was cast as Rolf in *The Sound of Music*. I was determined, of course, to make Rolf a star cameo turn. A dance instructor was brought in to teach me how to waltz with the girl who had been cast as Liesl for the big "You Are Sixteen" gazebo number, but the cul de resistance occurred when Mrs. Prentice rewrote the finale cemetery scene for me so that Rolf wouldn't be the bad guy and blow the whistle on the von Trapps. Instead, he sang a "Sixteen" reprise (with new lyrics written by *moi*) and then, with a slight tremor of his hand, triggered off *another* Nazi spotting the von Trapps.

That was the same year that I bought my first pornographic magazine. I had just gotten my driver's license and had become a great adventurer on my own, planning trips to downtown Atlanta to usher for matinee performances of the touring Broadway productions that played at the Fox Theater, a former movie palace near the Georgia Tech campus. I bought that first illicit magazine at a convenience store that was attached to a gas station on my way home from a performance of the musical *Grease*. When I went to pay for the gas I had just self-pumped, I noticed a rack of magazines near the check-out counter—plastic wrapped editions of *Hustler, Playboy, Penthouse,* and a magazine I had never seen before—*Playgirl*. I reached directly for the *Playgirl* and, without even acknowledging it, slapped a ten dollar bill boldly down on the counter and in my best good-ole-boy Southern accent said to the guy behind the register, "My sister is too embarrassed to buy this. Can you believe it? She wants it for a bridal shower." There was not an iota of a reaction from the guy over my purpose, and my bold, brazen action went unremarked. (I suppose the salesclerk was as bored with his job as he looked to be—even the junk food at this particular store looked like it hadn't been moved in more than a decade.) The salesclerk gave me my change and I walked swiftly back to the car, the magazine placed on the seat beside me, its contents driving me so crazy that I finally had to pull off to the side of a road once I had crossed the Chattahoochee. I tore the plastic cover off that magazine as quickly as I could, flipping eagerly through the pages to look at the pictures of the nude men, studying how many men were featured, which ones were hairy and which were not, who had the best body, and who had the most unbelievable equipment.

That magazine set a yearning into place that would take me a few more years to fully comprehend, but I know now, in retrospect, that that may have been my first confusing of sex with love. It wasn't *just* that I wanted to know this man's skin and hair and cock and butt and smells and sounds and tastes. I wanted to be *with* him, wanted him to *need* me and *want* me as much as I *wanted* him. I wanted to belong to him as much as I wanted him to belong to me, to know that when he scratched his neck to understand whether it was an itch or a reflex, to know when he woke at night if he was restless or worried or had eaten too much, to know when he kissed me or held my cock that he knew my name and understood what I wanted to feel while he was with me. I wanted to be with a man when he got up out of bed in the morning, with the same man when he went out looking for lunch or dinner, with him again when he wanted to watch a movie or even better yet, when he had tickets to see a big, brassy, never-seen-before Broadway musical. At that age I'd never imagined anything except romantic sex, had never fantasized about any kind of a guy except a seriously-involved-with-me-and-only-me one. It never occurred to me that sex could be, well, meaningless, functional or simply recreational. What I wanted, of course, was someone to love. And I wanted to feel as if I should sing about it in a Broadway musical.

Though it would be years before I would be able to articulate my desire for men to anyone other than myself, I had no such qualms of my love of the theater. In college, this appreciation grew and the people who became my friends were theater people—performers, designers, actors, singers, dancers, and choreographers. My life wasn't so much a slow, unfolding drama of acceptance and coming out as it was a long learning curve—a soaring arc of light that hoped to find a home somewhere on a stage, waiting for the right moment to belt out a show tune and bring down the house.

HOMETOWN SWEETHEARTS

In those days, New York seemed as far away to me as Tokyo does now, even though the guilt I felt then can still inexplicably rise in me as if it were only a few hours in my past. On Saturday mornings, I used to drive my Civic from the dorm parking lot at Emory University through the back roads of north Atlanta to a part-time job I had held since I had graduated high school, as a sales clerk at the jewelry counter at Sears in Cumberland Mall. It was a thankless job—polishing glass counters, arranging display cases of gold-plated earrings, ringing up sales of silver chains or writing exchange slips for Timex watches—but it put spending money in my pocket that I would otherwise not have had and would have had to work double-time on-campus to earn as much. When my shift ended, I would meet up with Annette, a girl I had known since my junior year in high school, who was usually spending the day shopping in the mall. We might have dinner together or go see a movie at one of the new multiplexes that were springing up all over Cobb County, and afterward, I would follow her in her gold Mustang back to the split-level house where she had grown up and where she stayed on weekends away from her own dorm room at the University of Georgia.

Annette lived ten minutes from the mall and only ten more minutes from the house in East Marietta where I had grown up in. Emory was roughly an hour's trip from my job and my hometown—a lot of time for an anxious college student to be stuck behind a wheel, particularly on a weekend, but Annette had a tug on me that I wasn't yet willing to sever. When we reached her house, we might spend a few minutes chatting with her mother or her younger sister Lisa, or playing ball with her black terrier in the living room, who loved to lie on his back and let me spin him around on the carpet. Then, Annette and I would go into her bedroom at the end of the hall, close the door, turn the stereo on softly, and have sex as if were the most natural thing for the two of us to do. Only on the longer drive back to my dorm room later that night would I begin to feel a deep shame stewing in my stomach, a knot of misapprehension which boiled up into the indigestion of *what-have-I-done now?* By remaining so close to my home and my high school past, unable to break this psychological distance even geographically by attending a college no further than an hour's drive away, the person I used to be was not allowing the person I wanted to be a chance to happen. And I was desperately realizing I was not happy with the guy I was pretending I was while this *other* guy was making up his mind what to do next.

Annette Tucker wasn't the prettiest girl in my high school class. She wasn't a cheerleader or a majorette, or even a member of the pep squad, a contingent of uniformed girls who sat in the bleachers at football games and waved pom-poms in the air. But then I wasn't enough of a jock or a good-ole Southern boy to attract one of those types of girls. I was a smart, bookish student, active in the band, editor of the yearbook, secretary of the Key Club, and a member of the National Honor Society the first year a student was eligible. I was the son of two Methodist parents, not as strict as the save-the-sinner Baptists in my hometown (who didn't allow their children to dance or drink). But because I was the second borne child and not the first in my family, instead of growing up rebellious, I grew up to be an overachiever. Annette was a girl in my eleventh grade history class who passed me notes now and then on a friendly basis without any kind of social designs, or so I thought at the time. I certainly didn't strive to date her, didn't look at her as a way to move into an upward social circle, nor was it ever my intention to bed her or use her to initiate or educate me in the ways of sex.

But Annette wasn't plain, either. She spent a great deal of time enhancing her appearance. There was something long about the lower half of her face and the fact that on the upper half she didn't seem to possess cheekbones. She decorated herself with make-up in the way a child might paint an Easter egg—big rouged cheeks, long spidery eyelashes, dark red lips outlined with thin black lines. Her appearance also relied on a well-planned ensemble of blouses and necklaces and matching skirts and shoes, and she spent as much attention sculpting her long brown hair into the then-popular style of Farrah Fawcett feathery wings. Annette wasn't tall, either, or, rather, she wasn't taller than I was, as many girls and guys already were, but she had a small curvature at the top of her spine so that she walked as if her shoulders were slightly slumped. I always wanted to tell her to pull her shoulders back, but I never did because she seemed so proud of her transformation beyond the ordinary polyester-suited big-haired women who roamed our suburban world.

"You didn't call me like you said you would," she would tell me in her thick Georgia drawl, when she found me at the mall standing beside the cash register waiting for customers. She would say this with a little huff of air in her voice or a tiny little stamp of her foot for emphasis.

"I guess I got busy," I would half apologize and never meet her stare. "I thought I said I would call you if I got time."

"So did you want to do something?" she would tilt her head to one side and ask in her sly way of making sure I did not already have other plans.

"Okay," I would answer unless I was busy and had made other plans, which somehow Annette always seemed to know in advance of my informing her of this fact. Annette seemed to endure every obstacle and exasperation I placed in front of her. If I *was* busy with someone else, Annette would always call or show up again at the mall the next weekend. She was determined to make me want to see her and, in this respect, she was a true Southern belle.

* * *

I didn't date Annette in high school. As it happened I only had a few dates with girls and most were met with disastrous, embarrassing results which I did not wish to repeat. I do remember disliking kissing Janet Terrill because of the metal braces and rubber bands in her mouth, and being confused while groping Nancy Blake's breasts when we were parked in her driveway, baffled about whether or not I was supposed to unhook the bra first before I felt her up. My first Junior-Senior Prom I took Charlene Williams, a cheerleader I had never spoken to before because my friend Andy Wharton had hooked us up. Charlene and I did not talk during that date, other than my complimenting her dress and presenting her with a wrist corsage when I arrived to pick her up at her house. In my recollection, that date ended before it ever began and is something to this day I still wish had never happened.

I did have a lot of girls who were my friends in high school, girls whom I had known since elementary school and junior high and who were an integral weave of my hometown fabric. I played duets (clarinet and piano) and went to state music festivals with Wendy Crockett, traded calculus problems with Marylee Blackstone, danced with Carolyn Lanier in our senior class production of *The Sound of Music*. (She was Liesl; I was Rolf). Melissa Chambers and I had known each other since she was six and I was seven—she was raised five houses down the street from the ranch style house my family moved into when I was entering third grade; our childhood paths crossed because our mothers' and older brothers' did as well. Melissa was affected and pretentious—but with a sense of self-irony that was rare in my hometown. She wore her hair in ringlets long after she had passed through puberty, but even at an early age she had a dark-skinned exotic look about her, as though Dorothy Lamour had been whirled up in a cyclone and plunked down in southern Appalachia. By the time Melissa entered high school, she thought of herself as a cross between an urban bon vivant and a would-be star, the kind of girl who felt she deserved to be plucked out of a chorus line and made famous. I loved spending time with

Melissa because she was so spontaneously crazy and wanted to grow up and live somewhere else other than the South, just as I did. She introduced me to tequila poppers and Slo Gin Fizz, taught me how to blow smoke rings, and made us converse with British accents. Everything was dramatic in her hands: the arrangement of flowers, the swell of music, the placement of candles around a room. I never slept with her, however; in spite of her wild streak, Melissa was a bit moralistic and, unlike my affair with Annette, I always feared that the news of Melissa and I "doing it together" would somehow make its way back to my house and haunt and shame me in ways I was not yet ready to confront. But I did continue to see Melissa beyond our high school graduation. When I wasn't spending time on a Saturday evening with Annette, I was usually with Melissa. Annette had learned to adapt to my passive-aggressive behavior in regards to how I viewed my relationship with her; my involvement with Melissa, however, was a continual source of exasperation.

* * *

My college years were abundant with cultural enlightenment outside of the classrooms. I met my first black, Jewish, and Asian friends at Emory. I ate bagels and sushi for the first time. I smoked my first joint. I also found myself hovering around the musical and theatrical organizations on campus, an environment that also brought me in contact with my first gay friend.

I didn't know John was gay when we met; we both sang second tenor in the Emory Glee Club, but our friendship didn't strengthen until we were both cast as dancing waiters in a production of *Hello, Dolly!* John and another student, a senior named David, choreographed a routine for us of flips, cartwheels, and athletic springs. John had been a high school gymnast and I did my best to keep up with him and not lose my balance on stage. But the heartfelt conversations we had off stage during rehearsals were what continued the connections between us—earnest admissions that only two young men full of dreams and new-found opinions can make to one another on their journeys to becoming friends, from preferred clothing choices, disliked professors, to favorite ice cream flavors of all time.

    I soon became aware that everyone had a crush on John. We were the same height, had the same abundant waves of brown hair, though John's could retain the highlights of the summer sun for months afterward, whereas my own would only redden and frizzle into split ends. John was also more sturdily built than I was: he had a lithe, athletic body in the days before everyone became gym-toned, which he displayed in shrunken T-shirts and faded jeans, augmented by flannel shirts when the weather grew colder. He was dark-eyed and dark-skinned, which he credited to his Italian ancestry, and the whole effect of being with him was like discovering a wild stallion who had run out of the forest in search of others in his herd. My own crush on John confused me every time we were together. I was wildly attracted to him and wildly terrified by that attraction. But instead of acting on it sexually I allowed John to educate me culturally. I went with him to my first gay bar, a nightclub on Cheshire Bridge Road in Atlanta named at the time The Magic Garden. I danced with John through a string of disco hits—it was the early Seventies and the sound systems in nightclubs were just beginning to change their rhythms—not just with the steady drum and bass beat, but with large superspeakers positioned in darkened corners which could deafen a dancer if he twirled too close to them. John served as my tour guide to gay life, explaining everything from the difference between "tops" and "bottoms" to the specific sexual acts the color shadings of back-pocket handkerchiefs meant. In those years, I did not admit that I was gay to myself or to others, only that I was open-minded and curious and found everything about gay life arousing. I didn't sleep with John or any other man in Atlanta during my college years for many of the same reasons that I had avoided sleeping with

Melissa. I did not want the news of it to reach my parents before I was ready to announce it myself.

* * *

It is hard for me now to pinpoint the exact moment that my vision of the world expanded and changed. John's tutelage during those college years was tantamount to my gay education, but it's not difficult for me to discover snippets of my gay self within my boyhood years. I remember in seventh grade being erotically aroused by the photographs of bodybuilders in the muscle magazines I had discovered at the newsstand of the local pharmacy, or even earlier, at age nine, watching my first live theater performance—a touring production of *The Unsinkable Molly Brown* and wanting to re-enact the songs and dances I had heard. Was a shy, lonely boy wanting a better body or to perform musical numbers in front of an audience an expression of a developing gay identity? Or was the notion that this was the way in which he wanted to be loved the outgrowth of a germinating gay consciousness? It's hard for me to psychologically separate those layers because they seemed to be so resolutely entwined in my own experiences. I can also remember when I was ten that I was furious with my parents when they made me attend church services instead of allowing me to stay home and watch *The Wizard of Oz* on TV—Judy Garland's performance already had an inexplicable psychic pull on me.

And I remember the year my body began to change—at age fourteen, I finally developed hair in my armpit (and acne on my face)—and I spent hours in the basement lifting weights and singing show tunes, and discovering, during breaks between my routines and repetitions, a slim volume hidden among my father's old tools and books, which cataloged with words and photographs the horrors of sexually transmitted diseases, including a chapter on homosexuality, a part that I read and re-read several times trying to make some sense of it. What happened then that made me recognize the difference between myself and the rest of the world? Was it my developing hormones or my curiosity over lives different from my own? What was it that sent me to the basement to fantasize about being someone else and not outside to ballfields befriending other boys?

Reading also broadened my awareness of different lives and experiences. Books took me to faraway lands, out into space, up into helium filled balloons, made me wonder what it would be like to be a boy swinging from a vine in the jungle or battling Nazis in Europe. Movies only heightened the possible adventure the bigger world could offer—*Dr. Zhivago* took me to Russia, *Lawrence of Arabia* to the Sahara, *The King and I* transported me to historical Siam (as well as introducing a new set of music and lyrics to learn). And television perpetuated this myth that other lives were more exotic and adventurous than my own—Sandy had a dolphin and a handsome dad; Will Robinson had a robot, a handsome dad, and a good-looking friend chasing his sister.

Religion must also be factored into the shape of my growing gay consciousness during these years. Over many centuries, religious theology and doctrine have constructed moral outlines, a guide of what is right and wrong, and no matter what denomination or religion of the world is examined, gay sex is not considered the natural, biological or moral choice a life should take. Every gay man confronts this awareness at some point in his development. In today's society, popular culture reflects those centuries of behavioral conditioning, feeding society romantic and sexual images of men and women, boys and girls, man and wife. Books, television, films, music, and just crashing around in the real world only solidify this perception for every subsequent younger generation.

But what religion also teaches are the recognition of one's true faith and the acceptance of the honest self. Somewhere deep inside me I knew as a profound, personal truth that my sexual attraction was toward men and not to women. I also understood that I had to accept it as the natural order of my own world if I were to accept myself as an honest man. In this bizarre and wondrous way it was religion that gave me the courage to believe that I should not be ashamed of who I was and find the faith to come out as a gay man to others.

* * *

College graduation arrived without any resolutions or admissions, however. I was aware that I was gay but had not had sex yet with another man, had not even been able to muster up a confession of my desires to any other person except within my own fantasies. John, by then, had been through several boyfriends, and had settled into a relationship with a dance instructor and moved into an apartment on Juniper Street in downtown Atlanta, within walking distance to his neighborhood gay bars. I envied him but could not act in that manner myself. Instead, I moved back home to East Marietta, into the bedroom I had grown up in, and went to work at Sears full-time while I went out on interviews in search of a career. I did not know what type of work I was looking for or exactly what my career path was to be—I had been an English major and thought about working for my hometown newspaper, only to be told in my interview with an officious director of personnel that I was overqualified for any kind of job he could offer me. I loved the theater, loved working on or around the stage, but other than a one-day role as a miscast Baskin-Robbins clown in the Independence Day parade and an unpaid internship building sets in Chastain Park for a production of *Shenandoah*, those types of opportunities were rare and difficult to find in Atlanta.

Melissa had transferred to a college in South Carolina and was not around the summer I returned home after college graduation, but Annette had also moved back into her parents' house and found a job with an airline as a stewardess, a job that seemed well-suited for her. She spent a considerable amount of energy trying to convince me to apply for a position at the insurance company where her mother worked. Her mother, though, was not doing too well. She had been diagnosed first with breast cancer and then with lung cancer. She no longer went to work, spending her days on the couch draped in bright floral moo-moos watching her favorite TV programs, waving to us as we made our way down the hall to Annette's bedroom to have a good time and not be too noisy.

Returning home after college was both a necessary and unnecessary mistake I had to make. Back living under the watchful eyes of my parents for the first time in four years, I was paralyzed by the psychological distance of the liberal environment of Emory I had left behind and the secretive interior life of East Marietta I now inhabited. During this time I came to know several truths about myself, however, foremost that if I were to live my life as I wanted to live it—as a gay man—which is who I felt I should become—then I would have to do it somewhere other than my parents' home and my hometown. I would have to leave home for a more gay-friendly environment.

I used my education and my love of books and theater to plan my escape and my eventual coming out as a gay man. I sent off applications to several graduate schools offering advance degrees in English or Drama—the University of Chicago, Stanford, Yale, and New York University, among them. When the acceptance letters came the following spring it was not a difficult choice for me to make. New York was not so much a destination I knew I was headed toward as it was a dream that I wanted to find. I had bought into all of the movies and songs and plays I had seen and heard and read and studied about love and romance and making it in New York (even though that kind of love and success belonged to young men who desired young women). I read *The New York Times* whenever I could find it at the library, studied the new advertisements carefully in the Sunday arts section, and memorized the names of shows and theaters and things that were important and vital and must-do in the city. I also knew all about Greenwich Village—its history of bohemians and artists and as a haven for gay men and lesbians. When the thought of finding myself living in Manhattan actually seemed like it could be a reality, I would palpably shake with anxiety because it could not happen soon enough.

Before I left Marietta, Annette hurled another road block in my direction hoping that it would change my mind. I had tried to stop seeing her just as she wanted us to become more serious. I know she expected me to give her an engagement ring, a sort of wait-for-me-while-I-have-this-one-quick adventure talisman, but, instead, I handed her a firm date for leaving for New York and was trying to let her know, in my best passive-aggressive manner, that this was the ending of us and the beginning of something new for myself. One day during the week before my departure, Annette called my house during dinner time, knowing she would reach me while my parents were also near the kitchen phone. She knew from past experience that whatever reaction she could provoke from me in our phone conversation would most likely be overhead by my mother and father. This was when and how she told me she was pregnant.

"Are you sure?" I asked her, when the news had sunk in and the blood had returned to my brain. Behind me, I sensed my parents, sitting at the kitchen table, bending their bodies toward me with some kind of concern.

"Well, there isn't anyone else," she said with her thick-winded sigh of exasperation.

"No," I said, turning toward my mother and father and shaking my head at them, as if there was nothing unusual to the phone call and certainly nothing to be concerned about. "Are you sure? Did you see a doctor?"

"Momma made me an appointment for tomorrow," she said. "But I know there hasn't been anybody else."

When I hung up the phone, I lied to my parents and told them that Annette was calling about her mother—telling me that she was ill again and likely to go back into the hospital for more tests. In my mind, Annette had played me a dirty card. The one thing I had carefully planned for was that this would and could not happen. I had always thought of myself as my greatest obstacle for escaping my hometown. I had never considered it could be someone else.

* * *

I was twenty-two years old and it was summertime when I arrived in New York City. I had taken the train from Atlanta to Washington, D.C., stayed overnight with a friend, and then taken another train the next morning to Manhattan. I can remember now, with a clarity that can still make me hyperventilate, those first moments when I nervously emerged from the steps leading away from the underground platform up into the busy corner of midtown—the mixture of awe, fear, anxiety, and excitement I felt as I clutched my meager possessions—a gym bag full of clothes, a portable typewriter, and a sleeping bag hoisted over my shoulder—and looked skyward at the towering skyscrapers around me. I found a room a few blocks away at the YMCA on West 34th Street, a tiny cramped space of mustard-colored chipped walls with a single bed, but, in a few more days, I had a job at an answering service on Seventh Avenue and an expensive apartment on a tree-lined street in Greenwich Village, which I decorated with crates and cast-off bookcases and furniture I found on the street.

It didn't take me long to find the locations of the gay bars in the neighborhood; I had arrived with a list of street addresses and descriptions that I had culled over the years from John and other gay friends. But I had not yet found the courage to walk inside any one of them. Somehow I was convinced that the men inside of these places would know I was a fraud and still afraid of admitting that I was a homosexual, that I was inexperienced and technically not even gay yet since I hadn't had a real, true-to-life, honest gay experience. But the Village was also a hot bed of gay activity *outside* of the bars. Openly gay shops and businesses were everywhere. Hundreds of clones, muscular gay men with bushy mustaches and dressed in jeans and T-shirts cruised Christopher Street at all hours.

Walking beside them, studying them on the streets, I came to understand how I was so unlike them even in my desire to become exactly like them. I missed the guide that I had had in John back in Atlanta, missed how he had effortlessly shepherded me through the maze of clues and signals as he explained the opportunities before me and the types of men I could expect to find. I felt, in those early, bleary wanderings through gay Manhattan, like I had arrived in Mecca without knowing how to pray.

I also hadn't been able to completely shake off my past. Annette had come to believe that my relocation to New York was only a temporary inconvenience and not a permanent break in our relationship. Her pregnancy had proven to be a false one—no rabbit died and her menstrual cycle returned to normal. By the end of my first month in New York, she had adjusted her flight schedule to accept more trips to New York and LaGuardia airport. And if the truth be told, I was glad to see her because I had not yet made any strong friendships in the city; she was the familiar face I found in all of this confusion that was swirling inside and around me.

When Annette arrived in town, we toured the city as tourists would—riding the elevator to the top of the Empire State Building or the ferry out to the Statue of Liberty—and I came to love the city much as I saw the joy of it filter through her skeptical eyes. Because Annette was also in the city on business, I ended up meeting her at the hotels her airline booked for her, sometimes in the grand and spacious ones on Madison or Park Avenues where they turned down the sheets and left chocolates on the pillows as bedtime treats, but more often at the industrial motel-like ones near the airport. Wherever I met her, however, Annette made it clear that she was perturbed by these new turn of events in our relationship and the fact that I was so geographically and emotionally removed from her. Though she did not distinctly state this to me, I knew this as a certain fact: Annette was ready for me to fail in New York so that I could return to Marietta and become serious about her.

"You're so difficult to reach," she said one evening when we met and I took her in the circle of my arms. I tried to kiss her but she held me at arm's length, searching my face for a sign I still could not reveal to her. "But I'm happy to see you again."

"And here we are," I answered, evasively, and kissed her lightly on the forehead. I picked up her bag and carried it to the back of a mini-van that would take us from the airport to her hotel. "Did you have a good flight?"

She laughed. "I had a terrible flight," she said. "Turbulence over Baltimore." Her smile was both cheerful and sentimental and I knew her mind was at work trying to solve the riddle of us. I told myself I would not think about revealing my sexual uncertainties with her yet; I had only been through the first round of classes and already I was juggling a lot: graduate school, full-time job, Annette, and experiencing the city as a new boy in town.

In the hotel room, we undressed and went through our familiar sexual motions. I was aware of the beauty of her body—her pillow-like breasts, the curve of her hips—and the way my own body felt and fit against hers. At moments I thought I felt a hardness and a constriction in her, a grave distrust and despair of what we were when we were together like this. I tried not to think about it, but somewhere within the core of myself, I realized I was doing something awful to her, and it became a matter of how not to let this fact become too obvious to her—I wanted her to find her own way out of our relationship.

We traveled through a network of Annette's cries, her fingers running along my spine, the tucking up of her thighs, her sighs becoming softer and more urgent. Then it occurred to me that we had made no preparations to prevent her from becoming pregnant this time—even after the scare she had recently forced us through. Not long before she had arrived for this visit, Annette had also confided in a phone conversation that she had stopped taking the pill because it was ruining her complexion—and I had forgotten to bring a condom when I set out from my apartment to meet her that day.

She disappeared into the bathroom when we had finished and I heard her turn the faucets of the sink and the water running against the porcelain. I lay there naked, with my socks still on because my feet were cold, and waited for her return. The thought of a child belonging to Annette and me washed across my mind and I felt suddenly trapped again. When she returned to the bed I let out a nervous cough to force my tension away. She curled her body up against mine and laid her head against my chest. I wanted us to stay there, secretive and silent, but something deep within me also wanted to keep moving. At last she asked me. "Have things changed more?"

"I don't know," I said.

She turned away from me, lying on her side, looking toward the door. "I don't know who you want me to be," she said. She ran one hand, impatiently, through her hair. "I need a reason to keep doing this."

"You mean very much to me," I said. "Is that enough reason? Is it enough that I don't want to hurt you?"

"Hurt me?" she answered. "That makes you seem so decisive, which you certainly aren't."

"I haven't been very nice to you, have I?"

For a moment everything was quiet and I heard the rumbling of a subway car a block away and sending a slight tremor up the walls of the building. I felt her waiting—everything seemed to be waiting on my decision or lack of one.

"It's not like I'm asking anything unusual," she said. "I only want what anyone wants. Is that what you want?"

"I'm glad you're here," I answered. "I wanted to see you. Let's have a nice time together."

She reached for her purse and retrieved a cosmetic case and she studied her face in its miniature lighted mirror. "My schedule could change in January," she said, finally. "I've asked for another route. I could do New Orleans-Atlanta-New York regularly now."

"What does that mean?" I asked.

"That I'll be here at least twice a week," she answered. "And if I want, I could base myself here. So I would be here on my days off, too."

The words fell against me like blows in the chest. I had changed my life so that it would not revolve around her and now she was thinking about changing her life in order to control mine. "But your mom's not doing any better," I answered. "You said that."

"Lisa's there," she replied. Her younger sister, still at home, could help her mother through the upcoming battles. "And I would be there as much as here because of the flights."

"And how would you feel about that?" I asked. "I know how your mother relies on you."

"Will you think about it, at least?" she asked, after a while. A faint something, a hint of redness in the eyes, suggested that she would cry later when thinking more about this. "Could you let me know if we can at least take a step forward?"

"Okay," I answered and kept my frustration hidden. Annette had presented me with another obstacle. Just when I thought I was escaping, once again she was trying to reel me back in.

* * *

For the first time in my life I was not a serious student. I found my classes at NYU tedious and boring, not capable at all of energizing me in the way a simple morning walk through the West Village could. I'd come to love being out on the streets of Manhattan—the smell of baking bread wafting down the street in the mornings, the agitated honks of taxis and trucks when rush-hour traffic overwhelmed the city. But by the beginning of October, my fourth month in the city, I had not made any new friends, had still not found the courage to become the person I wanted to be. And I became someone I truly did not like. When Annette's mother died suddenly one night in the hospital of a heart attack and complications from a drug, I did not return the messages Annette left for me on my answering machine. I did not send flowers to the funeral, did not fly home to offer her comfort. I did not even send a card offering Annette and her family my condolences. Those were things that I had been raised, educated, trained to do by instinct as a Southern gentleman and good-Christian servant and I could not do them now. I moved through my hours in front of a switchboard, connecting callers and delivering messages, as if I were the worst, most ungrateful person who had ever arrived in the city. In the evenings, I could not concentrate in class, would feel my eyes watering up with tears, and I spent the next hour or so with the palm of my hand pressed against my forehead. I could not call her at all. To do so, in my mind, would show her that I cared for her too much.

I'm not exactly certain what made me go to the library after class that evening; maybe it stemmed from a desire to remove at least one layer of guilt from my misery—I had invested a lot of money in my move, taken out a loan for tuition and seen it chipped quickly away to pay for higher-than-usual living costs that city life demanded from you, and I thought perhaps I should at least make a half-hearted effort at beginning to work on a paper that was due soon for one of my courses. I'd walked from the class room building out into the warm October night, around the perimeter of Washington Square, watching the leaves swish and shush above me and the city do its thing in the way only Manhattan can romantically do it.

Inside the library, I drifted from shelf to shelf, aisle to aisle, then waited for the elevator. I saw a librarian notice me as I entered the department where the theater manuscripts were kept—my course was on Russian theater and I was looking for material having to do with Chekhov or Meyerhold. The librarian looked unlike any other librarian I had ever seen: a big, stocky fortysomething man with bulky shoulders and thick forearms, more like a high school football coach than someone who might understand the Dewey decimal system. His brown hair was cut short and pushed back and upwards at the crown, and his face, long and squared off by a flat, wide chin, made me think of a handsome model I had noticed on a billboard on Broadway for a cigarette company. "Can I help you find something?" he asked me.

"I'm not really sure what I'm looking for," I answered. I caught his eyes and they worried me, so I deflected my gaze to the shelves behind him.

"The cinema department moved upstairs," he said. "They needed more space."

I gave him a wistful smile, wondering if he understood that I didn't want to be anywhere but here at this moment, staring at him, wondering how I could make him a part of my life. I didn't have any sort of knowledge that he was gay other than my instinct that he was, an internal suspicion that John had affectionately described as "gaydar" when we were out together back in those long-ago halcyon days at Emory.

Somehow I explained to this handsome librarian that I needed to find books on Russian theater and he stood up from his desk and said he would show me where they were located. I followed him across the floor, detecting the woodsy scent of cologne he left in his wake. He stopped in front of an aisle and outstretched his hand and said, "Down there." He paused and laid his hand on a shelf and asked in a most casual manner, "Do you speak Russian?"

My heart was beating quickly, as if I had run the last few steps instead of following slowly behind him. "No, of course not," I answered, as if he had asked me the silliest question in the world. And then out of nowhere a force pulled up into my chest, made my body freeze, and sent blood rushing through my cheeks. "I think you're attractive," I said to him, feeling a thin layer of sweat form on my upper lip.

It was truly a queer thing to say to a stranger who stood in front of you for the first time, and, in retrospect, it's easy for me to look back and laugh at this desperate, innocent, and needy young man that I was. But the librarian did not flinch and accepted my compliment, and, before he left to return to his desk, I had introduced myself and snared a date with him for the following weekend.

* * *

His name was Bob Kinnaman and he lived in Chinatown. I met him at his apartment on a rainy autumn evening, called him from the pay phone on the corner first so he could come downstairs to the street level and open the front door of his building for me. Upstairs, on the fourth floor, his apartment was large and spacious, the walls painted a deep shade of maroon and the rooms full of fluffy couches, oversized pillows, and vases full of long reeds and ferns. Everything seemed to happen rapidly once I was inside. He locked the door behind us and we stood before each other breathing hard. He pulled me against him and I tilted my face upward to accept his kiss. It was both strange and elating to taste him, to feel the hard scratch of his stubble against my own, to seek out the shape of his body beneath his dry clothes as his hands pressed harder against the wet chill of my body. When we broke apart, he led through the rooms of the apartment and into his bedroom, where we continued kissing and he unbuttoned my shirt.

I was trembling while my clothes were removed, something in my brain going, "No, no, no," yet something deeper sighing, "At last, at last, at last." As we landed on the mattress and he wiggled awkwardly out of his clothes, I was aware that I was filled with a level of lust I had not felt before.

His body wasn't flawless but to me it was beautifully necessary: a muscular frame maturing into middle-age, broad fleshy shoulders, a low hanging chest covered with dark swirls of hair. He positioned my arms around his shoulders and my legs around his waist so that we sat before one another like volumeless bookends and we could grope each other's bodies as we continued kissing. Slowly, his mouth branched away from my lips to moisten my forehead, eyes, earlobes, neck, and then the curve of my shoulder. In the gray light of the rainy city drifting into the room, the warm touch of his mouth against my cool skin was the most arousing sensation I thought I could experience.

He continued down the hairline of my chest, reaching my navel, pecking lower and lower until his lips reached my hardened cock. He nudged it with his nose and sniffed it like a dog, and slowly he ran the tip of his tongue along the shaft of it. When he took me into his mouth, I let out a moan; I had never felt so alive, so deep and stiff and sexual that the aching adventure of it pleasantly hurt. Only after he had retrieved a towel to dry the sticky fluids which landed against our bodies did I return to the complexity at work within myself and make an effort to leave.

"I hate it when guys just up and leave so fast," he said. His arms had found my waist and he drew us together, kissing my neck again. "It takes all the intimacy out of it."

I stayed there for a moment in his embrace, quiet but not calm. Inside me was raging a fierce battle. Even though I felt a relief that this had finally happened, a layer of shame was working its way through me—I had come to terms with my sexuality, but had not yet conquered the enemy troops of morality, religion, and society. I fidgeted out of Bob's grip and began searching for my clothes. I had narrowed the million questions crashing around in my brain into a single one and, as I found and slipped on my underwear, I blurted it out. "When did you know you were gay?"

He lay on the bed on his stomach watching me get dressed in the dim light of the room, his upper body lifted off the mattress by his elbows. "I always knew," he answered. "I never doubted it. I was having sex with guys when I was twelve. And you?"

In the darkened room, his smile was wide and luminous, and I wanted nothing else to understand the direction he had accepted for himself and make it a part of my own path now. "It doesn't seem so black or white to me," I answered.

"I didn't notice it was a crisis a moment ago," he answered, the tone of his voice almost snide with insult.

I could not find it in myself to confess to him that he was the first man I had ever had sex with and I was still at war with what I had left behind—in another town and city and state. Then it occurred to me that something that was not so obvious about myself had been obvious to him when we met in the library.

"Do you want to go for some Chinese food?" he asked me, when I was dressed. "We did make plans for dinner, too. There's a place downstairs Peter and I love to go to."

"Peter?" I asked. "Who's Peter?"

"My partner," he answered. "He's away for a month."

"You have a boyfriend?" I said, with the same exasperated tone that Annette would often direct toward me.

"He's cool with this," Bob answered. His smile now appeared both charming and secretive, as mine must have seemed all those times when I didn't want to let Annette completely understand who I was. "We could do this again, you know," he added. "I thought it was sweet the way you found me."

* * *

I must confess that there are others involved in the tangle of my life in these years. It was not simply a choice of seeing Annette, of Melissa moving away, of John becoming involved with another man, or of my desperate reach out to Bob Kinnaman in the library one evening. No, no, no, there are others who were ensnared in this web of mine (and I in theirs). If this were a work of fiction, the reader might toss the book against the wall and say that the author could not bring in a new character or reinvent his scenario this late in the story. But by carefully studying the design of this reminiscence, it is clear that I have left this opportunity open. So what happened was that the "friend" whom I had visited in Washington en route to a new life in New York also came to visit me in Manhattan during this time. Her name was Stacey and I had known her since college.

Stacey was dark-haired and dark-eyed, and had a tiny, upturned nose sometimes camouflaged by the thick-lensed eyeglasses she needed to wear. We met at an audition for a play, the same campus group where I got to know John better. During the spring of our senior year at Emory, Stacey had a role in a musical comedy I directed. At the cast party to celebrate the final performance of this play, I ended up drinking too much and kissed Stacey out of appreciation. She mistook my affection and, in the final weeks while the rest of the campus was gearing up for graduation exercises, she wrote me a letter and said she loved me and that it was tough falling in love with a friend. But she also wrote that she was what I needed. I knew she was wrong, but did not write this back to her. I was glad that graduation came around and offered us a distance between one another. I moved back to my hometown; she moved to Washington to begin graduate studies at Georgetown. We kept in touch with one another as good friends at a young age will do; she wrote me long letters about her new experiences in Washington, and I replied with short explanations of my big move to New York. So it only seemed natural to me to stop over and visit her on my trip northward and celebrate this new direction of my life.

It's hard for me even now to explain the course our friendship took without making myself look opportunistic or foolish. The sequence of events still make me shake my head and roll my eyes and wonder *how in the hell did I let this one happen?* In some respect, it could have been my excitement at beginning something new or a way to prove that my path might not be the right one for me to take. I was as much riddled with self-doubt as I was anxious about finding out who I could truthfully become. So what happened was that during my visit with Stacey in Washington we had sex together. It was not accidental but neither was it self-determined. It just happened the way that sex can happen sometimes between two people. I kissed her, she kissed me back, and we ended up in her bed together. The next morning, I said my good-byes and did not feel that I had to justify my actions with promises of love or other future visits or romantic dates or any of the other things that Stacey was now looking for from me because that was not what I was looking for from her. What had happened had simply happened and it had not occurred to make something between us change.

But by October, her phone calls and messages for a repeat performance had worn me down, and Stacey arrived for a visit I no longer had the energy to postpone. I met her at Penn Station and, after we had dropped her suitcase off at my apartment, we took the subway to Central Park, walked through the rooms of the Metropolitan Museum, had a late lunch in the café, then walked down Fifth Avenue back to the Village. By the time we reached my apartment, it was hours later and I was exhausted from trying to keep Stacey entertained. I also saw with a clarity that I refused to acknowledge when I was with Annette, the exacting and tremendous confusion I was causing her. Throughout the day I did not touch Stacey as a boyfriend or lover would; I was not affectionate beyond the boundaries of friendship. Back in the apartment, lying side by side on my bed, I knew she expected me to reach out for her, to make her feel wanted in the way she desired to be. Instead, I rolled over and made my confession.

"It's not that I don't care about how you feel," I said. "I do. And I want us to be friends with each other. But I just can't be who you want me to be. I'm gay. I want a boyfriend not a girlfriend."

"I don't know what you mean," she said, drawing back from me. The news seemed to strike her with surprise, even though we had friends in college who had already come out as gay, even though she must have heard rumors of suspicion of my own sexuality during the years I knew her and paid her no more attention than as a friend. "Then how could this have happened?"

I could not explain to her the difference between my sexual attraction toward a man and that toward a woman in a way that would not insult her, that what I felt with Bob Kinnaman was so natural and necessary and what I felt with her and Annette felt too forced and confining. "I've not told anyone else this," I said. "It's not a secret. It's just something that I'm ready to accept now. It's just that this is who I think I am."

She rolled over and started crying and though my instinct was to comfort her, hold her and say that everything would be all right, I did no such thing. I got up out of bed and left her alone with her unhappiness, though my shame and guilt at doing so overwhelmed and punished me.

I went to the refrigerator and found a soda inside it, drank it straight from the bottle like a boy alone in his house would do, and tried not to feel trapped and depressed within the spaces of my new world. After a while, Stacey stopped crying, and we ate dinner and fell asleep watching television. I did not feel any better when she left the next morning, nor, do I think, did she. But Stacey was the first person I came out to as a gay man. And this experience finally opened my closet doors and allowed me to make this admission to others.

* * *

I might have found the courage to have this same discussion with Annette had it not been for the fact that Lisa, Annette's sister, called to say that Annette was in the hospital. The exact words and phrases still blur in my mind when I try to remember these details—but there was something about too many pills taken one night, the inability of Lisa to wake Annette in the morning, and an ambulance ride to pump out Annette's stomach. The reason for this behavior was never explained to me—Lisa did not pass any judgment on Annette or me, though I am aware that my own behavior might have contributed a good deal to Annette's instability at the time. I called Annette a few days after I received Lisa's message, when Annette was more stable and had been relocated to a psychiatric recovery unit, and our conversation was kept short and vague, in order to keep it from scratching open her healing wounds:

"How are you?" I asked.

"Better."

"I'm sorry."

"It's not your fault. Don't blame yourself."

"Are they helping you there? Is there someone you can talk to?"

"Yes."

"Will you let them help you?"

"Yes. This won't happen again."

Annette's "accident," as Lisa had defined it to me, gave my own life a chance to change. It was during this time that I found the courage to finally enter a gay bar in the West Village that I had been pacing back and forth in front of for weeks. I met a man that night, and then a different man another night, and somewhere within a short space of time I learned just how complex and difficult gay life could be. Gay New York was at the height of its arrogance and glory; sexual venues such as the Mineshaft, St. Mark's Baths, and the Hudson River piers were thriving. It seemed clear to me that my desire to have sex with another man would therefore make me feel comfortable in the gay community, but the truth of it was I still did not know where I fit in even after I accepted the fact that I was gay. I learned that the gay world was (and still is) full of subcultures—leathermen, drag queens, bears, and guppies and on and on—and what I was doing was trying to figure out *what kind* of gay man I wanted to be. Gay life was also making me aware of the alternatives of relationships that I could expect to find, both temporary and permanent: friends who had once had sex with each other but searched for other partners, lovers who had sex with others but maintained each other as a primary partner, buddies who got together occasionally for sex and not friendship, one night tricks whose names were kept anonymous. And, like the life I had dreamed of before, I wanted to experience all of those things but not have them define me in any one way until I was ready to do so myself. At times, my thinking and behavior now made me feel as if as if I were not a very good gay man; "good" being defined by achieving a level of contentment in the relationships I was finding and accepting. But during this period, I never stopped believing what I wanted from gay life—to find a man who could be equal parts partner, lover, and friend. *I wanted a boyfriend, not a girlfriend,* I repeated to myself like a calming mantra—that much I knew from my experiences crashing and banging around in the greater world around me—gay, straight, or otherwise.

I kept in contact with Annette during these first few weeks of my explorations into gay life, checking in to make sure she was recovering, but also, in a shameless way, to make sure she did not desire any visitations. Then, the end of the semester arrived with papers and finals, and next, the giddiness of my first end-of-the-year holiday season in the city kept me occupied, running to see the giant Christmas tree at Rockefeller Center, the elaborately designed store windows at Saks, Lord & Taylor, and Macy's, and the crowds of people gathering in Times Square to watch the ball drop on a chilly New Year's Eve.

And, before I knew it, it was February when Annette called to tell me that she had moved to Louisiana and was beginning a new route for the airlines, flying from New Orleans to Chicago to Seattle. She did not say if the decision to change her route was self-determined or mandated by her employer, but she did express an interest in seeing me, and suggested that I could come visit her for a weekend. She had even outlined a strategy for this to happen before I had a chance to balk at the cost of such a gesture—she could fly me down on a free ticket as long as I pretended to be her brother. Something in her voice told her me that she had reached the same conclusions about our relationship that I had and that this was a way to give us both a sense of closure and begin the rest of our lives apart. So I accepted her offer and, a few days later, she met me at the New Orleans airport.

Annette now lived in Metairie, a suburb of New Orleans, and driving to her apartment beneath a gray sky and a vista of strip-malls, drive-thru-banks, and fast food stops, it reminded me of where we had grown up in Georgia. Neither of us offered much affection for one another that day—there was no kissing or hand-holding or even tender pats in our reunion—it was as if we were relatives, now estranged after years of not seeing one another and uncertain of how to act or react when reunited. At her apartment, a small, indistinct unit among a development of similar ones, Annette fixed us sandwiches for lunch. I waited until we had finished eating and were clearing the dishes from the table before I brought up the subject of us—I didn't feel that it was right to let the weekend begin to play itself out without this conversation occurring.

"Not all of this is your fault," I said. "I think you should know I'm gay."

The news did not seem to shock her in the way that it had Stacey. Her back was to me, her hands in the sink rinsing a plate beneath the running water. I was grateful for this because I did not want to meet her eyes. She tilted her head slightly down, then looked my way without looking at me. "Well, then," she said. "That makes some sense."

I would not say that the news turned things around, that we became best friends after that. But neither did she let my admission spoil the weekend—we had, after all, a history of good times between us; we were friends long before we had tried to become lovers. She also did not spend time quizzing me on how I had come to this new and open realization about myself. Nor did she hope to change my mind. But there were plenty of awkward moments for us that weekend, nonetheless—observing other couples when we walked through the French Quarter, choosing an intimate restaurant for dinner by mistake, the quake in her voice when she asked if I wanted to sleep in her bedroom when we returned later that night to her apartment.

"I don't think that would be wise," I said.

"No," she answered, and straightened her posture, once again avoiding my eyes. "That wouldn't do either of us any good."

* * *

Looking back on this confusing time in my life, I am aware that there were others involved whom I have not mentioned here. There were two other girls, both friends from college, whom I did not sleep with but who were too close in my life to consider now as just friends. There was also another girl whom I *did* sleep with at Emory. My sexual performance, however, was less than adequate—I had not even been able to get an erection with her—and I am surprised, in retrospect, that it did not have some kind of ramification on my social standing at college. There was also another guy from Emory who captured my affections in these years, and another guy I actually kissed in a dorm room but prevented us from going any further. My last night in Georgia before my move north, we flirted and danced at Backstage, a gay disco in Atlanta, until "Last Dance" by Donna Summers closed it down for the night. But I could not go any further with him and I left town with a deep regret that perhaps I could have made things work there. In New York, I would not complete my studies at NYU and receive a graduate degree, and the University would not provide me with any other further dates or sexual encounters, though it would serve to introduce me to another young gay man who would become my first friend in New York. And, in the haze of my memory, I also recall an older man whom I worked with at Sears who invited me over one night for drinks to see his new apartment. He took me upstairs to his bedroom and offered to give me some dress pants he said he had outgrown. I remember trying them on, my head light from a cocktail he had made me, and his hand kneading my crotch while checking the zipper and my ensuing erection and hasty escape. Now, of course, I wonder why I had let that and other opportunities pass.

I would never see Bob Kinnaman again or know what happened to him. John would rematerialize in my life—we would later become roommates in a succession of New York apartments. I would hear of Melissa's comings and goings for years from my parents and the last piece of gossip I heard from my mother was that Melissa had lost her once-slender figure and was still single and living in Marietta. I was invited and went to Stacey's wedding—she married a man she met while in graduate school in Washington. But it would take me until I reached the age of thirty-nine to tell my parents the truth of my sexuality. Long before that, however, I'd discover that "coming out" as gay was a process that never ended—every new job, new friend, new relationship would arrive with this baggage in hand needing to be unpacked and explained.

It would be twenty years after my breakup with Annette before I would again confront the impact I might have had on her life. I returned to East Marietta to attend my parents' fiftieth wedding anniversary. Before arriving at their house, I stopped at the mall where I used to work to find gifts for my nephews and nieces. Sears was still there, so were many of the stores and restaurants where I had met Annette after work. But Cobb County had become a tangle of ramps and perimeter roads, full of traffic congestion and delays and confusing signs and lanes which seemed to evaporate the moment you drove into them. On my drive home from the mall, I became lost and found myself accidentally on the street where Annette had once lived. The split-level house was still there but I knew that Annette and her sister had long ago sold the property. I stopped the car in front of the house and looked at it again, thinking I might notice some detail I had never noticed before or forgotten because of time, or, maybe, something I could convince myself that the new owners might have added. Instead, I felt the shame of my youth settle in my stomach and I revisited the troubled spaces I felt with Annette and how hard it had been for me to come to terms with my life within my hometown. I reminded myself that Annette's life had turned out all right without me. She had married, settled in New Orleans permanently, and had given birth to two boys—I recalled having received this news one year in an unexpected Christmas card that arrived in the mail to my New York apartment. We had long ago stopped any contact or correspondence with one another but, as I put the car into gear, for a brief moment I was a young man again trying to escape the will of a determined hometown sweetheart. I had always believed that I could find a space—both mental and physical—where I could accept my sexuality and live my life the way it seemed most normal and exciting and challenging for me. Those years with Annette had been full of my desire to evade, to flee, and to run away from what frightened me.

But they had also been full of hope. I didn't choose Annette because I had chosen hope instead. Hope was the only logical path for me to take, the only direction I felt where I could discover my true self.

ON A DAY I AM NOT MYSELF

This was a few years ago but not too many. I was at a bar and a guy approached me and said, "You look just like that guy."

"Who?" I asked. "What guy?"

He looked me up and down as if to convince himself that I was not who he had imagined me to be.

"That actor," he said. "I don't remember his name."

"Then I must not look too much like him," I answered, "if you don't know who he is."

"No, no, you do, especially in the eyes," he said. "Except his are brown. And yours are what, green?"

I nodded and the man continued. "You must know who I am talking about. He was in that movie that everyone liked. Your chin is a little stronger, though. You've got a better chin."

Over the years dozens of people have commented on my resemblance to other people. This has happened to me in restaurants, at bookstores and parties, and on the street. I have been mistaken for a magician, a director, a self-help guru, and a chef, but most of the time I am mistaken for one actor or another. I have never had anyone tell me, however, that my chin is stronger than someone I am not. It gave me a little bit of hope that I might be attracted to the man in front of me because he might be attracted to me, or at least the person he thought I was.

"I'm sure I'm a bit older than who you are thinking about," I said, since this resemblance thing has been going on for years. My mother once told me as a baby I looked just like the child on box of diapers. In elementary school, I was told that I looked like a boy in a television show.

The man stared at me silently for a couple more seconds, not willing to refute my age against the person I was not. I knew my comment was testing him and he was quickly losing whatever points he had gained by the strong chin comment. Finally, he said, "He's not a very good actor. I didn't like that picture."

He lost some more points with that, and, after staring at me for a few more seconds, I lost whatever interest in him I had been able to muster when he first approached me. I said, "I'm sure he's a lot nicer than I am too," and, with that, I walked to another corner of the bar.

I think I managed to have a good time that night in spite of that exchange. I met another guy who thought I looked like someone else, too. His opening line went like this, "I bet I could make you my favorite actor." And, as someone who has often wished he was someone else, that was a line I pretended to like for a while.

ACTORS

I never believed I had enough self-confidence to become a working actor, which was why, when I moved to Manhattan at the age of twenty-three, it seemed more natural for me to find an offstage job. I worked for a publicity firm that specialized in promoting Broadway and off-Broadway theatrical productions and which was owned and operated by two older women who were lesbian lovers (and who, in their own youths, had also wanted to be seen more on-stage than off). Because of this job in the theater, many of my first friendships in New York were with other gay men and lesbians who worked in the theater, and I soon found myself coming out in what felt like a comfortable and protective gay environment. So it seemed more ironic than serious to me when I was confronted one day by my two bosses because of a rumor they had heard that I was having an affair with an actor in a Broadway show (which the firm was also publicizing). In my recollection of these events, this was a low moment for all of the parties involved—the two women threatened to fire me on the spot if the rumor was true and, because I did not want to lose my job, I pretended that the actor and I were just good friends. In fact, I acted like the affair really was a rumor. My lie was accepted but, not to let the matter drop entirely, the women decided to pass along some words of wisdom to me which they said they had each learned the hard way from experience: Never become involved with an actor. He'll always stab you in the back for someone better. (Or, in their case, she will steal your spotlight if it can get her a better part.)

These words of wisdom did not stop me from sleeping with other actors after the affair with the Broadway actor was over. In fact, as I recall now, that affair was already over by the time the two women confronted me with the rumor and so, perhaps, my lie was not really a lie, after all; by then, I had moved on and was sleeping with a producer of another Broadway show (and one which my firm did not represent). However, I did understand the truths the two women had presented to me because the producer I was sleeping with neglected to tell me that he had a lover who was also an actor, a fact I learned through another of my theater friends and had to pretend like I didn't care about when it was uncovered for me. I have always wondered who stabbed whom in the back in this particular case: me, for leaving the producer by moving on to another actor, or the producer, for acting with me like it was the first time he was in love.

There was another man I dated who was not an actor but who was always acting when we were together. He went to great lengths to pretend he cared about me and even greater lengths to pretend he wasn't stabbing me in the back. He had once been married to a woman and so he was full of alibis that had worked with her but which aroused suspicion when they were presented to me. (I knew, for instance, that the flowers that arrived at his apartment one night while I was there were not from his secretary but from another boyfriend, and, that the weekend he told me he spent celebrating his brother's birthday, he really spent celebrating with another lover.) This man was a good lover but he was not an honest man, which is why he was an unconvincing actor to me but nonetheless magnetic and intriguing. (Some men are more attractive because they are bad boys than simply because they are good-looking.) Some nights we would lie in bed and I would listen to him describe how he had fooled his wife into believing that the nights he spent with his first gay lovers were really impromptu out-of-town business trips. This was also when I created my own ethical understanding about the way men acted, and how, in order not to go crazy myself from despair and confusion, I came upon this conclusion: If he cheated on his wife, he will cheat on a lover.

This is not to say that this is a good characteristic or a bad moral trait at every given time it occurs; circumstance can dictate how deep or detached the parties are emotionally involved. For instance, not long ago I met a Scottish man who was in town with his wife and his two kids. He was a tall, beefy fellow with a shaved head and an earring who had left his family behind in their hotel room and walked a half-block to the nearest gay bar in midtown Manhattan, which was where we met. He told me he was not out to his wife and kids and only fooled around with guys occasionally. Since it was clear to me while we were talking with one another that this was to be one of those occasions he would fool around with a guy, I had no problem with assuming the role of the trick and taking the married man back to my apartment.

Which leads me to remember another man that I slept with while I was working at the off-stage Broadway job. He was a patrician-looking sort of fellow with a penchant for wearing bowties and suspenders and he had a high-pitched voice which meant he was often mistaken for a woman when he called my office. Nothing about his body was womanly, however. He had a musky smell at his underarms and there was a grainy feel to his skin, and he had a big floppy dick which he liked me to sit on when I came over to his apartment. Outside his bedroom, however, he pretended that we had done nothing together inside that room, which made sense to me the day he confessed that he had a fiancée. I pretended I had not been stabbed in the back, or anywhere else, and that I was not even upset by the news; instead, I acted as if I had already moved on to another lover myself.

This acting strategy was not always able to camouflage my emotions. A few years later, I met a man at a time when we were both vulnerable. I had just finished watching a friend die and he had just moved to town after the breakup of a relationship. We were a terrific comfort to each other in bed, where neither of us had to pretend to be attracted to the mismatched personality of the other. (He was a playwright who was not at all in tune with his prejudices, in my opinion.) Our personal drama might have run longer had it not been for the fact that the playwright had only moved out of town to take a new teaching job and not to end his prior relationship. One day at the grocery store, I ran into him and his would-be ex-lover (who was in town visiting) only to realize, as the playwright stammered through a hasty explanation, that I had been cast in the role of the third wheel without even auditioning for the part. My anger was award-winning, however, and I believe I gave one of my finest performances as that of the wronged party.

A few years before, I dated an actor who made me into a different man, or, rather, he created someone while we were together who I could no longer recognize as myself. He did not want to believe that I was unhappy in my career, unable to afford my expensive apartment, or that I should expect a date to be anything more than a good time, and so there was no discussion of how those things in my life might be changed or achieved, and I was transformed into a person whose life was stationary and uncomplicated. Confrontation and displeasure were banned from our conversations, which meant, in my opinion, that communication between us stopped. My life was reduced to a string of one word-adjectives like "Wow" and "Nice" that were more appropriate to the superhero sidekicks found in comic books. In retrospect, I do recall he had a great body, though he had none of the other admirable traits of someone you might expect to be able to save you from your own life. As for who wielded the knife in this situation and who plunged it in first, I do not recall. I only learned, in this instance, that I was really as poor of an actor as the script demanded, and that it was impossible for me to create a character who could rise above the truths of himself.

There was another guy from my early working days on Broadway, however, who I always expected to have a different life than the one he found. Our jobs required us to talk frequently to each other on the phone and we soon began meeting in person for dinner after work once or twice a week.

He was tall, slender, had black curly hair and thick eyeglasses, and wanted to be a producer, not an actor. Though I had a crush on him, I always felt we looked like Mutt and Jeff when we were together, and, therefore, let this fact prevent us from becoming serious about one another, even though it was clear to me that there was plenty of chemistry between us. There was also the matter of his admission that he was straight and mine that I was not, and so we spent our dinners dreaming about how to produce a Broadway show and not about how to bed each other. When our paths crossed on the street more than two decades later, he stopped to say hello and mention that he was now married to an actress and no longer a producer but an agent for actors. Since I didn't ask the question of his profession or his sexuality, it struck me odd that he so hastily provided me with these answers after all these years, which led me to believe that perhaps he was a better actor than I was, since I was still unable to forget the exact spot where he had plunged the dagger in my heart the night he stated his preference for women and not me, in order to prove he could become someone I was convinced that he was not at that moment, or would be at any other moment in the future.

JULY

I could have spent it in the city. I had been invited to Maine. I had wanted to go to the south of France. Instead, on the last summer day of July, a cool breeze sighed through an open Southampton window and whispered across the sun-bleached hair of my arm as I shifted it around the waist of a man named Philip, my face pressed beside his tanned back, our legs entwined beneath a sheet. I wanted to sleep but couldn't, my thoughts kept tumbling to the moment when he would say it was time to leave. I ran the tips of my fingers over the curve of his shoulder, around his chest and back down again to his waist. He turned, his eyes were closed and his mouth open, and his breath blushed into the hollow of my neck. My hand paused at the small of his back and I adjusted my breathing so that we rose and fell in unison. His face was still, so I closed my eyes and tried hard to repress what I had locked up for many months, maybe years.

The house this morning was still too. Over the last six weeks it had heard many sounds, and had hidden many more behind its closed doors. It was too early to begin packing and cleaning. The evening had lasted late, till dawn for some, so the morning would surely not begin till afternoon. I pulled the sheet up over Philip and around my arms and stared at the old leather chair where I had discarded my polo shirt and jeans, and he, his oxford shirt and linen shorts. Beneath the bed were buried the underwear and socks, a towel lay quietly in the middle of the room looking lonely, used hurriedly somewhere in the night. Outside a bird was composing a tune out of short curled tones and staccato phrases. I lifted my eyes and looked through the window to see if I could spot the bird perched on a limb, but all I saw was the wind swaying the branches back and forth, then rushing into the room to lift a piece of paper from the desk and scurry it to the floor. The wind rushed in again and tousled Philip's short brown hair, and for a moment it made me happy. But I sensed that this bucolic scene would not be repeated any time soon, certainly not in a city where schedules, commitments, jobs, and other pressures made a habit of invading into life.

"I miss the old Jimmy," my friend Barry announced four months earlier at a small dinner party in his apartment. "You used to be so much fun. You don't go out anymore and you look like a mess." It was true to a point. A few years ago I might have seemed more festive. I went to the bars, I went dancing and, occasionally, I even went to the baths. I'd had a lot of good times with Barry. We were younger, of course, and I was new to the city and many of its ways, so each step taken was an enthusiastic one.

But then I withdrew. Not from any particular reason. Maybe from worry, maybe from the current health panic, or maybe from just becoming insecure with myself. I concentrated on other things like a career, my TV set, old movies, and books. I exceeded my average weight limit and sprouted an unbecoming beard. I declined invitations to parties and eluded friends. I wanted to be and finally was, ignored. But most of all, I think, I wanted to avoid meeting new people. I didn't want to be vulnerable.

So when the members of this small dinner party started discussing plans to rent a house for a month during the summer in the Hamptons, to my shock and theirs, I agreed to be a part of it. Walking home that evening to my apartment, a six-floor walkup on a busy Village street, I told myself I had no expectations from this house. Well, maybe one. I wanted to escape the suffocating summer temperatures of the city. And maybe I would get a chance to relax, get a tan, work on that novel I had been telling myself should be finished by now, and maybe, just maybe ... No, not that.

JULY

And so the summer began. I shaved the beard, cut the hair to a short wash 'n wear crop, and shed a few pounds. The house was situated half between Southampton and the North Sea, a rambling Tudor Gothic off a semi gravel-dirt-sand path nestled deep in the woods with not a neighbor in sight. My housemates for the six-week rental were friends of Barry, most of them roommates from his previous Hamptons' escapade. Craig was a high school music teacher from Long Island who had just joined a gym the year before and was anxious to show off his newly developed physique. Keith was a Wall Street headhunter who, by the time summer came along had just found a lover, Daniel, who danced in a Broadway chorus line. Warren was an entertainment press agent who rattled too much about his clients, and Barry was, well, Barry, the *bon vivant* of our group. I was the youngest of the lot, just turning into my twenty-eighth year, the others, except for Barry, having passed the Great Divider of Thirty.

I must admit the beginning weekends were a mixture of frenzy, confusion, amusement, and adjustment. I enjoyed rediscovering the Hamptons. The landscape was not new to me; I had explored it thoroughly four years before. Yet I still approached it with a caution, aware that everything must be kept in order and perspective. On sunny days when my fellow housemates would scramble off to the beach in search of beautiful men, I would bike to the bay or the nearby lake and swim. Now and then I would join them at the beach, judging and worshipping the perfect physiques, falling silent when the sun melted across a flat washboard stomach reposed on a nearby towel. On rainy days we grouped in the living room and played gin, crazy eights, a noisy game of Trivial Pursuit, or raced into town to line up for a movie matinee. After dinner, nights were spent at the bar, arriving late, drinking too much, and then dancing it off with each other or with friends from the city. Still I felt an anticipation clouding the air wherever I went or whatever I did. Every so often it seemed as if I was caught up in a surreal version of *How to Marry a Millionaire*, where the topic of conversation was limited to three subjects with minor variations: Weather (Was it nice? What was the forecast?); Food (Where to eat? After, of course, What to eat?); and mostly Men (Where to find them? and Where to meet them? Never, What to say to them?).

But for the most part I was content. I lived through the quirkiness of the roommates, the house guests who trampled in and out at odd hours—invited and unexpected, the disastrous informal and undercooked house barbecue, and the annoyance of the long trip back to the city. I even survived a fashionable East Hampton cocktail party where the only thing that was biting were the mosquitoes on the lawn.

I've been told that when you're not looking for something, there it is. It was the usual night at the bar. It had been a glorious day, one of those really rare occasions when sun, sand, and attitude had meshed perfectly and flowed gracefully into the evening. As the midnight hour approached, the bar began to get crowded. I was at my usual corner inside the disco drinking my second rum and coke of the night, away from the accumulating traffic of men outside chattering, gossiping, and ogling one another underneath the striped canopy. The dance floor wasn't crowded yet, just four couples and one guy. I leaned against the wall, lit a cigarette, and watched. Watching, I recognized two types of dancers in front of me: those that danced to their partner—eyes connecting, and shoulders, hips, and feet tilting to the same pulse, and those that danced with their eyes closed, enrapt in the music—allowing only a momentary acknowledgment of who or what they were dancing with.

Soon I started a third rum and coke, and I waited for my housemates to wander inside, ready to dance. I was not observing the crowd, instead my attention tilted to the spinning display of overhead lights. A guy standing by the bar ran his hand briefly through his hair and paced toward the door. Instead of exiting, he stood beside me and smiled and asked if I would like to dance. Numbed and surprised, I responded with a quiet, "Sure," and headed toward the vibrating lights. I don't remember what song it was—a lot of them have a habit of sounding identical, the syllables and tones so recurrent you never know if you're sliding from one song to another. But we moved down the steps and began dancing—he with his eyes closed and me smiling when he wasn't looking. I did, however, shyly inspect who I was dancing with. He was attractive, probably just turning into his thirties. Taller than me by about four inches, he had wide shoulders that sloped gently down to a firm waist, suggesting an offspring of a swim team. He had a classic composure, dressed in a comfortable blue polo shirt and tan shorts which ended just above the knees. He danced simply, just moving back and forth on athletic legs, in docksiders without socks. His face was both strong and gentle, a sturdy WASPy jaw, not-too-sharp nose, thin, kind lips, and when he opened them, generous cool blue eyes. I giggled at myself as we stepped to the music, through the crush of favorites and on until it cleared. We stopped as quickly as we had started when he announced he had to find the restroom. Great, I speculated, even Mother Nature is not on my side. He left and I headed toward the bar.

A little later I noticed him on the other side of the room and decided that on my way outside I would stop to speak. Perhaps the oddest thing I did that summer was to thank him for asking me to dance. "It was nice," was the only phrase I could find to elaborate, and followed with "I have to go outside, it's too hot in here." That was true, because at that moment sweat was soaking into my T-shirt and I nervously patted away the stream of perspiration from my forehead.

To my astonishment he followed me outside and we started a conversation that included such reliable Hamptons' subjects as, Wasn't the weather great today? What was the forecast? Are you renting or guesting? Where in the city do you live? and I silently thanked him for ending this pale barometer of existence mercifully with another "Do you want to dance?"

"Sure," I replied again. And we danced and drank and went through some more minor dialogues. He was an advertising executive who worked on Madison Avenue. He lived on 63rd Street but was staying in the Village, only a few blocks from where I lived, subletting his apartment uptown for the summer. He was just out for the weekend, having opted not to do a summer share this year, and was staying at a guest house in East Hampton with two friends who were lovers.

In spite of the alcohol, the atmosphere, the circumstances, and the discourse, our talks seemed natural and relaxed, mildly probing yet politely avoiding. By four am that morning we had not covered a lot of territory, but nevertheless I responded to his sincere and uncomplicated manner, and as I bought the last round of drinks, I asked if he would like to come home with me.

Sex was not easy and resplendent that evening. We were both a little too inebriated, and after a few false starts, we opted to sleep before any further action. By morning our seductions resumed, but he left early, having to meet his friends in East Hampton, and I scribbled my name and phone number on a yellow scrap of paper and said in a groggy morning voice that I hoped he would call.

"Maybe we could get together for a drink in the city," he said.

"That would be nice," I answered.

I watched from upstairs as he drove away from the house, the wheels of the car sputtering bits of dry gravel into the air. As they pounded back down to the ground I winced at the examination of mistakes I had made. In my self-assurance of not seeming desperate, I had neglected to do one important thing. I did not ask for his last name and phone number. I had not completed and defined his existence. I could taste his warm breath against my lips, feel the way his arms had embraced my body, I rehearsed the sound of his voice reverberating through my soul, and decided that it wasn't just a one-night score. Indeed, I had a cause to be elated, and my housemates were shocked, ecstatic, and jealous.

In the weeks that followed I was not terribly disappointed when he did not call. Something far worse happened; I looked for the situations and emotions to be repeated. At first, I fled to the bars in the city during the week, hoping find him—to talk, to keep the momentum going. But he was never there. Instead of lamenting, I pushed with such an abandon to become acknowledged by any man I could snare. In the city I offered to buy strangers who would not look at me a drink, just to be able to communicate with someone. Most of them said no. In the country, I asked them to dance and a few said yes, but nothing ever progressed to anything beyond that, not even small talk. Gradually, these efforts subsided and I threw myself into the sun, running to the beach, the bay, or the lake. I became serene again, basking in the glow that a felicitous summer could at least include a brief encounter.

Finally the last week of our house rental arrived and I took time off from work. To show my independence from the others in the house, I rented a car. I kept a careful distance from the mainstream of men flowing between the beach and bar and only once let my guard down, at the insistence of my companions, to attend an afternoon beach party where my only tomfoolery was to get so dead drunk that it took fourteen hours to sleep it off. The weather cooperated with my plans too, proving that July can be an explanation to the meaning of a legendary eternal summer of mind. I often sat on the beach reading, turning the radio up loud, or just reclining, watching as an incredible tan matured. I lingered at the shore, close to the water's edge, until last of the light dissolved into fevered hues of scarlet, indigo, and amethyst. The house was also busy that week, with final attempts by everyone to grasp an indelible remembrance of our Hamptons summer. The last rush of guests invaded, and I dodged and dipped amongst them, pausing only for a bewildering conversation with a stunning blond man about morality, abortion, and the Jesuit religion.

And when the weekend approached and the weather turned sour, dispositions turned rancid and everyone fell to arguments, nagging one another or brooding alone in silence. On the day the rain stopped, the countryside remained entombed in a hazy fog and Barry and I drove to the beach trying to escape our claustrophobic spirits. We sat for a long time atop the dunes without speaking. Barry is my oldest friend from the city and with those types of friends many things can be communicated without linguistics. I curled my toes through the wet sand, building castles with the arches of my feet, and soon was surrounded by a mist so thick I could scarcely see him next to me. We recounted many events we had shared through the years, and reflected on a lot of choices we had made in our separate lives. Yet, I convinced him and myself that even if certain decisions had been different, the road would still be the same.

"But there's something else disturbing you, I can tell," Barry said over the sound of a braying gull. "There's still too much distance."

"My independence seems crushed," I sighed, lifting my face into a gust of wind. "I hadn't expected to feel the way I did about Philip and it all came too quickly. Instead of being able to dismiss it, I still keep looking for someone to replace him, to complete the picture."

I clutched at the sand and brought it slowly up to my nose, deeply inhaling the smell of brine, then tossed it aside, mentally trying to count the number of grains which remained firmly between the whitened knuckles.

"If you had one wish what would you want?" Barry asked, his elbows digging into the sand.

"Just to be happy," I paused, then added, "One wish would not be enough."

"I'd wish I could be straight," Barry offered.

"It would be easier," I agreed. In the distance a dog barked at the ocean.

That evening the clouds rolled away and the breeze swept away the mist and dried the puddles. Back at the bar, I leaned with one shoulder pressed firmly against the wall, my mind still hovering around its somber thoughts. As faces floated by I spotted a familiar one, more tanned and composed than the time I had last seen him before. I held myself in reserve, arguing whether or not to speak, and then what to say if I did. He was dressed in white, white shirt and white shorts, and as I approached I lost my nerve but turned too late, for he had recognized me. We started over on a few conversations and he explained that he was just back from a vacation in Bermuda with friends. And we danced again, this time the music screaming out words of desperation I tried not to hear. As the night progressed we explored each other further and the ease and comfort returned. He explained a foreign film, I recapped a best seller; he described a trip to Greece, I recounted a childhood in London. And finally we effortlessly slid into talks of parents, family, mutual friends, careers, and the future.

"I'm terribly embarrassed," I stated in a momentary lull. "I never got your phone number," I apologized, as if it had been all my fault.

He smiled, "How old are you?"

I paused for a moment to remember, then teasingly replied, knowing there was nothing to lose, "How old do I look?" and realized I had instead set myself up.

"Thirty-two," he guessed.

"Yes," I lied.

"I just turned thirty-four on Monday," he said dryly and I could tell the subject was an unfortunate one.

"Then let me take you out for a birthday dinner, to celebrate," I replied. He agreed and we set a date for the following week in the city, and with that I received his full name and number.

And we danced and drank as before. I felt lucky this time, kissed by mystical god.

And that's when I awoke with the breeze blowing across my arm, the wind sighing, the bird singing, and my thoughts tumbling about the room. The sex had been more passionate and varied than before. He left and I cleaned the house, washing the last bit of sheets and towels and began packing to return to the city. It was just Saturday and in my original scheme of design I had planned to leave for Manhattan early, but decided it was now worth to stay one more night.

That night was another mistake, for he avoided me at the disco with a fervor, finding others to dance with, others to talk to. I did the same, making it seem deliberate on both accounts, yet watching too closely to see if he would look for me. It's funny how Fate plays her hand, and as the morning light broke in the distance, I left for the city, more depressed than I had started the summer.

Back in the city, the evening was hot and uncomfortable, and I awoke many times during the night, to wipe away the sweat or think about what I was going to say to Philip, hoping to avoid being melodramatic as I pictured explaining to him what he had meant to me that summer. Yet as the night grew darker and the shadows that echoed from the street disappeared, I became frightened, not understanding why I could feel so deeply for someone who was really a stranger.

I phoned him Monday morning and we made plans to meet the following evening for dinner, the dinner I had promised for his birthday. I felt sure before I heard his voice on the other side of the phone that he was going to back out for some reason, but he didn't. He actually sounded pleased that I had called.

I was relieved. I wanted to end these confusing emotions gracefully, at least to myself. That day and the next I felt tired and heavy as if someone were now placing their hands firmly against my chest, pushing down hard with all his strength to stop my breathing. We had agreed on a Japanese restaurant in the Village that I liked, where the decor is stark and dimly lit by colored lights and the waiters could have passed for the Olympic gymnastics team. He was a few minutes late when the appointed time came around, yet I didn't mind. I had prepared to be stood up.

We commented on how different it was to see each other "out of context" of the Hamptons and how different it was not to be "East," as he liked to say. Our conversations were again easy and relaxed, more than I had anticipated. In fact, it only reminded me of how fond I had grown of him in such a short time. When dinner ended and the conversation died down, I felt a flutter in my stomach, as if I had remembered something too late, and a thousand emotions and expectations argued within my heart.

And that was when he confessed and said he was dating someone he had met on the train ride his last weekend "out

East." I was not smart enough to know if this was a lie to let me down easily or if he was telling me the truth.

    I smiled at him across the table and thought about sitting on the beach, arms folded around the knees, back hunched against the setting sun. I gazed out to the ocean and watched the water break against the pebbles and shells and disappear beneath the sand. The sky was clear, like his eyes across the table, and I watched a gull soaring overhead and tried desperately to spot a ship somewhere on the horizon. But it was too late in the afternoon. And I thought a brief moment about the month of July, and how it had been a mixture of sunshine and sunburn, of rain and tears. I paid for the check. It was time to go. This was another person I would have to learn to outgrow and leave behind.

PASSING GRADES

I recently turned thirty and one evening, after a celebratory dinner in Chelsea with a friend, I headed home to my Village apartment. Strolling casually by myself along Seventh Avenue, I passed several couples—male and male, female and male, female and female—linked arm in arm and enjoying the gentle autumn weather. I was not disarmed from my euphoric state by these happy and content couples. (I see them every day.) That happened when I passed an attractive man walking in my direction—a tall, handsome guy dressed in a suede jacket, cotton shirt, and jeans, himself probably just in his early thirties. And he was alone. He glanced in my direction for one of those brief moments and, as I swept my eyes up to meet his, he looked abruptly away. It was that brief visual exchange that disrupted my contentment. I began to worry if I was still capable of making passing grades.

I am not referring to the types of grades we got in high school or college, those academic marks my mother always frowned about when I warned her that I might be receiving a "B" instead of the usual "A." I mean the grades the causal glances mark, those curious little asides that linger for a half second as you continue down the street, step on a bus, shower at the gym, or stand in a crowded bar. The ones that can serve as a prelude to so much more.

My roommate, who is a month younger than I and also now in that peculiar third decade, is still capable of receiving high marks in this department. I have witnessed men, women, even children stop on the street to admire him. But then he has one of those bodies that time seems not to weather, just to define and chisel a little more perfectly each day, regardless of how much hair he might have shed from the top of his head. Still, my roommate is not immune to this "test." Although he receives high grades, he administers strict examinations. I constantly listen to his stories of dismay about dates—one was too tall, another too old, one too bald, and even one too young. There is always something a little too "too" about all of his prospects which, given a little time, might become an admirable characteristic. And so it was, in that brief moment on Seventh Avenue that I wondered, too, if I was not only flunking tests, was I also flunking others?

And then one night not long after that my roommate announced once again that he was desperate to meet the ideal man. But this time he had a solution: He had decided that he was going to meet Mr. Perfect/Mr. Right through computer dating. (This from someone who could get anyone on the street interested by just standing still.)

"I want a monogamous relationship," he announced. Another bizarre statement, I thought, from someone who often settled for something quick and safe and had been through several unsuccessful monogamous relationships. I listened as he filled out the questionnaire and eavesdropped on his phone conversations as a computer dating service began to arrange his first contacts.

His dates were brief and unfortunate. One date barely spoke English, another guy was too spaced out on drugs, another never showed up. The worst was the young boy who paid for his dinner in quarters, and then had to borrow money when he found out that he didn't have enough to pay for his portion of the bill. And none of my roommate's contacts were quite up to his physical attraction standards. "I specifically requested *Very Attractive* on my form," he ranted around our apartment.

I could not help thinking that my roommate might be overlooking something. Was he grading his dates on attractiveness, as we all so often do? What about sensitivity, caring, creativity, and a whole slew of other important attributes that should be graded?

"He just wasn't right," my roommate growled as we loudly discussed the subject.

"You're taking a bad date out on me and that's not fair," I answered and sulked into my room, ending the argument. Then I remembered an incident of my own and began to sympathize.

I, too, had once graded someone rather harshly. It was right after an unrequited relationship had turned sour. I had convinced myself into believing that the man I was seeing was someone I could fall in love with and he man was not allowing the relationship the opportunity to work. One night, in an utter state of confusion over the matter, I crept into the shadows of a bar. I stood there silent, with a gloomy disposition, oblivious to all distractions, until a man in his mid-thirties who stood at my side interrupted my contemplations. He was tall, and though not unattractive, not altogether handsome, either. A real average-looking guy. As we talked, I found this average-looking guy warm and understanding. This was a genuine person, and on the one date we had, to see a movie, he was attentive and caring, and ready to be patient as I attempted to rebound from my previous unsuccessful relationship. Yet, I subsequently avoided him. There was something missing between us, some little chemistry that did not ignite within me. As I recall now, I had not given this guy a passing grade in physical attraction.

What is it exactly that I'm after, that perhaps my roommate is also seeking? I will admit that the first thing that draws me toward a man is his physical attractiveness, though I do not desire any particular category or trait; for me it could be something simple—the way a strobe of light illuminates a profile, a wisp of hair that is blown out of place, a shirt slightly askew but firmly defining a shoulder. I sometimes wish I could settle for a brief physical encounter. But those days are gone for me. Those momentary opportunities were once satisfying by themselves, like a Chinese take-out meal. Quick and easy, and if nothing else materialized, could soon be forgotten.

Now I find I want more. Not only must prospects pass a physical evaluation test, I also grade them on other things. Perhaps the greatest barometer of evaluation I use is the characteristics I admire in my friends. Does this person possess the humor, wit, adventure, intelligence, and affection of my friends? Can this man sustain me for more than one night? Although I am thirty, I do not feel that much older than I did a year ago. In fact, I feel better. My friends tell me I even look better (but that is what friends are for). And I find it a relief to be chronologically thirty, instead of worrying about what it's going to be like when I get there.

A few days ago, I met a friend for a drink. He was about to leave for vacation and suggested a bar we both used to haunt. "And bring along your roommate," he added. "I haven't seen him in months." It was a genuine request. My friends like my roommate because my roommate is my friend.

We met as planned, and the three of us laughed, chatted, and gossiped in a dimly lit corner. Eventually, my friend left to catch his flight. My roommate politely disappeared to cruise the crowd. I was suddenly left alone, leaning against a wall, feeling in a good mood.

A handsome young man standing next to me turned and spoke. "The guy you were talking to before, does he come here often?"

"Occasionally," I answered, and turned to study this guy.

"What's his name?" the young man asked, before he had asked for mine.

"John," I replied. "He's my roommate."

"Was he a gymnast? He's got one of those bodies."

"He was in high school," I answered, and sipped my drink. "But the rest is from the gym."

Perhaps the subject will change, I thought. Perhaps this guy is using my roommate as a pretext to begin a conversation with me.

The young man continued to pump me for details. "How old is he?"

"Thirty," I answered.

"Is he seeing anyone?"

"Perhaps you should ask him yourself," I said, and placed my empty glass on the counter and disappeared.

I don't remember much more of that evening. That brief encounter sent me fleeing to other bars and other dimly lit corners, where I moped and guzzled more beer. It was silly for me to be so dispirited, really. Thirty wasn't that old, after all. I was still young. I still felt young. And I could get a guy to notice me if I really tried. I had everything in front of me but didn't care. I drank that night until my money ran out, then finally trudged back to my apartment, alone. The truth was that I had flunked someone's physical evaluation test.

But the next morning I awoke ready to take on the demands of another day. Surprisingly, there was no hangover, physically or emotionally. As I stepped outside and walked again along Seventh Avenue, I hesitated for a brief moment as I, myself, passed a grade on a handsome man walking in my direction. It was nothing to get upset about, I decided at that moment. Physical grading will never disappear and the hands of time cannot stop them. But I did remember that it is a road traveled in both directions. We not only pass grades, but offer ourselves up for examination. Passing grades is just one of those little things one has to live with, like each year growing a bit older.

INVITATION TO DANCE

There is something wonderful about the way a man dances—the way the hips move back and forth or in and out, the shoulders shift to heavy rhythms of music, the feet twist in a way not possible when walking. There is something wonderful about watching a man dance—the eyes darting to follow an attractive figure spinning and twirling between colored spots of light which shoot down from a black, smoky ceiling. There is something wonderful about dancing with a man—eyes, shoulders, hips, and feet balanced, connecting to a synchronous beat. There is just something wonderful about dancing, enrapt in the magic of music and motion.

In the decades since I first acknowledged a preference for my own sex, there are few things that I still enjoy as much as dancing. For it was in the milieu of the disco, those dark cavernous rooms overflowing with stunning physiques and alluring smiles, that I learned what it was like to dance with another man.

Back then, in the heady disco era of the Seventies, dancing served for me and many of my friends as an introduction to gay society. For many of us just coming out in suburbia, our trips to the city disco palaces were propelled by curiosity. It was our first attempt to investigate this culture and open our understanding of what we were trying to be. It was an opportunity to contemplate the lingering glances, to see if what we felt was unique or if there were others who shared our proclivities. Most of us became enchanted, suspended in the carnival of blinking lights and throbbing sounds where handsome men advanced and retreated, paused and primped, cruised and waited. And we watched, lightly rocking in syncopation to the music on the heels of our feet until we decided to join in the dance. And when we made our decision, we patiently sifted through the quasi-intimate conversations, wanting to hear or speak only one phrase: "Do you wanna dance?" The answers which followed could open or close bedroom doors.

It was in this dancing world that we began to define our conceptions of sexy and sex. Even more, it created many of our illusions and fantasies. Dancing with a desirable man between a rousing drum break and the swell of synthesized violins lifted us into a dream of who we wanted this man to be and what he would mean if he remained when the music stopped. It was a chance for us to imagine the future, where all this dancing was leading, what could possibly be next.

It has sometimes crossed my mind that now, somewhere beyond thirty, I would have moved on to something else. But the image of coming out in a world of dancing men has forever shaped my consciousness. I have fallen in love many times with dancing men.

So why, if dancing means so much to me, did it suddenly become so intolerable? Perhaps because I began to take the dancing too seriously. I am not referring to the study of dancing, for the lessons which taught me where to pivot the feet, when to swivel the hips, swing the arms and dip the shoulders, and how to harness the pirouette, heightened the performance of dancing and produced the self-confidence to remain on the dance floor. I mean the obsessions dancing generated, the rituals it demanded, the excesses it provoked, and the expectations which resulted.

It was the obsession to float in a sea of desirable men—men with "sculpted profiles" and "chiseled torsos which glistened with sweat" when T-shirts were removed and tucked into the back pockets of tight jeans. It was the ritual of what to wear, when to arrive, what attitude to assume, and when it was time to shove the clenched fist toward the ceiling in time to the pounding tempo. It was the excess to maintain the good time—the magic, the beauty, the high—through whatever drugs or drinks we wanted to try. It was the expectation that participating in this frantic revelry would guarantee an even better time in bed, which in turn could lead to an even greater expectation—finding myself with a boyfriend, finding myself in a relationship of commitment and caring, one conceived in love and happiness. This was what I wanted—sometimes as far-fetched of an ideal to other dancing men as, well, a trip back to suburbia.

I never realized the tremendous despair this world was breeding until one morning when I hit the street alone at five in the morning. The dancing hadn't stopped, but that night I had never started. I was waiting for something to happen, something or someone to make me start.

A few years ago, at a time when I was going through a particularly dry social period in New York, my job sent me on a hopscotch path to many of America's major cities. In New York I had discarded all my expectations of one-night-stands; I wanted something more permanent. If that wasn't possible, then I would be content to spend an evening with friends or alone. And it was a time our world was becoming more cautious. Carrying this attitude out of town, my curiosity returned. The same curiosity which had led me into this culture was nagging me back. I was curious about what the rest of gay America was doing.

They were still dancing.

But I never discovered if they were dancing the way we had been dancing, or if they were dancing with some newfound attitude. For when I returned to the disco and stepped out on the dance floor again, I discovered the most important secret about dancing today: Dancing is just a simple joy. Dancing, I could release the frustration, forget the pressures of the job, the schedule which could not connect with another person's. I could forget about the rent and the bills. I could ease the heartbreak of knowing friends were dying, had died, or were scared about dying. I could forget about the plague that haunts us all and disrupts our lives. I could forget about sex. And relationships. At last, the expectations, obsessions, fantasies, attitudes, rituals, excesses, and illusions had disappeared, replaced by simple motion. Dancing became a physical pleasure, not a philosophical quest.

Today my friends don't understand my passion to keep dancing. They don't go out dancing anymore; it resurrects too many memories for them of what our world used to be. They miss it, though, the way we used to dance.

But I have not stopped dancing. Now, I dance because it makes me feel good. That is what I tell my friends they must now learn. I know what I like, and I like the feeling I get from dancing. A feeling like being kissed for the first time. A feeling of muscles vibrating inside my skin. A feeling of motion pushing me somewhere forward, leaping over the hurdles of life.

I know I will never stop loving the way a man dances, *or* dancing with a man. And I know one day my own steps are going to slow, the rhythm become more guarded; I cannot fight the process of aging. But now, sometimes late at night, if the blues begin to seep into my body, I can fight back. I turn the lights down low, plug my headphones into the stereo and twirl around the room—happy, just to sweat and pirouette, dancing as the music spins.

THE LAST MINUTE FRIEND

It was 7:49 p.m., Saturday. I had showered and dressed in a clean shirt and jeans. I had no plans for the evening, so I sat on the small couch in my apartment and waited for the phone to ring. Someone would call. Someone would want to see a movie, have a drink or go out for a bite to eat. Someone would know I was not busy. Someone usually did. And they all knew I rarely said no.

At 8:01 I became restless. I could wash the dishes, clean the tub or water the plants, but I did not feel like moving. Instead, I decided to wait. If no one called, I would fix myself a drink, watch TV or read a magazine. If the evening passed without a call, I might fix another drink, turn on the stereo and sit by the living room window and stare at the wall of apartment windows across the courtyard. I could watch my neighbors entering and leaving their sanctuaries, lights blinking on and off at their commands. Behind the flower pots scattered on the ledge of the fire escape, between the laundry fastened to plastic wires that stayed out for days to dry, I could witness other lives. Directly opposite my window I could watch a girl, hair in rollers, talking on the phone. Next door, behind a twisted black grate, an old man would be silhouetted against a blue wall, worriedly smoking a cigarette. One floor beneath and two windows to the right, behind red venetian blinds, I could see a bed. Sometimes, on nights like this, I would just stare and wait, watching to see if the man behind that window added a companion sometime in the night.

My apartment, a six-floor walk-up on Bleecker Street, offered a variety of views from each of its windows, so different and startling fom each other that when I had first stepped inside the apartment I was able to overlook the cracked tiles on the lopsided kitchen floor, the makeshift shower atop a dwarf-sized tub, the over-painted door frames that reached up to a crumbling plaster ceiling, and the tiny alcove which could be used as a second bedroom.

Here, I lived in a bright spacious bedroom, and through my bedroom window I could contemplate the statue of a saint recessed into the steeple of a church across the street. The face on the statue was indiscernible, but the palms of the man were clasped in front of a flowing gown and a cross rested over his heart. Underneath, the word "Humilitas" was etched in the white cement. This was a window which would not inspire hope, would not encourage desires and would not allow dreams to overshadow life. It was a view that showed a way to survive, promising insignificance in a city of significance.

It was now 8:17 p.m. and the phone had not rung. There hadn't been any calls all day. Nothing for my roommates Debbie and John. Nothing about the party I had missed last night. Nothing to do with my public relations job, where I would usually show up on Saturdays to make up for mistakes I had made during the week. But not this weekend. I had only been out of the apartment an hour this afternoon and when I returned no one had left a message on the answering machine. Nothing from Bill. Not even a call for Kim, a transgendered sex worker who had mistakenly advertised her services with my phone number in the back pages of a tabloid which someone in Ohio was usually thumbing through.

I stepped toward the living room window, but tonight the wall of apartments was dark. Inside, the refrigerator was empty. Debbie had cleaned out the leftovers before leaving to visit a great-aunt in Connecticut. John had finished off the last of the cheese and crackers before disappearing on a date with a waiter that so far had lasted two days. And I wasn't hungry. Habit was sending me searching for something to do.

I thumbed through my address book, longing to find someone I might call. Steve was still in Atlanta; Karen was floating in a pool in Florida. Barry was at his parents. Mark and Kevin were out of town. There were names I dared not call and names I knew I would never call. There was even a list of names I could never call again. Maybe it's too late to call anyone, I thought, and closed the book. It might only prove I was depressed and alone, and oddly, tonight I was afraid of showing that to anyone.

Turning out the lights in the living room, I went into the bedroom and stretched out on the bed. I tilted my head and stared at a photograph of the rooftops of Vienna which hung on the wall. Gray, brown, and red clay shingles topped the buildings beneath a bright blue sky, spires jutted to heaven while the white-framed windows below were dark and empty. My eyes wandered to the black space of the window and strained to find something in the agnostic void. If only the saint would stretch out his hand and offer comfort, but I knew not to expect a miracle from chiseled stone. An attack of anxiety, as abrupt as a lightning bolt, made me jump from the bed and grab a jacket from the closet. I bolted out the door, hurrying down the endless flights of stairs, and into the street. Maybe something will distract me. Please, if there is a God, don't let me be alone with myself tonight.

When I reached the street, I jammed my fists into the pockets of my jacket to break the gusts of wind, took a deep breath, and slowed my pace. As I started down Bleecker Street, I stopped briefly to watch a cat settle into a nook of the pet store window, then walked quickly past the flashing neon sign that hummed "Reader and Advisor," avoiding the stare of the heavily jeweled woman who drooped her chin into the folds of her neck. Colorful bins of apples and oranges lined the sidewalk outside the greengrocer, the smells which drifted from the buckets of flowers made the city seem like it really was spring. Across the street, the antique clothing store where I had bought my jacket, tonight displayed exotic hand-embroidered gowns.

I turned my eyes toward the pavement as I stepped past the line of customers outside the pizza parlor. I thought for a moment about sitting in the cafe on Cornelia Street but decided the espresso I would probably order would only make me more agitated and unable to sleep.

On Seventh Avenue, a black stretch limousine was parked at the curb, the driver blowing smoke from a cigarette through a crack in a window. At the intersection a few steps further, stacks of papers atop wooden crates at the newsstand were bannered with headlines and photos of subway violence. I stopped and wondered what was left to do. Any other time I was alone I might go to a disco or a piano bar, a crowded room of men dancing and singing could often lift my spirits. Sometimes I would walk to the gym and work out, then sit in the steam room till I was finally overcome with exhaustion. In the last three weeks I had exercised off about seven pounds. Now I wore contacts instead of my glasses. Ray, a friend who worked at the salon on Christopher Street, had recently cut my auburn hair short around the ears and neck, the long thick strands which he had left on top had not even begun to thin or recede. Ray said I had never looked better. He still looked more like twenty-five than thirty-four. If times had not changed, I knew I might drift toward the baths, spending the evening enwrapped in an anonymous man's arms.

Beyond the liquor store window that was taped together, I paused at a clothing store and studied the airbrushed bodies of mannequins wearing strapless gowns. Below, in the corner, a "Help Wanted" sign leaned against the glass. Behind me two young men in baggy cotton shirts laughed at one another as they passed by, and I turned and followed them for lack of anything better to do.

* * *

The door was slightly ajar and the light from the hallway slammed into the darkened room in the form of a single beam of light, creeping along the polished floor till it bent upwards to sit on the bed. I hesitated before entering the room, studying the pale, withered body which lay motionless underneath the white sheet. A white gown stopped just above the thin, fragile elbow of a man, the rest of the exposed arm punctured by tubes and needles and the prodding hope of a miracle.

"His friend went downstairs for coffee," a nurse said when she passed me standing beside the door.

I entered the room and the beam of light disappeared as I flipped on a lamp. I sat in a chair by the window and looked out into the night. The view was another wing of the hospital; the other windows were dark or concealed by drawn blinds. I turned and drew the chair closer to the bed and its motionless occupant. Behind me a dresser was covered with flowers, arrangements in baskets and vases cascaded toward the floor. I tried not to stare at the virulent lesions which ringed the thin neck of the man in the bed, but the short purple strips seemed to have been beaten into the body, whipped into the flesh by an insensitive master.

"She let me go home early today," I whispered softly to the man. "They were so jumpy because the weather was so nice."

I leaned forward and touched my fingers to the silent man's chest. It looked as though the breathing has stopped. I felt my hand lift and fall lightly atop the body, and I withdrew my arm and placed it against the side of the chair.

"I brought a book to read," I grew stronger. "I thought about bringing a magazine but then I was worried you might have read it already. I even thought about bringing a Bible," I tried to laugh. "A Bible? Can you believe it? I mean, even if we could make any sense out of it, would you believe it? You know, I don't even remember what religion you are. Or if you even had a religion. Did you? Sometimes, like this, I don't think the Bible has an answer, and I don't know it well enough to find a passage of comfort. I was never that kind of a religious person."

"But this is a really good book," I explained and held the book as though the man could look at it. "You might have read it before. And I'm sure you know the story. Still, it's one of those books you can always read again. And it sounds really nice out loud. It's one of the few twentieth century books that do."

I opened the book and began to read, slowly and deliberately, careful of my enunciation and phrasing, though knowing I might be the only one listening to the sound of my voice. I read of a world where all people are not equal, as told through the voice of a man reserved of judgment. My lips and throat became dry when I reached the end of the first page and I stopped. I had lost the desire to even turn the first page. Perhaps my choice of reading material was wrong. Suddenly I did not want to read a story about shattered dreams and romantic hopes, a tale of desire defining reality. "Please tell me if you were happy with your life," my voice cracked as he spoke to the immobilized figure. "Did you know all the things you wanted to know? Did you feel everything you were supposed to feel?"

I knew there would not be an answer and I left the chair and returned to the window. "It's not fair," I said. "I want an explanation first. I feel like someone's firing a gun while we float in a pool."

* * *

I hovered uncertainly outside the door. Many times I had hesitated before. When I first moved to the city anxieties had caused my hesitation. I was afraid of finding myself on the other side of the door, worrying about spending an evening alone. Tonight, I hesitated from a different sort of fear, the fear of knowing no matter how long I stayed on the other side, when I left I would be leaving alone.

Inside, I felt as though I had been wedged into a mirrored sardine can, packed tightly between the bodies of denimed men and soaked in smells of beer and cigarettes. There were a few men huddled in groups, chattering and laughing, but the majority stood silent and alone. I squeezed between two guys who eyed each other with expectant glances, caught the bartender's attention, and paid for a beer. I found an unoccupied corner of a wall which vibrated from the pulsing rhythms of the DJ's music and leaned against it; next to me a guy in a sleeveless T-shirt rippled his arms and made me feel like a teenager in white socks, out of sync at my first formal dance. I noticed a group of young men looking in my direction, and decided their glances were directed at my flexing neighbor. Maybe he's a porno star? I wondered. The porno star was obviously the subject of several conversations, but the men in the room seemed either mildly curious or gravely intimidated and only shifted closer as new arrivals jockeyed for positions.

As I sipped my beer, an inexorable expectation lingered at the back of my mind, the belief I could still find a relationship with another man, a relationship based on something more than fashion and physiques. I knew times were different, but I hoped my own desire had not been altered. Surely there must be something more, I thought, than this undeniable passion to connect with another man's body.

"See anything you're interested in?" a voice behind me asked.

I turned and smiled. "Hello, Philip," I said and patted the man on the shoulder. "You're looking good."

"Not as good as you," Philip smiled. "You must have noticed that half the men in this bar are cruising you. And the other half are cruising themselves."

I shifted his back against the wall to make room for Philip to stand beside him. "It's hard to believe we're still doing this," he laughed.

"Welcome to the Decade of Illusion," Philip said and waved his glass in the air. "Today you can look sexy. You can be sexy. But the question is, is anyone still having sex?"

"Somebody must be having a good time," I said and sipped his beer.

"Virgins," Philip sighed. "Virgins are having a good time. The rest of us are getting drunk," he jiggled the ice cubes in his glass. "And the best thing an older man can get today is what he can give himself with his own hand."

I focused my attention on a dark-haired man on the opposite side of the room. Jeans hugged a slender waist, a plaid cotton shirt caressed the wide shoulders. What would it be like with him? I wondered. Would it be possible to share something more than just sex? Could he be sincere and trusting? Affectionate and witty? Does he possess the qualities I admired in my friends? Barry's humor? Kevin's charm? Not long ago that might not have mattered. I would have been satisfied and content with just an evening of sex.

"Is that all you wanted?" I asked. "Sex?"

"It was all I needed," Philip said. "I never took someone home and said, 'Stick around, maybe we can throw a dinner party together.' But if he did stay, that was great. At least for a while. Then one of us would get restless, and that was the end of it. We always wanted something more."

"Something more or someone else?" I asked. "Something more was what we couldn't keep for a night. Someone else was what we always went after. Didn't you think you might fall in love someday?"

"Who needed to think about love? I was satisfied with the blond salesman from California in the afternoon and the Italian lawyer at night," Philip said. "And you know something? I don't regret any of it. How can I? How can I suddenly feel guilty about something I didn't know about? I can't walk around thinking, 'Why did I ever sleep with that guy from 76th Street?'"

I watched the man in the plaid shirt and jeans move to another corner of the room. I turned and noticed Philip had also been looking at the man.

"And you?" Philip asked when I returned his stare to the man in the plaid shirt. "Why didn't you ever settle down? Everyone always thought you'd be the perfect catch. And look at you now. The rest of us are fighting our middle-age bulges, and you look younger than the day we met."

"I always thought I would know when I was there," I said. "When I wouldn't have to look any more. I never knew it was something you had to work at, and something that had to work both ways."

"Why didn't it work?" Philip asked.

"One of us wanted someone else," I said.

"The other wanted something more," Philip replied. "I should have loved you."

And I could have loved you, I thought, and headed toward the bar.

* * *

I lit a row of candles. Though the night outside was warm, the church felt cold and vacuous, and I rubbed my hands slowly over the flickering flames, the heat momentarily dispelling the chill from the tips of my fingers. I dipped a finger in a puddle of hot wax that had formed at the base of a candle. There was a prickling pain, as though I had been stabbed with a needle, but when I checked my hand I noticed the skin was unmarred and I rubbed the drop of wax against my thumb until I had worked it into a tiny, supple ball.

The church was almost empty, a few women wearing scarves around their lowered heads were scattered throughout the pews. I took a seat in the back of the church, but kept turning to the left to watch the light of the candles lick the gray stone walls, rising in spontaneous leaps toward the bottom of a darkened stained-glass window. I was surprised I had decided to visit the church, for years I had looked at it from the window of my apartment and wondered what the interior was like, yet walking past it at least twice every day, I had never considered stepping inside. This time I had not approached the church deliberately. I was on my way to my apartment, when I had noticed an old woman climbing the steps toward the church door. Feeling I was not yet ready to be home and alone, I followed the woman inside.

Before I entered, I knew the sorrow I carried would not be dispelled, yet I hadn't anticipated the chill and the silence and the bleakness of the church carrying me deeper into my thoughts. Sam had been the first to die. Sam and I had only been casual friends. We had met eight years ago at a party in the East Village. Over the years we had never made plans to see one another, but occasionally our paths crossed at other parties, the beach, and sometimes at a bar. Sam had died almost two years ago, and the reason, his friends said then, was he did everything excessively. One of his friends said he smoked too much, drank all the time and could never get enough of the young boys he picked up loitering on Christopher Street. Another friend gossiped that it was the steady stream of drugs that infected him. Everyone said that even though they were far from being saints themselves, they all agreed they were never as obsessive as Sam. What had happened to Sam would surely not happen to them.

When Gordon died, I was startled at the realization of the abrupt transformations that were occurring in my life. From the small stage of the off-off Broadway theater where Gordon had appeared in a play, I told a gathering of friends about a trip we had taken to Provincetown one summer. Gordon had spent a week romancing a couple from Canada, breaking them up and then putting them back together. As I explained, it was both heartbreaking and hilarious to watch, and though my voice was tinged with a fond nostalgia, what I failed to mention and kept locked in my thoughts, was the knowledge that such an adventure could never happen again without the fear and guilt of possible consequences. And I wondered silently, too, what had become of the couple: Were they still together? Were they in love? Had there been others and how was their health?

I had not even been aware Cliff was sick. We had briefly worked together in the publicity office, but after he left to take another job we often spoke on the phone and met for drinks. It was Cliff's father who called and said he was cleaning out the apartment. Cliff had left a note about some books he had borrowed, and he wanted to be sure I got them back.

There had been other friends and other funerals. A week before he died, Mike said to me that now it seemed like life was intruding on death. Sometimes I felt I couldn't remember what it was like before. Sometimes, when I stood too close to a strange man in the subway or at the gym, I would catch myself staring too intently and wonder why it was I must now think before touching. Sometimes I simply closed my eyes and imagined I was in another place and another time: the man would undress and turn toward me, the next sensation would be skin against skin.

When Mike died, I thought I would finally feel relieved. I had accompanied him to doctors and hospitals, picked up prescriptions and vitamins, and waited through chemotherapy and blood transfusions. Bill, Mike's lover, never once gave up hope, reading all the information he could find, he would spend hours hounding doctors on the phone. While I helped them with their cleaning and cooking, Bill kept Mike amused, every inch of their apartment was crammed with some kind of distraction, from video tapes and compact discs to a miniature electric train that circled the floor. Every day we made sure Mike got out of the apartment; toward the end they had to carry him in a wheelchair up and down three flights of stairs. What Mike left behind, I found, was not the memories of ten years of friendship. Somehow, when he died, Mike left behind his pain. I had watched Mike's healthy features fade: at first the once taught muscles disappeared, then the skin began to pale and the dark black hair fell out. And gradually Mike's eyes grew larger and larger, till I was afraid Mike would not be able to bear the weight of them. And what was left, I realized, was not the release of relief nor the recollections of the young man I once knew, but the image of the man who now haunts me, a disrupted figure suddenly turned old, a man who learned too soon what it's like to die.

I felt through my jacket but the pockets were empty. In my jeans I found a quarter and I pulled it out and let it fall to the floor. The sound of the coin sent a discordant clatter through the church. Somewhere I had heard if you threw a coin to the floor of a chapel, an angel would slip and break a wing. I wasn't trying to cause immortal harm; I only hoped if someone divine was listening to my thoughts, that now He might understand why I felt the pain.

I left the church quickly. Zigzagging around a band of boys huddled over a box and a deck of cards, I was back on the sidewalks of the Village. A gust of wind whipped around the corner of a building and carried scraps of paper furiously skyward in a whirlpool of dust. I twirled around in the wind and the colors of the glaring neon signs and the people who rummaged through the garbage blurred into an abrupt and beautiful kaleidoscope. Beyond the noise of traffic, the honk of a taxi cab and the thunder of the subway beneath his feet, I heard the siren of an ambulance screaming into the night.

* * *

It was as if my head had been stuffed with cotton. I squinted at the bright lights of the coffee shop and the balls of thin white cotton seemed to have been dunked into a thick, heavy syrup. Lights blazed from every corner of the store so I could not even locate my own shadow. Lights so vivid and brilliant, I thought any minute they would singe the white tufts of threads, ignite the explosive syrup, and blind my view of the trays of donuts behind the counter. Honey-dipped, lemon-filled, cinnamon, chocolate-covered and more. A whole universe of sugary choices in a shop that never slept. I propped his elbows on the shiny steel counter which reflected more beams of light and ordered a bag of glazed donuts.

There were only three other people in the shop. An old man in a bright orange parka rubbed his hands over a bowl of dark soup. A woman in full evening makeup with a raincoat thrown over a nightgown mashed a slice of toast into a yellow puddle of eggs. A young boy with a shaved head and studded metal clamps across his forearms sipped a cup of coffee. Each was alone, adrift in their own little fantasies, as silent and oblivious of one another as the pitch black night outside the torch-lit shop of dreams. A man with a stubble of gray beard handed me a bag and folded his arms together, his eyes growing vacant and thin, as if they too had been dipped in a sugary film.

Twisting the key into the front door lock of my apartment building, I jiggled the metal frame lightly, waiting for the unknown, metaphysical force which would slip the tumblers into place. I never knew how long this twisting and jiggling could take. Sometimes it would be a simple and clean snap, other times it would take pounding and jabbing to connect. This was a door which would open, though it could never be prejudged as to precisely when.

Tonight the key snapped quickly and I slowly ascended the six flights of stairs, the heavy syrup that clogged the cotton sifted deeper and deeper into my body with every step. At the top floor I unlocked the apartment door and flipped on the light. The digital clock which hung on the exposed brick wall informed me it was precisely 2:47 a.m. I walked into the kitchen and ate three donuts quickly, tearing each into strips before shoving them into my mouth. I wiped the table clean and threw a handful of sugar flakes into the sink, watching them dissolve when they touched droplets of water. I turned out the light and stumbled to the bedroom in the darkness, flopping onto his bed without undressing.

"Is Kim there?" a husky voice asked when I lifted the ringing phone in the dark.

"No," I grumbled, awakened from a cloudy sleep. I looked at the clock on the night stand which read 3:29.

"Is this the right number?" the voice asked.

"No," I replied and listened to the static crackle through the line. "It's been changed."

"Who's this?" the voice asked curiously.

"I'm sorry. I'm not what you want," I informed my gentleman caller.

"Doesn't matter. What's your name?" the voice warmed.

"Jimmy."

"Are you alone?" the voice whispered.

"Yes," I whispered.

"What are you doing right now?" the caller inquired gently.

"Thinking...," I drifted, his eyes looking in the direction of the stone saint illuminated by the street lamps outside his window.

"About me?" the husky voice asked.

"Perhaps...," I replied. I turned away from the window and found a pillow to support my head, then slipped a hand slowly and deliberately between my thighs.

ROCK HUDSON'S VACATION

When Rock Hudson died at his home in Los Angeles in October 1985 at the age of fifty-nine, his death created a transformation in the public consciousness of AIDS. Though he was the first major public figure to openly acknowledge that he was suffering from the illness, his last days were not without sensation and scandal. Speculation about his health began earlier that year when he appeared thin and frail during a taping of a cable television program hosted by his former co-star Doris Day. News reports during the summer had him collapsing at a hotel in Paris where he had gone to seek medical treatment and, soon thereafter, stories began to appear of the actor's secret gay life in Hollywood. Not long after that, and only a few weeks before his death, Hudson released a statement at an AIDS fundraiser in Los Angeles that read: "I am not happy that I am sick. I am not happy that I have AIDS, but if that is helping others, I can, at least, know that my own misfortune has had some positive worth."

Rock Hudson's closeted gay life was not so secret to many people; like the sexual activity of many other gay entertainers (Liberace, Tony Perkins, and Montgomery Clift), Hudson's homosexuality was generally known and accepted in the entertainment industry and gay community and, in the days before media "outing," protected by the goodwill of both. Five years before his death from AIDS, I met Rock Hudson at the opening night party of a Broadway musical that I was working on as an apprentice publicist. The black-tie affair was at an Upper West Side restaurant near Lincoln Center. Hudson and his partner at the time were friendly with two women I worked for and I was introduced to the actor while he was seated at a table with his friends. One of my bosses was also seated at the table and as I leaned down to whisper a question in her ear, she turned to the man next to her and said, "Rock, this is my assistant." I tilted my head and my eyes met his briefly. He smiled and I blushed, but before anything else could be said, my boss was standing up from her chair, pushing me out into the room, and giving me instructions to assemble the cast for a photograph. I was twenty-five years old that year and still a wide-eyed newcomer to New York City and the Broadway theater, and I did not let the opportunity pass to find some kind of a detail of the man who was an American icon which I could pass along to my friends and family. In my recollection of that night, I realize exactly how young and boyish I was, amazed simply by the actor's towering height when he stood up from the table to leave the party. He was heavy-shouldered and six-foot four, and it was clear to me why he had made it in Hollywood—he still carried the handsome ruggedness that had made him a legend.

I am not even a minor character in Rock Hudson's story. My meeting is not revealed as any anecdote in any biographies of the actor or the reminisces of his friends. He was never an idol to me. I didn't think much of the films he made with Doris Day—there was always something so implausible to them—though I came to admire his films more in the years after his death, my favorite being *Giant* because of its epic quality. Rock Hudson was more a part of my parents' generation than my own. And, as I recall, the year that I met him I was more enamored with the likes of Richard Gere and Jack Wrangler.

* * *

I must backtrack, however, to explain how I found my first job in the New York theater. After college, I moved from Atlanta to Manhattan with the dual purpose of attending graduate school and exploring my attraction toward men away from the scrutiny of my family and a hometown girlfriend. At New York

University, where I was studying in the Drama department, I met my first gay friend in the city, an editor for a show business trade paper who was involved with a man who worked as a theatrical publicist and whose office was looking for a gofer. At the time, I was working a few hours a week as a telephone answering service operator used primarily by actors and the money I had taken out in loans for graduate school and my move north was quickly drying up. I thought a full-time job would help get my finances in better shape and, if the truth be known, the lure of working in the professional theater was too heady to resist. I loved the theater and desperately wanted to be a part of it. As a young man in Atlanta I had performed in summer stock productions, built sets for productions that played the Civic Center, directed large scale university productions, and toured shopping malls, high schools, and retirement homes singing with a cabaret troupe. My interview with the woman who co-owned the entertainment publicity firm was brusque and brief. I was hired on the spot, not because I was young and eager and smart and came with theatrical experience and a recommendation, but because I could spell and type without too many mistakes. (This was the era of carbon paper and bottles of white-out, three copies of everything typed at once.)

My daily duties at the new job included canvassing the newspapers and magazines that arrived in the office to find tearsheets and clippings that mentioned clients and shows the agency represented. I was so naive to the business of show business that I was not even aware that the city sported three daily newspapers or that there were such things as theater critics for television networks. I was taught how to fold a printed press release and the correct way to insert it into an envelope (headline side up), as well as how to seal only half of the flap on the back so that it would be easier to open by the recipient. The two co-owners of the agency, their one associate, and I sat in the same room with our desks facing each other so that our interactions were both effortless and annoying. I was to answer the phone before it reached its second ring, even if I was talking on another line. In the mornings, I made coffee before anyone else arrived, and at lunch time, if there were no pressing engagements for the owners with a producer or a reporter, I brought back pastrami or tongue sandwiches from the deli across the street. At night, I delivered ticket requests to the box office and messages to back stage doormen of the theaters where the office had shows running or clients performing. I typed names on envelopes, licked rolls of stamps, and carted bags of mail to the post office. It was one of those jobs that makes you question why you went to college in the first place, and so it was no surprise that I surprised myself and dropped out of graduate school because I felt that, well, as silly as it sounds, I was learning a lot more from working in the theater than I was by studying it in a textbook.

The main partner of the agency, the taller and older of the two women, was a mannish lady with a penchant for long mink coats and cowboy accessories—pointed toe boots, large engraved belt buckles, and Stetson hats. She had worked in the publicity business for more than thirty years and was full of a wisdom she felt necessary to direct toward others, particularly me, since I was in such close earshot of her booming voice. She had originally hoped to be an actress, but during rehearsals for a show she tripped on an imaginary flight of stairs and broke her collarbone and, as luck had it, ended up working in a publicity office where she began by typing, answering phones, and reading the papers, just as I was doing. Years of smoking had left her with a hacking cough and a deep, phlegmy rasp, which she would transform into a girlish tone when on the phone, trying to place a story with an editor or columnist. Her partner was a short, younger Italian woman with manicured nails and a teased hairstyle that made her pale face seem surrounded by a pair of large, dark raven's wings. She was the novice publicist of the two owners, but the sharper businesswoman when it came to keeping the office running and the books balanced, and she spent hours refusing to take phone calls while she punched the keys of a calculator with the eraser tip of a pencil, the chug-chug-chug of its motor spitting out a long ribbon of paper.

I did not know that these two women were lovers when I first began working in the office, but it was not difficult to realize it after a day or so of their temperamental activity toward each other. They were big New York City creations—butch and femme—two self-made successes with a few family pedigrees thrown in, who shared an apartment on Park Avenue, a summer home in Connecticut, and a Mercedes Benz which they housed in either east or west side garages, depending on what side of town they were on at the time. In addition to their celebrity clients and Broadway productions, they had a Rolodex of high-profile friends, gay and otherwise, culled not only from the theater community but also from the fashion industry and the media. On New Year's Eve, they threw an annual party where black tie was *de rigueur* and the likes of Rex Reed, Ann Miller, Lana Cantrell, Liz Smith, and Ethel Merman might be spotted and which, once I had paid my dues in overtime hours, I was also expected to attend, even though I was decades younger than most of the other guests.

I soon found that there were other young gay men working in the support industries of the Broadway community training to become company managers or house managers or press agents. Many of them became close friends when we began to gossip of the bizarre behavior of our employers or clients. We would swap tickets to each other's shows the same way straight boys would swap baseball cards, and invite each other to opening night parties where we were not expected to work because we were not there for a client but could, instead, find ourselves locked in the embrace of a waiter in the stall of a downstairs bathroom for a few brief minutes of unexpected pleasure. It was a heady time to be young and gay and working behind the scenes. My story, however, and my years of working in the theater, is not that of someone who might have bartended at Studio 54 and found sex and drugs and a kind of celebrity for himself. It is the story of young man trying to understand a quirky business and who is always overworked, but aware that there is something special around the next corner that he has never before seen or done or known about, so he puts up with a little more than he might have if he was older and wiser. One night, for instance, I *could* make it inside the velvet ropes of Studio 54 and watch Andy Warhol's coterie arrive because a friend of a friend had passed along a VIP ticket for that night, or another night, I might have to work and show up late at the theater to escort a press photographer into a backstage dressing room when Robert Redford congratulated the cast. The list of people I worked with and met is extraordinary for its time: Truman Capote, Kathy Bates, John Travolta, Eve Arden, Geraldine Page, Celeste Holm. Harvey Fierstein sent me a Christmas card. Elizabeth Ashley pressed a bandage against my forehead one evening after I had been injured while preventing a mugging. I once had a conversation with fashion designer Donald Brooks about the shoes I was wearing, a pair of gray suede platform shoes I had brought with me from Atlanta.

I've often avoided talking about my work in the theater because I felt that it could easily overshadow other aspects of my life. I am also somewhat embarrassed by this past obsessiveness of mine to belong and be a part of the theater, as well as the large amount of faith that I invested in it, hoping it would lead me to find myself, and which is why, when the novelty of this job wore off, I found that I was fighting a cynicism that was bitter even by New York standards. And it's hard for me to admit, too, that I invested a great deal of time and energy trying to prove myself in a career in public relations that I soon discovered I was ill-suited for, whether it was in the theater or in a corporate environment. But that is not to say that those years were without fond memories or deeper discoveries about the direction I wanted to take my life. This, too, requires a bit of backtracking to explain.

* * *

By the end of my eighth month working in the publicity office, I began a three-year apprenticeship to join the union which represented the theatrical press agents and managers. It would be a long struggle for me to complete this because I had added up the pluses and minuses and found my heart was only half in the job. The apprenticeship was low paying, my bosses were jealous and vengeful and, while I continued being the office gofer, I was now juggling added responsibilities—writing press releases, setting up interviews, helping with the details of opening night performances and parties. Occasionally, there would be some other person brought in to help out in the office, but generally the budget was small and limited and the new help that was found was not necessarily interested in starting at a rung that was well beneath the basement floor. The associate who had found me the job was gone before I began my apprenticeship, and another associate packed up his bags when a show he was working on folded; another came in and found no problem with having the young kid do his work for him until it was time for him to leave as well, which left the agency essentially a three-person operation—the two older women (the bosses) and myself (the hired help who kept things going).

You may notice that I have not identified my employers by name. It would be years before I could acknowledge the damage to my self-esteem they had caused. Sometimes I think that I watched my youth disappear during this time—I always seemed to be working, dragging myself into the office on weekends to update a list of press contacts, repair a release I had fudged, or cover an event that was happening at a theater. I was also rock bottom poor. The money I earned from my apprenticeship was not enough to pay my rent. I often walked thirty blocks to work to save money that a subway fare would cost. Many days I skipped lunch. I was lucky that I answered the phone at work so I could hang up on the credit card companies tracking me down about missing a monthly payment without my bosses knowing how bad my finances were. As I look back on those years, however, I do see that I had dates and affairs (though no one serious emerged), and I explored gay life with my friends with the same curiosity I was investing in the theater. I went to the bars, beaches, and the baths, hitched trips with friends to Fire Island and the Hamptons, took buses to Provincetown and Atlantic City, but it always seemed that I had this job to come back to that I didn't like but everyone else thought was wonderful. At times I wished I were older because then I thought I might be able to take my life more seriously and that others might regard me as someone other than the kid who worked in the office. For a while I grew a beard in hopes that it would make me look older, but the truth of it was, I looked, instead, like a boyish man impersonating an older one.

It was during this time that the two women I worked for began talking about a vacation that they would be taking around the upcoming end-of-the-year holidays. As a rule, they did not take vacations and loved to remind me of the fact when I dreamed of taking one myself. (There are no holidays in the theater, my bosses liked to tell me, only added performances.) The women did, however, maintain a three-day work week during the summer months, which essentially gave them four consecutive days at their country house. My work schedule during those summer months remained the same, however, always available and always on call and always trying to cover the fact that they were not in the office and not available to take anyone's call.) Their upcoming holiday vacation was a Caribbean cruise on a private yacht with several friends, among them, as I recall, Claire Trevor, Ross Hunter, and Rock Hudson and his partner. At the time I thought it was a luxury to have them out of the office. They were eager to get away from the relentless pull of the theater and work and I was eager to see them go. My bosses were big drinkers and I imagined their celebrity friends to be as well, and when the day of their departure arrived, I visualized them lounging in recliners and sipping exotic drinks, attended by smartly dressed sailors and cabin boys. *Bon voyage*, I said to them on the phone. (And please don't bother me while you are away.)

By then, the day they left for their cruise, I had fully recognized the mistake I had made in continuing with this publicity job, but I was also becoming aware of who I wanted to become. I had decided I wanted to be a writer. I did not see my own life as something to write about, so for inspiration I had become enamored with the idea of writing down the anecdotes of a friend who was an itinerant actress and musician and her travels with a small group of musical performers around the country. I was writing my first novel. I had started reading more to learn the structure behind fiction, started constructing my friend's anecdotes into tales and then stories and chapters of a novel. And I could not get this idea or this desire or these characters out of my head until I had put them on paper. They pursued me down the street, waited with me while I delivered messages or asked questions about interviews and held press tickets in my hand. I recall one day being tugged away from my responsibilities in the office and toward the typewriter by one of my characters chattering away in my mind, and I started typing away at my desk, only to be asked in a suspicious tone by one of my bosses what the hell it was that I was so furiously at work on. I made up a lie, telling her that I was writing down some column ideas I had heard. (After that, in the office, I only wrote notes on scraps of paper while answering the phones, everything typed up later at home.)

So when my bosses left for their vacation with Rock Hudson, my immediate reaction was *Hooray!* I would have more freedom to write in the office. Of course, I was grimly wrong. Anyone in a small office (or large one, for that matter) who has ever covered for someone who is on vacation knows that it is usually twice the work load to assume. And, in my case, since I was covering for two absent bosses and trying to keep a business running, it felt even harder. The phones showed me no mercy during this vacation—I was constantly trying to retrace my bosses' steps and cover their tracks—they had left me a list of clients who they did not want to know they were out of town. For two days I said that my bosses were at meetings, or at a rehearsal, backstage in a dressing room or not back from lunch. I hated lying. I wasn't a very good actor, though I had managed to fend off Jerome Robbins and Bobby Short, among others, set up an interview with an actor and the *Daily News*, and help an out-of-town critic get press tickets. One small-time producer, however, wasn't buying my lie and demanded to speak with my boss. After his third or fourth phone call to the office, when he stopped short of calling me an ugly name, I called the number of the coast guard that I had been given to use only for emergencies, and was patched through to the phone aboard the ship. A man who I assumed was the captain answered the line and I asked to speak with my boss (the butch one). While I waited for her to come to the phone, another man came on the line and asked, "What's the weather like in New York?" It was unmistakably Rock Hudson. "Cold and stormy," I answered, wondering if he was aware that I was also talking in metaphors. "Well, let's hope it clears up before these two try to catch a flight home."

The next thing I knew my boss was on the line. She was not in a good mood. I had obviously disturbed her for unimportant business. When I told her about the continuous calls from the producer, she let out a string of expletives. She sounded a bit drunk, but then she wanted to know everyone who had called the office while she was away. I went down the list I had been collecting. When I reached Jerome Robbins, she interrupted me and said in her little girl voice, "Jerry called? When did Jerry call?"

After I had given her an answer and the phone number Jerome Robbins had left, she reverted to the booming voice of an ogre that I had come to expect and received a dressing down because I should have known to call her about Jerome Robbins and not the small time producer.

As I moved through the remainder of the week with a frantic skill, it occurred to me that I had to find a way out of this "career" and change the direction of my life if I wanted to become a writer. Here I was in my mid-twenties, already facing a mid-life crisis.

* * *

During the second year of my apprenticeship, a small story was published on the back page of the first section of *The New York Times*. It was a news report about a type of cancer which was being found in gay men. I remember that it triggered a lot of thoughts and questions within me, foremost the notion if my desire to have sex with a man instead of a woman was biologically determined. At this point my story takes a similar route of other gay men in the city during these days. We worried, we read the news, we talked with friends and compared potential symptoms and confusions over the concept of "safe sex." The theater community was one of the first and hardest hit by the first wave of the AIDS epidemic. I worked or attended early fundraisers at cabarets, discos, art galleries, theaters, and even a performance of the circus. I can remember when the phone would ring in the office and the conversation would be over a sudden change in casting because an actor was in the hospital or gossip about whether a certain director or producer might be ill. And many of these remarks were about people I knew and worked with on a daily basis.

The analogies that have compared the early years of the AIDS epidemic to trying to survive in a war zone were apt. Some days I felt it impossible to control the direction of my life because each piece of news that arrived was like another bomb exploding. And, as the truth became more grim, I carried around a depression that was difficult to shake off.

As it happened, the years passed and I completed my three-year apprenticeship and, not long afterward, I held a union contract for the office for the national tour of a play. While this new position allowed me some opportunity to travel to other cities and be outside of the office for days at a time, it did not remove any stress I felt from the job nor did it change my dislike for the profession of being a publicist. My bosses had also reached a change in their own thinking about my role in the office; they now expected me to bring in new clients, something that they had clearly not championed during my prior years nor had even bothered to discuss with me. When the national tour suddenly closed due to a lack of sales, I found myself back in New York and without a job because the office was without enough clients to support paying all three of our salaries. Within days, however, I was fortunate to find a job in the corporate sector, helping publicize, among other things, spray paint, motor oil, and fast-food hamburgers. This was another odd fit for me and when, a few weeks later, another theatrical contract was offered me in a different (though still small) entertainment publicity firm, I returned because I had not found a sense of self-confidence in any other place beside the theater. This, too, was another unfortunate decision for me to make; I went to work for a man I had known socially through my theater friends only to find out that he maintained a nervous, hyper-officious alter ego in the office. He made the butch and femme look like school girls.

Throughout all this I did not lose my desire to be a writer. I had long since finished the itinerant actor-musician novel, sent it out directly to a list of editors and publishers I had culled from press clippings, and had a large folder of rejection letters that did not so much disappoint me as to challenge me to become a better writer. And so my life in the city became a daily routine of odd contrasts, walking uptown to Times Square from my office near Macy's, for instance, to cover an interview in Judith Ivey's dressing room, only to leave a few minutes later so I could sit in a small neighborhood park in Hell's Kitchen and read a book that I hoped held some new clue for me on how to be a better writer, before the next duty at the theater called me back to Broadway or the sun set and I was forced to return to my tiny, expensive apartment. I refused to allow these two personas to overlap though it was often hard to keep them separate. I told very few people about my writing because I was afraid of being mocked and losing my passion to continue. And I was continuing to write about working in the theater, but now my stories were closer to my own experiences. I had written a short story about an actor who was trying to hide his illness, loosely based on a client I had known while I worked in the publicity office. I knew it wasn't ready to be published, so I enrolled in a writing workshop that was being held on the Upper West Side, hoping to find a way to make it better.

This was the point I was at when the news of Rock Hudson's death came to me. It wasn't difficult to glance back and remember when I met him at the opening night party or talked with him during his Caribbean vacation with my former bosses. It almost seemed like an idyllic time in my mind; since then, the ground beneath me had shifted and trembled with and without my own uncertain steps. In the wake of Hudson's death, the media would begin to change their coverage of AIDS. Elizabeth Taylor, his longtime friend, shocked that no one even wanted to mention the word, went into action and helped form The American Foundation for AIDS Research, at a time when then-President Reagan steadfastly refused to even acknowledge the crisis.

And in truth, I believe that Rock Hudson's death did not change anything in my life that was not already on that course before it happened. But it did make me realize that what had been a part of my former job in the theater was not necessarily going to be a part of my future years in the city as a would-be writer. I never really lost my love of the theater, but during these early years of the epidemic, it just grew into a smaller and less important part of myself. AIDS would further impact me in ways that I could never imagine. It would take me a few more personal crises to find my own voice on the page and the way to the stories I felt I should tell. But one other thing that became resolutely clear to me at this moment: There was no going back to what had once been—things had changed and I had to find a new way to survive.

ISN'T IT ROMANTIC?

One of the most romantic evenings I ever spent was a night two years ago with my friend and roommate John. We were both thirty-one and depressed. He had just broken up with another boyfriend. I had not had a date in several months. We sat on my bed watching a science fiction movie I had rented entitled *Space Camp*, I believe, and drinking lite beers and eating pistachios. We laughed a bit between moments of boredom and talked over the ramble of action and dialogue which jumped out from the screen. I was tired from a stressful day at work and the beer had easily made me relaxed. I was wearing the black sweatshirt and loose fitting white cotton pants I wear when I sleep. It was cold in the room and the windows of our Chelsea apartment had been poorly constructed and winter air seeped through the sills like puffs of breath. John was in jeans and a blue cable sweater which was a present from his now defunct boyfriend and he was wearing no socks. This was not an unusual night for us. We had done this many times before. Yet, when I looked away from the TV momentarily, the flickering images against the darkness were so much like candlelight it made John's short hair seem blond and then thick and black. I suddenly felt buoyant, enchanted and content. I have always thought John was a handsome man. Then he slipped his bare foot beneath the calf of my leg to keep it warm.

For years I have always imagined and fantasized that moments like that would lead to something else. You know what I mean? From romance to sex to love is the way it goes. (Or is it from romance to sex to love? I'm not sure exactly what the progression is now that this decade has become so confusing.) It's true that I loved John... still do in fact, but that sort of love stems from years of friendship, and sex with him wasn't on my mind that night. It rarely is when we are together. We have been friends since college, some fourteen years ago. But the feeling I had that night, the ethereal weightlessness I imagine an astronaut experiences in space, I can only describe as romance, as inadequate as it may seem.

Other romantic times: With my friend Karen one evening atop the observation deck of the Empire State Building. We were still in our early twenties and we had both recently moved to Manhattan. Below us the lights of the city shimmered for miles against the cool summer night, promising us years of adventures and experiences ahead. With my friend Joel after we spent a morning hiking at Acadia Park in Maine and we stopped to catch our breaths as we sat on a cliff which overlooked a serene mountain pond. With my friend Debbie one night as we walked down Bleecker Street and paused to listen to two street musicians playing a baroque duet. And again with my friend John. This time in Washington D.C. where he had just moved. It was a warm spring afternoon about two weeks after the cherry trees had bloomed and we had walked from the Smithsonian to see the Jefferson Memorial. The pond in front of the memorial had an immediate magical effect; the water was covered with fallen white and pink petals.

Each time the feeling was the same. The lightness, the tranquility, the mental clarity with all the edges out of focus. And sex was not a thought or a result. Romance is a powerful emotion; too many times it is tangled with love and sex. I have tried many times to analyze precisely what triggers this feeling in me. Most often it is initiated by something visual, usually spectacular or fascinating. But there are times when I realize romance is deeper than aesthetics. It's a matter of timing and depends upon a variety of factors; the right spot, the right attitude, the right companion, the right events which proceed the moment.

Even the dictionary which lies on my top bookshelf offers little help with understanding this type of romance. Forget the references to narrative verse or prose, forget the adventures of knights and chivalric heroes. It is not fabrication or imagination, exaggerated, idealist or fanciful as this particular book tries to explain. Even the movies cannot accurately capture this feeling. They can stimulate it, even to such an excess it can take your breath away, but the result it produces is a yearning of sorts, why can't life be like that? I ask.

Romance in reality is never how it is imagined. I will be the first to admit though, I have fantasies on the subject. I have always dreamed there is a handsome man just around the corner. Someone capable of sweeping me off my feet with attention, presents, and yes, love. Perhaps that makes me a bit of a sentimentalist. But I am also a realist. I've been unattached all of my adult years and I know that kind of romance doesn't happen as often as it does in movies and books. For me it's a little like believing in ghosts and witches and horoscopes and crystals. But again that's not the romance I'm trying to describe. I mean the romance without any strings or expectations attached.

Surprisingly, one of the most romantic times I ever had was by myself. Three years ago I was in Paris for four days and I spent most of my time seeing all the things a tourist does in Paris: the Louvre, the Eiffel Tower, the Latin Quarter, Montmartre, the Champs Elysees and Note Dame. And what I had heard for years was exactly true. Paris is romance. Everything from its monuments to its sidewalk cafes. But I learned one valuable lesson from that trip. I would never go back to Paris alone. Romance is something you want to share.

I do not know if my friends have felt the pockets of romance I have had with them. I do not know if the vividness I experience had the same recognition for them as it did for me, but I have an intuition it did. Last year my friend Kevin and I went to see the circus at Lincoln Center, something we had done many times during our friendship. But this time Kevin was sick. He had been diagnosed with AIDS nine months earlier. He had Kaposi's sarcoma, had lost a great deal of weight and had been unable to work for almost a month. He had trouble walking and was afflicted by inexplicable pains in his lower back and legs. That night the ground was slippery and it was covered with snow that had melted and then turned to ice. Kevin refused to use a cane and we walked slowly toward the entrance of the circus, our heads lowered to the ground, cautious of our steps. It was cold. A brittle wind blew around us and my hands were shoved into my coat pockets. I glanced up for a moment, noticing the white lights in the trees near the entrance to the circus. And then Kevin slipped his arm around mine, his hand resting on the inside of my elbow. At first I thought he needed to balance himself or slow down the pace. But then he said as he looked ahead, "Isn't it romantic?" It is a moment I will never forget. He knew exactly what I was thinking.

Perhaps what this means is that romance is one of those forces I will never have the capacity to understand or explain, right up there with gravity and electricity and why my car runs on expensive gas instead of water. Perhaps romance lies more within the heart than the mind. But one thing I do know. I like the feeling. I like the moments.

THREADS

Thursday, June 23, 1988. The day began hot, humid. The fan perched on the windowsill offered little comfort; before getting out of bed I was covered with a thin layer of sweat. The radio announced optimistically today's temperatures would be milder: high eighties instead of sweltering nineties, but even after shaving and showering I couldn't stop sweating. It felt like the kind of day that makes me vow every year I will never spend another summer in Manhattan. Walking to the subway I noticed everyone seemed to be moving with sluggish, irritable steps. I could feel the sweat on my back, underneath my arms, behind my knees, streaming in pencil thin lines down the sides of my face. Even the Empire State Building, which bisects the skyline from this block of Chelsea, seemed uncomfortable and sullen, lost in a haze the color of cigarette smoke.

By lunch time, however, the sky was overcast: strips of blue-gray clouds shadowed the intensity of the sun, though the wind which whipped between the buildings of upper Times Square was ironically dry, the type I have always imagined belonged in the Sahara. Summer in New York City can be irritating: stifling, overcrowded subway cars, sidewalks that reek with the smells of urine and dried beer, the deli that always seems to have a broken air-conditioner on the day you want it to work the most. But it can also be a feast for the eyes: tourists wandering around in tank tops and shorts, messenger boys atop bicycles speeding across town in tight, spandex pants, actors and dancers with knapsacks slung across their shoulders, reciting lines to themselves as they head toward auditions or rehearsals. At noon, businessmen in white shirts and tailored dark suits stream through the revolving door of the building where I work, adjusting sunglasses and checking watches before dashing off to appointments. The construction workers of the new buildings which spiral skyward every block of this section of the city sit on the short, black walls surrounding the fountain and subway entrance of the courtyard of the Paramount Plaza. They have thick, tanned skin and wear tight, faded jeans, heavy dark workboots and T-shirts which cannot possibly have been ripped that way by design.

Crossing 50th Street at Seventh Avenue on the way to get a slice of pizza, I see the worker I look for every day hoping he has removed his T-shirt and stuffed it in the rear pocket of his jeans. Today he does not disappoint me; his body does not fail to stun me: a wide, solid chest and razor sharp abdominals, a tattoo on his left shoulder that reads USMC and biceps the size of the grapefruits they sell a block away at the Korean market. Amazing, I think, such energy at repose, a product of a profession of physical labor and an avocation of going to a gym. I can only stare at him so long without becoming self-conscious or risking a sneer. Looking skyward, I think if it rains later I will have a reason to change my plans. After work I am meeting my friend Jon at his office seven blocks from here. Together we're going to see the Names Project Quilt at Pier 92.

* * *

Three months ago my best friend died after having been diagnosed with Kaposi's sarcoma a year before. The day he called me and told me the results of his initial biopsy I said I would leave work and meet him, stay with him if he needed, do anything I could to help. He was choking over the phone, crying, saying he felt so ashamed, why had this happened to him? Then suddenly he pulled himself together, his voice returned to its regular intonation, and he said he had to get back to work, he would be all right. That night he went to the opening of a new Broadway musical.

I was the only one he told at first; though I did not feel privileged by being entrusted with this secret, I honored his desire to keep it quiet. I think what ennobles his life to me now, particularly his last year, was his inability to perceive himself as diseased. He treated his illness as though a cold or a broken leg, something that one day when he awoke would be better or healed, not something that was consuming him day by day, depressing him, immobilizing him. He kept up his normal, frenetic, crazy New Yorker pace for as long as he could, working long hours as a publicist and then attending film screenings, plays, and parties. And he continued to write, as he had since I met him nine years before, plays which had been produced in small regional theaters, plays which he never felt had been given the productions or recognition they deserved. Three months before his death one of his plays finally reached off-Broadway, and as he struggled with rewrites and revisions, we both knew but never mentioned, that this might be the only chance he was ever to be given.

Things did not get better. The medications got stronger but he grew weaker. After his second hospitalization the friends, family, and co-workers he had not informed were told. When things took a turn for the worse, in January of this year, he stopped working and lost the mobility he cherished, and though he was surrounded by a network of support and did his best to maintain his sense of humor and sharpen his wit, he still flashed through moments of frustration, abjection, and embitterment.

I have not been able to forget him a single day since his death. I am reminded of him by articles in the newspapers, reports on the six o'clock news, by his friends and mine calling to ask me how I am, by the details I have to attend to as the executor of the small estate he left behind, details which can be mundane, annoying or time consuming such as sorting through bills, writing letters, or photocopying his death certificate. And on the sidewalks, walking, where I think my actions, my movement will pull me away from his life and back to my own, I see reminders of him in the people who pass:

one man has his mustache, another his profile, others his gold wire-rim eyeglasses or his out-turned walk.

We were born the same year, six months apart but in different parts of the country. We grew to the same height, the same weight and could have worn each other's clothes if we wanted. But there were other, more important similarities which connected us as friends. We shared not only the same profession, but the same persuasions and aspirations: a love for the theater, movies, traveling, and men, and though our tastes were never identical, our passions kept us linked. We were introduced to one another in the lobby of a Broadway theater; we had both moved to Manhattan right after graduating college, leaving behind our suburban roots, and finding employment as apprentice publicists though dreaming of careers as writers. We were awed by the challenges, possibilities, and expectations of New York City, yet we were inspired to accomplish every conceivable goal, as young men in their early twenties with a lifetime ahead of them often are.

Today in *The New York Times* Canadian officials reported Soviet diplomats had tried to snatch U.S. Navy secrets, the Mets won but the Yankees had lost three in a row, and the Presidential hopefuls were in Los Angeles, Louisville, and Boston. A feature story announced The Paris Ballet would be presenting Swan Lake next week at Lincoln Center, a one-man off-Broadway show adapted from the novels of Becket was reviewed, and another article explained that an insect, smaller than a flea, was damaging millions of acres of forest in Vermont. A fire in Egypt killed forty-seven people, ten died in Burma riots, and a car bomb in Beirut killed two. Yet when I reached the obituary page, near the end of the last section of the paper, I felt a mild, morbid relief when I noticed there was no one listed I knew and the youngest man who had died was fifty-seven, killed in a sail boat accident when he was struck by the boom.

And throughout the day, as I sat behind a desk, typing, answering phones, and attending to the business that pays my rent, I keep reassuring myself I'm not the only person my best friend left behind. There is his mother, his sister, two nephews, a niece, his lover, and other friends, most of them who knew him longer than I.

* * *

After work I am surprised to find the afternoon sky startling clear and bright, the oppressive heat of the last few days has disappeared with the clouds. In fact the weather feels so nice, so comfortable, it is the kind of summer afternoon I wish I were spending at the beach. I meet my friend Jon at his office on 43rd Street and together we walk across the west side toward the pier. Our walk is slow and relaxing, by the time we reach Tenth Avenue there is little traffic on the sidewalks or streets. We tell each other about our day: I mention the new telephone system we are installing in the office; he tells me his boss is going crazy because of her high-fiber diet. Together we discuss our plans for a trip to Pennsylvania over the Fourth of July, next weekend: I mention I would like to drive through the Shaker countryside, he tells me about a restaurant a friend recommended in New Hope. As we draw nearer to our destination, our steps quicken, our eyes scan every building and person in sight. Now when we speak our voices are sharp, clipped whispers, notations edged by agitation.

Earlier today, a friend had warned me over the phone that viewing the quilt would be worse than going to a cemetery. Another said I would feel every conceivable emotion. Before leaving my office, I made a trip to the restroom and slipped some toilet paper into my pants pocket. As we wait to cross the street beneath the elevation of the West Side Highway, my friend loosens and removes his tie.

At the entrance to the pier, a white concrete building which is normally used as a passenger ship terminal, we ride to the second floor in an elevator that I estimate is larger than the bedroom of my apartment. When the doors open we follow those ahead of us, men and women of varying ages, into a lobby filled with tables and exhibits, pamphlets, registration books, volunteer workers and other visitors. We are handed programs and presented with the facts: this quilt weighs over 11,510 pounds and currently contains 3,488 names, although today space allows only 1,696 to be seen. Spread out, it is bigger than three football fields and includes the names of brothers, fathers, sons, mothers, daughters, lovers, and friends. It is the nation's largest community arts project and is designed to memorialize the thousands of Americans who have died from AIDS. New York is only one of the stops on a twenty city cross-country tour.

We walk through a doorway beneath a handwritten sign that says "Entrance" and enter the main room. My first impression is this room is enormous and bright; sunlight streams in through windows, outside it shimmers across the Hudson River. Inside it is crowded but quiet. And what begins with a sense of curiosity, as I begin to assimilate the first few panels which I look at and read, is quickly overtaken by a feeling of awe. The fabric panels of the quilt are six feet by three feet and have been sewn together in blocks of eight or thirty-two. The main section, draped atop the floor, stretches the length of the 775-foot pier. On either side are blocks suspended from the ceiling, creating alcoves to display even more panels, placed evenly between these fabric walls on the floor.

But it is the names that command the attention. As we follow the white canvas walkway which borders the perimeters of the panels on the floor, statistics suddenly become people.

Some panels are simple, containing only a painted name on plain fabric. Others are more elaborate with hand-stitched designs or needlepoint, or names spelled out in sequins or bordered by feathers. Some are personalized by clothing: a plaid shirt, gym shorts, boot laces, a leather vest, one, even, displays a jock strap. Others hold records, photographs, and quotes. Each panel contains only a single name of someone who has died. For me, the hardest to look at are the ones which contain only first names, the ones that read Mark, Bill, Mike or Steve. These are the names I collected years ago on scraps of paper at parties, bars, the gym, and the beach. They make me wonder if this is one of them now. Or is it the friend I haven't seen or spoken to in the past few months, the one I didn't even know was sick?

It is hard not to keep my eyes moving from panel to panel. And when I look up I notice we have not even made it a third of the way down the room. We are surrounded by other viewers, and I am not surprised to discover they are mostly men and women my age, mid-thirties, their heads bowed, motionless, as if in prayer. The tableau reminds me of those large cathedrals I visited seven years ago in Europe, the ones with plaques and epitaphs lining the walls of the transepts where people are buried beneath the floor. Here, at the quilt, it is as hushed and solemn, yet what was there, in Europe, was viewed with a calm sense of reverence, is here magnified with anger, shock, compassion, and grief. Here, footsteps move so slowly and carefully their sounds cannot be detected; silence is broken only by the shutters of cameras. Ahead a young man in a blue polo shirt and jeans sits crosslegged on the walkway in front of a red silk panel that spells D-a-v-i-d with silver block letters, his head is buried in the palms of his hands. Though I strain to hear but cannot detect any sounds from him, I know by the way his back heaves with short, jerking breaths that he is crying. Behind him, I am suddenly astounded by the sight of a woman pushing an empty stroller; beside her a man carries a baby, less than six months old, in his arms. On the other side of the panel an elderly woman with a cane touches the frame of her eyeglasses and leans to read a name. This is something that has hit us all.

Behind each name is the story of a life, someone who struggled with this disease and lost. Behind each panel there are many stories: Who made it? Who helped? Why this color, this fabric? What does the design remember or represent? Who cried when it was finished? Who recognizes the name as they walk by? And each of us brings our own stories to the quilt, our views, opinions, knowledge, and experiences with this disease. And we are united, sewn together as it were, by our thoughts of families, lovers, friends, and co-workers: some dead, some sick, some worried. This is our Gettysburg, our Vietnam Wall, our Tomb of the Unknown Soldier. Yet those wars are over, this one continues. All of us are frightened this could be happening to us next. The quilt grows larger every day.

When we reach the center of the room, a crowd of people surround a block of yellow canvas on the floor. At the edges are boxes of tissues and black felt tip pens. Here, the words "New York" have been painted in large, cursive purple letters. Shoes have been slipped off and left on the walkway, their owners kneel atop the yellow canvas and write, covering the empty spaces with remembrances. This canvas is full of writing: names, notes, signatures, and messages, hardly an untouched space, signed the way, years ago, we covered the pages of a high school yearbook. Now, standing here, watching a young man who looks hardly out of high school uncap a felt pen and write, I feel angry and guilty. Why has this happened? Why is it continuing? Was there anything I could have done to stop this? Was there something I can do now? At my best friend's funeral his mother said to me that what I had done was miraculous, the way I had helped make his last few months as comfortable as possible. The way when he could no longer leave his apartment, I brought him food, made sure he took his medication on schedule, arranged doctors, nurses, and friends to visit. The way when he was frightened and scared I tried to reassure him he was not alone by leaving work early or taking a day off, many times staying at his apartment overnight. The way when the depression would overcome him, I would entertain and distract him with videotapes, games, magazines, books and records. But now I feel that wasn't enough, and fearing I might abruptly lose my outward display of emotional composure, I turn and walk away.

As we approach the end of the room Jon sees someone he has not seen since college. He introduces me to his friend, though I remain silent and listen to their whispered conversation. As their talk progresses from reminisces and old friends to present day careers and activities, my eyes again roam through the crowd. All at once I see several familiar faces: a friend who works five floors beneath mine, a teller from my bank, a couple I see at the video store on my block. In the distance I spot an actor who has made a fortune from furniture commercials and who once appeared in a showcase of one of my best friend's plays. Behind him is a former patient of my former psychiatrist and a guy whose name I have never known, but whose tight physique I always admired at my old gym and which I haven't glanced at in over two years since I moved to a new apartment.

A man my age with a neatly trimmed black beard and wearing an old straw hat stops beside me and stares into my eyes. I look at him, confused for a moment, till he smiles and I recognize him as my friend Bryce who I once worked with booking guests on a late night local cable TV show. We hug, pleased to see each other alive in this room, and he tells me in the three years since I last saw him he has moved from Provincetown to Santa Barbara and now back to New York, where he has been living on the Upper West Side for the last two months. He apologizes for not having called, then his eyes narrow and he rocks his legs nervously, and says, softly, his best friend died this morning. I answer I am surprised he is here of all places, but I understand why he is. I know exactly what he is thinking and feeling. "How could I stay away?" he says and stops rocking and then looks at the ground. "I have it," he adds and I know not even to ask, "Are you sure?" Instead, I slip my hand around his elbow and lead him to a corner of the room, near a window, gently pelting him with questions: Do you have insurance? Are you working? Have you started treatments or medication? Do you live alone? Who is your doctor? Who knows and who is helping? He answers my questions politely, without embarrassment, but then adds in an exasperated voice, "I think it was the radiation treatments that killed him. He was fine till last week. When are the doctors going to learn you can't cover a bullet hole with a Band-Aid?"

Jon approaches and now it is my turn for introductions and I manage it with only a little awkwardness. As Jon and I part to continue viewing the quilt, I tell Bryce I will do what ever I can to help, that he must never hesitate about asking or calling, and though I start to write his name and new phone number on the back of my program, I stop just in time, finding a piece of paper in my wallet instead. We exchange numbers, embrace again, and as we part I tell him I will start by cooking dinner for him one night next week.

As I walk away, traveling the length of the room toward the exit, Jon slips his hand into mine, and though I am no longer looking at the names on the panels, I am aware my eyes have started to tear. Last week a friend told me it can take up to two years before the grief finally subsides. Yet I know I can never forget my best friend; he is the one who introduced me, four years ago, to my friend Jon, the thread that binds us together today. We stop again in the center of the room by the yellow panels and Jon unclasps his firm grip as I hand him my program. I slip my shoes off and step onto the panel, kneeling and pressing my knees against the fabric. I reach for a felt tip pen, open it, and write without faltering:

KEVIN
MAY 23, 1955—MARCH 18, 1988
I WILL MISS YOU EVERY DAY
LOVE,
JIMMY

WHY I LIVE WHERE I DO

In the evening it takes me about an hour to commute from my temporary job in Princeton, New Jersey to my house in New Hope, Pennsylvania. I have tried many ways in hopes of finding a quicker path—interstates, state highways, rural backroads, and country side streets. The route I have finally settled on, though not the fastest but certainly the least travelled, is a two lane country road with a number of winding curves and potholes larger than I ever saw when I lived in New York City. I lived in Manhattan for a decade, up until the end of last year, and most days I could be home by subway in just over ten minutes. Walking, I could make it from my office to my apartment in less than thirty.

Now, on my drive to the cottage I am renting in this part of the country, I drive past vast open fields of beige grass, pastures where race horses graze, dense forests or brief pockets of tall, slender trees, following the road as it bisects a valley or suddenly climbs a modest hill or the side of a mountain. Many times a deer will leap in front of the car; at night I can see the glare of the eyes of raccoons and possums which scurry along the roadside, hauntingly green or amber from the reflection of the headlights. This drive also takes me through a number of small towns, the type that has a Main Street, an Elm Street, large Victorian houses, a painted white church, and two stop lights, very Americana, exactly as Hollywood movies portrayed for many years.

Many stores are closing by the time I drive by. Through dimly lit windows I catch glimpses of clerks lowering shades, an elderly man searching through a shelf, a mother grasping simultaneously a paper bag and the hand of a child. And for a moment I feel a stillness, a melancholy of sorts; I miss the pace of the city, the crush of people heading home as others head out for evening adventures. I miss the contact with other people, not words or introductions, but the exchange of glances and shared thoughts. And I miss the delis and coffee shops and bagel counters that never close. I miss the immediacy of trying to find a taxi on a wet, rainy night.

The melancholy lifts a bit when I reach my new home. Entering the cottage, I have just picked up the mail. Sometimes I feel as if I have waited all day for this moment. I have always hoped, even as a New Yorker, that the mail will bring some unexpected good news; amid the bills and discount flyers I search for a letter or postcard from someone I haven't heard from in a while, perhaps even from someone I've lost contact with over the years and just heard that I had moved. Sometimes the news is good, sometimes it is disturbing, most often my expectations are in vain and I end up pausing briefly to thumb through a magazine or a catalogue that has just arrived. Yet when finished with the mail, I approach the answering machine and its awaiting messages with the same kind of blind optimism.

The evening ahead is usually a simple one: a frozen dinner, a TV show or perhaps a rented video, a chapter of a book, or an attempt to start a fire if it's really cold. I have few friends here where I now live. And the ones I do know are usually only here on weekends, commuting from Manhattan to their country homes. One friend, who, with his lover, also happens to be my neighbor and landlord, calls midweek to check up on his house and to see if I have met anyone new. He is constantly worried about my life as a single gay male in his early thirties; he is afraid I will become bored and want to move again. For a while I worried about it to; I have never been someone who was able to meet people easily. Slowly I have been introduced to new people: through friends of friends, personal ads, a local gay support group, and sometimes at one of the three gay bars exactly two miles down the road from my cottage. But my friend always queries me if any of these new acquaintances were "interesting" or "possible." He is convinced it is now time for me to find a lover.

In truth I think I have reached that age where I am finally comfortable living alone. This is hard to explain to someone who has been in a long term relationship, even harder for someone who might have courted several boyfriends and romance. My friend says I am perfect lover material: smart, moderately attractive, healthy, and domestic—so what is my problem? The problem is not a problem as I see it. Yes, I will admit there are moments of longing, sometimes even a fantasy of having "another half." And there are a number of men here I find I am immediately drawn to: the teller at the drive-in window at the bank, the young man at the dry cleaners, the bartender who hands me a drink on Saturday night. But a relationship is not something I will ever jump into headfirst again; my previous attempts were disastrous. A relationship, I believe, must be nurtured slowly and carefully, like friendship. Sometimes when I am overcome with an attack of anxiety at this very realization, I tell my friend I am considering getting a dog just to have some unabashed affection. "No," my friend answers. "You can borrow mine."

I have friends who were supportive of my wanting to leave the city, saying they had been trying to do it for years. Others were confused, some were amused and said I would be back. "Once you've lived in New York City it's in your blood," one friend said. Yes, I think that's true. Perhaps that's the cause of my shifting moods.

When I first moved to Manhattan I had just graduated college. I found a small apartment in Greenwich Village which an architect, demented I'm sure, designed so that none of the walls met in ninety degree angles. I lived alone and the rent was high, but the city was full of exploration and escapade. The streets were always busy, the bars crowded with available men, and I was becoming acquainted with a whole new group of friends: young, educated, witty, well-traveled, and searching for love.

I can't put my finger on when things started to change, a disenchantment began to settle around me. I believe, I truly do, it was long before AIDS made us change the way we live and look at life. Perhaps it was after my first mugging; today I still sport a small scar above my left eye. Perhaps it was from my failed attempt one summer at romance. Perhaps it was from a job that offered little rewards, monetary or otherwise, but demanded a great deal of time and involved a lot of stress. Perhaps it was a need I feel every few years or so to keep changing. In the ten years I lived in the city I lived in four different apartments with seven different roommates. For years I contemplated about returning to graduate school or moving to Connecticut or Boston, Seattle or Washington, D.C., or anywhere with a beach. I felt a need to keep moving, a restless urge to keep living and experiencing. I have heard stories about people leaving the city over the most minor of inconveniences: the closing of a favorite restaurant, the rising cost of going to the movies. But for me, I think, the final straw was watching a close friend die a horrible and painful death from AIDS.

I did not move here to escape AIDS, forget my former life, recapture my youth, find a more promiscuous lifestyle, or wipe the slate clean. Every day I am concerned about my health, every day I am reminded of my previous years by the news of someone sick or dying or dead. But I did move here because I thought it offered something I had never experienced before, a chance to make a change, though how or in what direction I'm not sure. Sometimes I think my move was rather impulsive. Though I had heard about this area I had never visited this side of the Delaware River until two months before I moved here, and then only at the invitation of my friend who had just bought a house. And my decision could still allow me the opportunity of returning to or visiting New York, when and if I ever wanted.

I learned a lot though while I lived in New York. I learned about wanting it and making it and having it and getting it and not getting it; I learned about sex, dating, romance, love, and death. And I don't regret any moment of it. I only wish sometimes that what I know now I knew back then. But isn't that the way life goes?

I can't say my new home is my Walden. Yes, there are ducks and geese and a pond less than a minute from my doorstep, and plants I think I will never know the names of. And above is a huge, open sky that on clear nights, of which there are many, I can see, if not identify, every constellation imaginable in this hemisphere. Here I have a cottage with two bedrooms, larger than I could ever find and afford in the city, on an acre of land. But every day I still buy *The New York Times*. And today, I still live alone, as much by choice as by fate. The truth about your life is not always easy to accept. And sometimes you don't learn anything about yourself until something makes you change.

HAIRCUTS

As far back as I can remember the top of my father's head was bald. What hair he had started where most men's ended, a dark brown ring circled the back of his neck. My mother said it was because my father always wore a hat when he was young, but that never explained why my brother, too, went bald at an early age. When we were boys, my father used to drive me and my brother thirty minutes into the countryside to a small Southern town, parking the station wagon in front of a barber shop that was part of a general store. My father said it was the last of a kind, a dying breed; suburbia was expanding and we were learning to use the word "mall." My father would get his hair cut first: the barber, Andy, and my father were on a first name basis, and Andy knew from experience exactly how my dad liked to have his hair trimmed. My brother, four years older than I, would go next. I would watch in part amazement, part horror, as the brown hair fell from his head onto the light blue smock. My brother, even at an early age, was a tough guy; he thought the crew cuts Andy gave us looked sharp and felt neat. I would go last, sitting on a telephone book to make my head higher than the back of the swivel chair, and watch, with tears welling up in my eyes, my reflection in the mirror and the hair, which I had begged my father to let me wear long, disappear, leaving a child who looked too much like his father: a soft round face and a fuzzy flattop, with hair so blond it was white, making him appear as though he were bald.

Some people are capable of outgrowing their childhood fears; they are able to conquer their terror of dentists, heights or water. Today, however, I am still terrified of getting my hair cut. I suppose that's why I let my hair grow long in college. I suppose that's why the few years the shag look was in I found I could cut my hair as good as anyone else could. I suppose that's why I prefer to go to a stylist instead of a barber. I suppose it's a silly thing for an educated adult male to fear, but too many times I have come home from a haircut and canceled all appointments for at least a week.

Where I live now, a rural town in Pennsylvania, there are barbershops on almost every corner. They are as popular here as gas stations were where I grew up. Now I find I am driving a few extra miles in search of a salon and a decent trim. But I also realize, even though I am hesitant to admit it, that now it is not the actual sound of scissors and razors or the smell of bay rum and talc that frightens me, it's the man I recognize and don't recognize when it's over, the one who's suddenly confronted with the question: Will the hair that's been shorn ever grow back?

Let's face it. One of the prime images of youth, right up there with health and skin tone, is a full head of hair. Over the years I can remember hair being the topic of many conversations. In junior high, a girl said she liked me because of my hair. I once dated a guy who, after spending an evening of running his fingers through my hair, asked me what type of shampoo I used. Many times when I and my friends were still in our early twenties, we talked often about what we would try when the time was needed: minoxidil, transplants, and weaves were okay, toupees definitely were not. And we each wondered what our pattern would be: Would it begin from the front, the side, or, aghast, would we end up looking like monks?

More than anything I have watched myself age through my hair. I am the same height and weight and physical frame I was in high school. Yet my hair is completely different. In high school my hair was light brown, thick and wavy, and I trained the front bangs to fall away from my face in a flip. Then I discovered the layered look and in college, as my hair became darker, I let it grow long and straight and wore it in a quasi-page boy style. For a while I added a mustache and then a beard. Now, clean shaven, I wear my hair short and simple, a modified businessman's haircut. And yes, today it's a little thinner, the texture different, the color almost black. And I've discovered the sides grow faster than the top; if I'm not careful I sometimes end up looking like Bozo the clown. Though a stranger would not notice my hairline is receding, it is definitely not in the same position it was a few decades ago. I've been lucky so far I guess, considering I'm a good candidate if baldness runs in your family and is carried in your genes. And I've accepted the fact that the way my hair grows will never be the same as before. But I still hope I will have the chance to turn gray before I go bald.

A friend of mine says a man's hair is a barometer of his vanity. If that is true then I can say I haven't owned a comb in years, though I have come to rely on conditioner and a hair blower more than I wish to acknowledge. Even more important today is the way hair has become a statement of one's personality. In the Fifties it was short. In the Sixties it was long. In the Seventies it was groomed. Now, at the end of the Eighties, it can be whatever color and style imaginable. Take a look at any magazine. The models immediately tell you who they are (or are trying to be) by the way they wear their hair. It seems more than ever hair is like a piece of clothing, a statement of fashion, providing you have the hair to do it with. And if you don't, there's even a solution for that. And let's not forget about the enormous market of cosmetics and treatments for men who have thinning hair. It's enough to make any man worried and confused.

But why does something so regular, normal, and commonplace as a haircut still frighten me? Perhaps it's from years of watching myself change in mirrors, the long-haired youth becoming an adult. Perhaps it's simply a sense that I have little control over the outcome. No matter what explicit instructions I give these days, I always end up with a stylist who wants to cut my hair into some sort of scooped back pompadour. Perhaps it's from finding the man in the mirror isn't the man he was a few years ago. That he himself had changed long before his hair style did, but only now did he finally notice it.

Ironically, the way I wear my hair today is much like my father did when he was this age. If it touches the ears, I feel a bit unkempt. But I like it that way. It's a part of who I am today, a man who is different from his father in many ways. And though the drain at the bottom of the bathtub seems to need cleaning more often than before, the man in the mirror isn't really worried about losing his hair. He's not afraid of change, he's not afraid of aging. What he is afraid of is a barber will do it for him.

DESPERADO

It's been four days now and everybody says the first three are the worst but today feels even worse than yesterday and all I want to do is to go back to bed because if I sleep I will not want to eat, not want to drink any more water, not want to chew any more gum, not want to exercise or go to a movie or to the grocery store or to a bookstore or to the mall or, especially, anywhere to have a cigarette, I have chewed a ball point pen to shreds, I am all out of my favorite sugarless bubble gum and now I'm chewing on a paper cup and my tongue is numb, feels like gravel and the headache won't disappear so I lie back down on the bed and try to fall back asleep but I can't because every limb of my poor, destroyed body feels as if it has been dismembered, filled with sand and then sewn back together with metal threads, all without any sort of anesthesia to ease the pain and I'm tired of taking deep breaths because the breaths make my chest ache and when my chest aches I want a cigarette more than anything else in the world, and the desperation makes me start crying and I don't even have any more energy left to jerk off—that, at least, makes my concentration focus on something other than eating or drinking or chewing, but I'm scared that I'm going to balloon up into a huge blimp and then I will never find another boyfriend, never have another lover, never, even, have another date in my life, and I will die alone here in the country and it will be months, years, before anyone discovers my body and all because I didn't have a cigarette when I wanted one, my life has been reduced to tears because of *one lousy cigarette* and now I feel the depression beginning to overcome me again, not at all like the other depressions I have known living in the age of anxiety, because now I know that there's no such truth to the saying that depressed people sleep and dream more, because if that were the case then I'd be dead asleep right now instead of wanting to be merely dead, and since I can't fall back asleep I have to work my way through this, *will* work my way through this, and I turn on my side, pull my feet up to my chest so that I am in a fetal position and rock, rock, rock, just to keep the body moving, doing something, till the exhaustion hits and I can fall asleep again but now the brain won't turn off and I think maybe I am *not* depressed, maybe what I am is *legally insane* and someone will come and find me after all and put me into a hospital and at least the drugs will help ease the pain, ease this depression—why didn't I even try to get some nicotine gum to get through this, or one of those silly patches for my shoulder, I don't know why I'm doing this to myself, I *enjoyed* smoking, smoking was *therapeutic* for me, I could think *clearly* when I smoked, I could *withdraw* into a cigarette, not like now, now I seem to be wearing every possible emotion outside, like a skin or one of those horrible tan raincoats that's too wet and won't come off, I thought stopping smoking was supposed to make you feel *better*, but I'm nothing but bruises and sweat and a broken down wreck, even my car is in better shape than I am and all I want to do is get out of bed and lead a normal life but I can't move, nothing feels the same, everything smells, tastes, looks, and sounds different and I'm scared and I can't remember *anything*, I can't even remember the last time I spoke to someone on the phone to confirm the fact that I am still alive and not merely being punished for all those sins of my former lives and now I can feel my chest hurting again and soon I will start hyperventilating and then I'll start crying and it's so hard to stop the crying now because anything can make me cry, and it's been four days now and everybody says the first three days are the worst but today feels worse and all I want to do is go back to bed but when I lie down I start thinking again and I remember about everybody dying and here I am trying to live and then I start crying—if only the crying would stop, if I could just learn to how to control the crying it would ease this frustration, that would be a step in the right direction—but I can't get the crying to stop, everything, today, feels so *desperate*, nothing will stop the crying, except, of course, a cigarette—but then that will just make me feel worse—guilty, unhealthy, and desperate all over again, so I just cry, *desperately*, now, because I don't *have* to change, I *want* to change, but why didn't someone warn me that change is not easy, *change hurts*, why didn't someone tell me I have to *suffer* before I can feel *better*?

CAUTION

When I first moved out of Manhattan I bought a used car and began driving a lot—to work, to the grocery store, to the dry cleaners, to the video store, and yes, even to the gas station. It wasn't that I had stopped driving when I lived in Manhattan: who needed to own a car in the city? My driving then was limited to rental cars for vacations, a weekend trip out of town or whenever I decided to visit my parents. Now, driving on a daily basis, I find a great deal more thought and effort and energy is demanded, not only of myself but of my car as well. Now, living in a rural area of Pennsylvania, I worry about things like when should I get the oil changed, what is that horrible rattling noise under the back seat when I make right hand turns, and why does the battery light keep blinking every time I stop at the light before the bridge which spans the Delaware River?

The first three months I lived in the country I was extremely nervous about driving. I never went as fast as the speed limit allowed, drove with both hands tightly grasped onto the wheel, and was constantly checking the rear and side view mirrors. I signaled a mile before I made a turn and I tried, whenever possible, not to drive at night. I am aware that there were many other factors involved with my anxiety: a new job, a new house, few friends in the area, an inherited poor sense of direction, and a general bewilderment over whether or not I had made the right decision of leaving the life I had established in the city. But driving was something I had to do here in the country: it was necessary to get from one place to another. And though I was overly cautious behind the wheel, there was still the thrill of sometimes being lost, sometimes discovering a new road or a faster way home. Driving in a new place could be adventuresome. But I also considered my caution well heeded. After all, I had heard reports that there were approximately 1,100 deer killed by drivers every year in the county where I now live. Then again, I have always been a cautious person. I am careful with credit cards, alcohol consumption, and shopping on an empty stomach. I worry about getting enough sleep, catching a cold, and flying in planes. Some days I tell myself my caution is too excessive. I can be apprehensive about anything, from blind dates to falling in love. These days my caution also extends to sex.

Perhaps the earliest recognition of my sexual caution sends my memory back to high school. As a teenager I was wildly attracted to men, especially the high school jocks, but as a bookish boy I studied too much, focused my energy on music lessons, and hung around girls whom I thought of as friends. I didn't understand my hormones: why I could watch the basketball team for hours, why I dreamed of the wrestling team at night. In retrospect, because of my caution, because of my hesitancy at just approaching and befriending these boys, I realize it took me years to come to terms with my homosexuality, years to get the courage to step into a gay bar, years to act upon my instincts and sleep with a man. I was scared at every step And each time I moved a little closer to the action, thought about it a little more, I worried I would be hurt or disappointed, was acting shamefully or was mentally unbalanced, or make others, particularly my family and peers, feel repulsed, ashamed or embarrassed and I would consequently suffer from their disapproval. But the more men I met, the more men I dated, the more self-esteem I acquired, the more self-confidence I felt about my decision to be gay, that there were, indeed, other men who thought and acted like me. And once I felt comfortable with my homosexuality, I realized there were many other decisions still ahead: primarily what to want, need, and expect in a relationship, not to mention where to find the right man.

Three years ago I met a man in a bar. We had spent about an hour cruising each other from opposite ends of the room. After three drinks and waiting for him to make the first move, I got the courage to walk over and sit beside him at the bar. After another drink, I felt brave enough to introduce myself. We talked a bit: my words slurring, he eyeing me with a mixture of interest and suspicion. And we discovered we had a few things in common: we had both finished reading the new book by Edmund White, we had both just seen and liked the new Steve Martin movie, and we each shared an interest in Broadway musicals. We were the same height, the same weight, wore glasses, and soon learned we were the same age, born only nine months apart. And though each of us considered ourselves writers, although of different genres, we both complained about those unknown forces of economics which made us earn our living by other means. That night we exchanged phone numbers and he walked me to the steps of my Chelsea apartment, and I kissed him lightly on the cheek before going inside alone. He called the next day and we saw each other seven times. Our dates usually consisted of a movie, dinner, and then drinks. Our conversations covered almost every topic, from politics to movie stars, from families to summer weekends with friends. We talked a lot about what it meant to be a single gay male in his thirties and what it was like to still be dating at this age: the awkwardness of first steps, the confusions about how to keep the other party interested and entertained, and, yes, the cautiousness about sex which had become ingrained in our thoughts. Yet in spite of our talks and the connections which could link us as friends, we never progressed beyond those parting pecks on the cheek. Looking back on it now I knew my caution had made me scared: scared of starting something new, scared of making changes in the way I lived, scared of finding myself in a relationship with the wrong person. Scared of the possibilities, perimeters, and expectations of sex. Had our meeting happened a decade earlier, we would have gone to bed with each other after that initial encounter at the bar, and whatever would have progressed beyond that one night would have been determined by the sex. And I feel both embarrassed and ashamed and disappointed in myself that it took me seven dates to decide this man was not the right person for me and we would not be the kind of couple I wanted to be a part of: all this caution before sex even became a part of the picture.

Sex is still on my mind a lot these days. It is one of the question marks right up there with what exactly is the proper amount of cholesterol, fiber, and exercise. How much sex do I require? How much do I want and need? For years I considered sex as a means of beginning a relationship: the exchange of intimacy a stepping stone to dating, romance and falling in love. But the more sexual experiences I had I realized that wasn't necessarily the case. And so I let sex become enjoyable because it was sex, because, as a friend of mine once said, the human skin needs to be touched. But then times changed and so did I. I felt I needed something more, and something was a relationship based on strong friendship, compatibility, and companionship. And I fell in love with a man who offered me just such a relationship. But the sexual chemistry between us was missing. The spark wasn't there. Sex, in fact, was infrequent and unfulfilling. And again I knew I needed something more; experience told me I needed out of that relationship. When I mentioned this to a friend he remarked that sometimes there are things other than sex which bond a relationship. But something in my gut told me that this was not right for me, that this was not what I wanted. And I told my friends so. After all, I said, the main reason I am homosexual is because I prefer sex with men.

A date once told me that we, as gay men, place too much emphasis on sex. Yet another friend of mine, a noted psychiatrist, says that the admission of one's own homosexuality is in itself an emphasis of one's sexual need. But what I told them both is that sometimes the need for sex and the need for love get confused. I recently met a man who told me he had three boyfriends, all sexual relationships, and he wanted nothing or expected more from any of them. I asked him what about love, what about the need to touch someone's soul or to have your own heart touched. He answered his life was full of love: from his mother, from his uncle, from his friends, even from his cat. But he did admit he would some day like a relationship that combined both sex and love, but right now, this was what worked for him. I told him I had been in a similar situation not long ago, an intense sexual affair that was clearly not going to go anywhere else. I mentioned that after two months I couldn't continue in that sort of a relationship. What worked for my friend did not work for me. What I wanted was both sex and love from the same man.

And so I keep thinking about the possibility of sex and love together, keep meeting and dating men, keep having sex. I still believe it's a possible combination: sex and love. And I am not a promoter of promiscuity, in fact, have never considered myself promiscuous. Because of my cautious nature, I am also an advocate of healthy, safe sex. But AIDS and the fear of it have not erased our sexual needs. Though no matter how much I have mentally or physically changed over the years, no matter how many times the heart has been broken or disappointed, somewhere in the back of my mind, the actions of what I do and with whom I do it with are still considered important thoughts, ways, means of finding love.

So what I guess I'm trying to say is what every parent shies from telling their children. Sex has an incredible power. Sex is a vivid, human desire. And caution must extend beyond the possible transmission of viruses and disease, or, in heterosexual cases, unwanted pregnancies. Sex can be an intoxicant: there have been periods where I have binged, periods where I've abstained, periods where I find it's not necessary and periods where I'm so horny all caution and rationale seem to disappear. Yes, sex is an impulse, an attraction, a passion and a requirement. But for me it's also more; like a car, it's a way of getting from one place to another. And I'll admit I've made a few wrong mistakes, been lost at times, taken a few wrong turns and had a couple of accidents. But had I not done so, I would never have discovered the things I like: the things I want and the things I need. And I feel lucky that my cautious, skeptical nature has kept my expectations rooted in reality. As Confucius said the cautious seldom err. Yet if I were able to get him on the phone today I would tell him that caution keeps us comfortable but seldom makes us happy. Sometimes we have to take chances—like moving to a new place. Adventure and knowledge are what keep us learning. Life, after all, is a road of experiences, and our bodies, like an old, used car, need a little attention, some repair, and a lot of fuel in order to reach its destination.

SOMETHING FROM THE RAIN

I remember the afternoon, years ago, that Geoff called me at work and said, "I need to get away. Let's go somewhere this weekend." And by the time I got home it was raining.

Geoff wanted to go somewhere anyway, and though it was still winter we decided to drive to the beach. It was dark when we arrived and found a hotel room; I was so tired from working all week and then driving for three hours that I fell asleep in the chair watching TV, my sweater and shoes still on.

The next morning it was still raining and we lay together in bed, watching cartoons. Geoff held me from behind that morning, his face pressed against my shoulder, the stubble of his beard tickling me as something on the television made him laugh.

In the afternoon we walked into the empty resort town, stopping for lunch at a diner which had a jukebox which played old surfing tunes from the Sixties. It felt so odd to hear such buoyant music while watching the winter rain. I remember looking out the window at the rain on the ocean and thinking water unto water, water unto water, trying to sort out some natural cycle I didn't understand.

The rain did not bother Geoff; he smiled and said it looked neat as it disappeared into the waves. Geoff refused to use the umbrella I brought that weekend. Or the cap I offered him. And his sneakers were never dry both days. But he never complained. He said the rain was good; it made everything feel clean.

On our last day there, I walked alone on the beach before Geoff got up. The rain had finally stopped and I found a small wooden hand mirror, unbroken, washed up on the shore, glimmery and brilliant against the dull, gray winter sand.

Geoff remembered all this differently, of course. He had a cold Saturday morning and the decongestant pills I gave him kept making him drowsy. He didn't remember the cartoons or the mirror I found but he did remember the diner—the service was lousy and the lady behind him kept blowing cigarette smoke in our direction—and he recalled, quite vividly, the pink flamingo-shaped salt and pepper shakers on our table and his rattling them in the air as though they were maracas.

The next week, when Geoff's cold got worse, he called and asked me if I could bring over some orange juice and more decongestants. I didn't realize, in those days, that this had something to do with the different ways people behave when falling in love. Though he would never admit it, Geoff had another motive for calling. I know, now, he wanted to be sure he saw me.

BETWEEN THE LINES

I started crying before I woke up because I had a dream about Peter and I was still so shocked from reading the paper yesterday and seeing that he had died, I never knew Peter that well but we had worked together on several shows and we had many mutual friends and it made me scared again because I didn't even know he had been sick, and if he was sick then it might mean that Michael is now sick or not doing well or suffering and I knew Michael *very* well but hadn't heard from him in a couple of years, mostly since I moved away from the city, and now I'm afraid to call him, afraid to hear more bad news, more than I could read between the lines of the obituary since it didn't even mention that Peter had died of AIDS, just after a long illness, and it didn't even elude to Michael only that Peter was just thirty-six, and now I'm afraid if I call Michael he will ask me if I am coming to the memorial service in the city next week and I will hear my own voice falter on the phone or grow tiny and far away and I don't know what I will say, I haven't even thought that far ahead, I mean, I should go, I *must* go, but the timing is bad because everything is crashing and crumbling again in my own life and I'm scared of going back to the city, scared of being the object of other people's attention, scared of being asked how I am and how is life out in the country, and I know when they ask the questions—all my old friends, those that are *left*, I mean—they will search my eyes and see no matter how well I can pretend that things are going better now, they will still see the unhappiness, I've never been able to mask that, and I know, sitting there at the service, I will start crying because I can cry just from a whiff of flowers these days, I have no control left over my own emotions, I mean, I started crying before I woke up this morning, which means I was crying in my sleep and it's no longer because of Geoff or Clarke or Kevin, or the frustration from a lousy social life, and it's not just because I can't stand my job, or because I'm now thirty-four years old and have less money than I had when I was twenty-four years old, and it's not just because I'm lonely, stuck out here in the country in this self-imposed exile without even cable TV, and I'm not going crazy because I want a cigarette or a pill or a drink, it's because I'm scared and I don't know what to do next, and I'm afraid of making *more* changes and feeling guilty—like I ran away when I *didn't*—I had to do this for *myself*—but now I wonder how did I ever get here, what have I done, how did all this happen to me, and then I wonder if it's like Debbie said—that maybe no matter where I am I will be unhappy—but I hope that's not true, it's just that I'm still learning who I am, still deciding what I want and feeling guilty for being *alive*, so once I pull myself together, stop all this crying, everything will get better but then there are all these disturbances, this *agitation*, like Peter dying, which makes me even more frustrated and I started crying this morning before I woke up because I *wanted* to know the *details*—how long had he been sick, how fast had it happened, what medications had they tried—and because Peter was such a handsome man—I couldn't imagine him sick, didn't want to visualize him as being ill—and he was such a nice guy and so young, and I know I should have been there and now I have to cry, I *really, really* have to cry but what I am afraid of now, again, *today*, is that the crying will *never, never stop*.

HOW DOES MY GARDEN GROW?

In front of the cottage I am renting in rural Pennsylvania is a small patch of land not much larger than the size of a terrace of a Manhattan apartment. This parcel of ground is full of weeds. It is surrounded by a tall brown fence on three sides and is considered the front yard of my property; a path of slender bricks bisects it to my front door. The back yard, almost an acre of land, I share with my neighbor, who is also my landlord. It is considered common property between us, but since all of the property belongs to him, my neighbor keeps this part of his grounds immaculately groomed. Though he has never mentioned anything to me about the state of my front yard, I know it is a sore point with him. But I cannot, in any sort of way, bring myself to do anything with this land. I cannot bear to pull up these weeds. And I do not own a lawn mower. To be honest, I have become fond of the state of its disarray. In fact, I find some perverse pleasure in waiting to see how tall I can let my weeds grow before he says something to me, or fall comes and they begin to die and wither and collapse of their own accord.

Oh my. How did this happen? This is not at all the sort of person I am. (I am otherwise a very neat, very responsible, very organized, and very orderly sort of guy, a Libra, after all, which means I have to maintain some sort of rationale and balance in my life.) So why doesn't this bother me? I have several theories on the matter. Here are a few:

Last spring, my first year living in the country after living in Manhattan for a decade, I tilled the front lawn, got rid of all the weeds, went to the grocery store and bought several packets of seeds marked "Wildflowers," "Country Blossoms," and "Assorted Flowers." I came home and threw them around my front yard and waited for them to grow. For months, I waited and waited and I never saw any flowers. I was very disappointed. In fact, I felt defeated. So this year I have let the weeds grow the way they want to grow.

But that's not the only reason. At the time I first plowed my patch of land, I was dating a man who was a horticulturist by vocation. He filled the inside of my cottage with plants and flowers, but he refused to help me with my front yard. It would be, he said, as though I were taking advantage of him. I, of course, did not see it that way, but I cleared my patch of land all by myself—that means without any help from this particular boyfriend—and planted the seeds all by myself—which means the whole process was carried out with a little too much resentment. But, in the end, I was very proud of myself for having done it. I felt I had accomplished something new. And while I was waiting for the flowers to grow, waiting for some sort of acknowledgment from this man of a job that I had done well, waiting for our relationship to blossom, too, I might add, he told me he wanted to date other people. As if they understood the metaphor, as well, the flowers I had planted never even sprouted out of the ground. And inside the cottage, all of the plants and flowers the horticultural worker gave me that didn't die I hacked to pieces, threw out, or burned. So I really had no other choice in the matter. I had to let the weeds grow in the front yard out of spite.

Another reason is rebellion. As a boy I hated mowing the yard. It was my least favorite chore. My older brother got to mow the flat front lawn. I got stuck with the hilly, rocky back yard. I can remember hating mowing the yard, crying mowing the yard, swearing and cursing mowing the yard, and one day mowing over a bee's nest. So I had to assert my independence. I had to let the weeds grow.

Another reason: I have never had much success with growing plants, indoors or outdoors. I have killed more plants by overwatering, underwatering, indirect sunlight, and too much heat exposure. Every indoor plant I've ever come into contact with is now dead. The only plants I still have in my house are fake—silk floral arrangements and pressed floral portraits which my mother made and sent to me for decoration.

One other reason: I am afraid of poison ivy.

Still another reason: In this area of Pennsylvania where I am living now, there are huge homes and estates that are beautifully landscaped and maintained. My neighbor hires people to mow his portion of the yard. They mulch, weed, spray, water, plant flowers and shrubs for him. The man who owned the house before my neighbor did was an avid amateur horticulturist. All around the yard there are strange, rare plants surrounded by chicken wire. My neighbor wants to maintain these plants; in fact, he is even trying to learn what kind of plants these are. The first thing my neighbor does when he comes home from work is to walk around and survey the condition of his yard. Every time I walk around this portion of his yard I only feel a bit more ignorant. I realize how very little I know about plants and how very little I will probably know in my lifetime. It is a horrible feeling, I might add, like taking a driving test and not knowing how to start the car. (And so the weeds grow.)

And I can give you another reason. I work all week. When I'm not at my job, I spend my free time grocery shopping, cleaning, washing, banking, driving back and forth from who knows where, doing laundry, and trying to write. When I do have some free time for relaxing, I would rather read a book, watch a movie, or take a ride on my bike than pull up weeds.

Another good reason: I am too poor to hire someone to do it for me like my neighbor does. (And I am too polite to ask my visitors to pull up a few sprouts up before they come inside the house for a visit.)

And a final reason: I don't understand why these weeds grow or where they come from, just like I don't understand how or why I get myself into some of my other situations or problems. And if you wanna know the truth, I personally don't see anything wrong with dandelions growing throughout the lawn—I think they look colorful and pretty. But I know my neighbor doesn't agree with this. He keeps hoping I will weed. If you ask me, he must believe in miracles. But then, I guess, so do I. Every morning on my way to unlock my car, walking through my front yard of weeds, I keep a careful, close watch for something wonderful to happen, something like a flower to break through all this mess.

DATES

First there was Jim. We have in common the same first name, the same birthday (though he was a year younger), the same type of car, and the same amount of brothers and sisters. (A little too frightening, if you ask me.) He lives in Philadelphia, so I drove down there after work and met him for dinner. He was nice and charming, a little shorter than me and had thick black hair, a black mustache, and a fair complexion. I found him attractive, and, yes, I spent the night with him and it was nice and comfortable but no, I'm not really sure if I want to see him again. I found him a little too flighty for my taste.

And then there was Evan. Evan answered my ad too. He lives close by, across the river in Lambertville, and is a commercial artist. We met for drinks at the Swan Hotel, where I had first met Geoff. I was very hopeful about him. His letter had said that he had just moved to the area from the city and was looking to meet someone after just breaking off another relationship. And I wasn't real disappointed in him when we first met. He's taller, a little pudgy, tiny black eyes, and curly reddish brown hair. He was a great talker, very up to date with movies and theater and music, and it was nice to compare notes. As we began talking we discovered we have a mutual friend in Manhattan in common, a musician I used to work with, so that broke some of the ice between us. But he kept staring at my hands the whole time we were talking. And then finally he said he thought I should think about doing some modeling. He said I had very handsome hands; he liked the way the hair grew on the backs and around my wrists. And then I asked him if he could tell that I bit my nails. He said yes, but a good manicure could solve that. And he was really serious. He gave me his card and we've spoken a couple of times on the phone. I know this sounds awful, but I found him a little too old for me, as if of another generation, and he had a terrible sinus problem and kept sniffling through drinks. I plan to see him again, though. If anything, I find him interesting and there is enough in common to possibly be friends.

Chris was twenty-seven and very good looking. He is a graduate student I met in Princeton. He had also answered my ad. He has that dark preppy look, brown hair, ice blue eyes, and the most beautiful skin of anyone I have met so far. He was rather refreshing to be with—he was so optimistic about his own future. We spent the weekend together. But I've been afraid of calling him back. He made me feel old and jaded and cynical, more so than I really am. But he was nice. He was really nice.

And Ted. Ted I met through the dating service—Ted I spoke to for six hours on the phone before I met him. We went to Flemington for dinner. He's something of a real outdoorsman type. He's over six feet tall, blondish brown hair, very heterosexual looking, and likes to fish and ski. After dinner we went bowling. But then at the bowling alley he started to chain smoke, and he turned very competitive. He was so *into* beating me at bowling. I'll remember not to do that again on a first date. It showed not only his ugly, unsportsmanship side, but my immature, pouty personality because I kept losing. (No one likes to lose, you know, and I do it enough in real life to have to keep repeating it in games.) He keeps calling me though to get together again. But I don't know. I just don't know....

Sal was a mistake. The minute I saw him I wanted to leave. And so did he, but we stuck it out for a couple of hours. Sal was about six feet, Italian (olive-toned skin, black mustache, brown eyes), well built, and had a scar running diagonally across his face. He had answered my ad and we met at a movie theater in Doylestown. I could smell cigarette smoke on him right away and then, as we were trying to make chit chat, he told me he used to do drugs. I didn't run away from him because

I thought he might pull a knife or a gun on me and chase me down. And I wanted to see the movie. By the time I left, with an impolite good-bye, I was so afraid of him I was shaking. It was not pleasant.

And then last weekend there was Rick. Ricky, Ricky, Ricky. Rick was very, very sexy. He was Barry and Mitchell's house guest for the weekend. Rick is an accountant in New York City, but don't let that fool you. I knew the minute we met that we were both interested in one another, but I never in my wildest dreams would ever have thought of inviting one of their house guests to spend the night with me! I was just on my way out the door to go biking when he came over to the cottage with Barry and Mitchell. He has blue eyes, fair skin, a nice body, and is very hairy. And he's a real looker. Very, very handsome. And he knows it. As I went out the gate on my bike Rick made a comment that he thought I had great looking legs. (They actually do look pretty good right now because of cycling so much.) There was a lot of chemical's flying around that afternoon we met. He kept staring at me and I kept staring at the crook of his neck. (That's the favorite part of the body for me, and he had a fabulous looking one.) I met up with Barry and Mitchell and Rick for dinner and afterward we went to the Cartwheel. Rick was cruising everyone in sight—he's just coming out and he looked like a little boy let loose in a toy store. Barry and Mitchell left early so I stuck around with Rick for a bit longer. I was interested in him, interested in people seeing me with him, and interested in seeing if I could meet anyone else myself. Finally I was tired of watching Rick chase after this blond and I just wanted to go home and go to sleep. Since Barry and Mitchell left early I was to give Rick a ride home if he didn't hook up with someone else. Fortunately, he was ready to leave when I was. When we pulled up at the house, we got out of the car and both paused in the driveway, looking up at the stars. We both commented on how nice the night was, the weather had cooled a bit since the afternoon, and then he walked over and put his arms around me. It was really romantic and sexy and fabulous and all I can say about

Rick was that I had a wonderful time, several times that night. I really needed Rick bad. I've spoken to him on the phone once since then, but he lives in Manhattan and he's seeing someone, and, well, you know the story, so the dating just continues....

THE CHILD IN ME

About two miles from my house in Pennsylvania is a creek which flows into a canal which runs beside a river. At the junction of these three bodies of water is a national park where a certain man and his troop of soldiers crossed the river over two hundred years ago on a cold December night. In the last year I have been to this park at least once a week. Here I have spent afternoons hiking the wildflower trails, sitting on the large stones by the river and reading, or climbing to the observation tower perched atop the mountains which surround this park. I have biked to the old covered bridge, waded in sneakers down the middle of the creek and watched my reflection in the water of the canal ripple and blur as a fish jumped up suddenly for air. I have been here alone, with my parents, with friends, dates, and potential lovers. I have had picnics, taken naps, listened to my favorite cassette tapes and played Frisbee, backgammon, and pinochle on the grass. I have watched a full set of spectacular seasons come and go, fallen in love with one man, broken up with another, lost four kites in the giant trees beside the canal and waited patiently one humid October morning for the geese to arrive from Canada.

The first time I came to this park was shortly after I moved here. I had taken a wrong turn while driving home and ended up there by mistake. But instead of turning around I followed the road as it curved through the park. I stopped the car, walked to the war memorial and then down to the river. Here I discovered a view I had seen many times since moving out of Manhattan: a river, a country road, and a cascading mountain slope covered with lush green trees. But this time I noticed as I looked out across the river that I felt a difference. I felt comfortable; this place seemed right. I realized this was the first time I had regarded this view as a part of my new home, not as a tourist looking at something astonishing and beautiful.

The next time I came here was two weeks later with a friend. I showed him the view and then we walked along the canal, stopping to eat oranges we carried in a knapsack near a pasture of grazing sheep and horses, This time I discovered I liked being outside. For a decade I had shut myself up in tiny New York apartments, going outdoors only to get somewhere else: to work, to a store, to a restaurant or to see a movie or a play. What was odd and yet so special about that day, was the same way I had noticed once on vacation in Colorado, that above me was this huge, vast open blue field of sky.

I've discovered many things last year: what it's like to have your sweat evaporate on an early morning, what it's like to fall in love, what it's like to have your car break down on a deserted country road. I've learned how to repaint patio furniture, start a barbecue, plant a garden, and repair a broken heart. I've learned it's possible to get a sunburn on a clear winter day, why it is important sometimes to cry, and how to tell the difference between poison and Boston ivy. And I've realized many things about myself, that I am protective of the people I decide to maintain in my life; attentive, jealous, and possessive, sometimes, I fear, a little distractingly so. I've realized I'm up front and honest about my emotions, but also at times moody, intent or intense. And I've decided what I want and expect and need in a relationship, but I have also discovered I make myself too vulnerable every time I meet an interesting man. And I've made a few conscious changes: I no longer smoke, drink less caffeine and alcohol, exercise regularly, and prefer to wear my hair cut short. But the most important and wonderful thing I have discovered this year happened when I started dating after a self-imposed hiatus. I discovered the child within me, and I will never let him disappear again.

The child in me likes to bike, eat ice cream, go to the zoo or bowling. The child likes to play card games, solve crossword puzzles, watch music videos and make kites. The child likes to sing, dance, roller skate, ride horses, and eat cotton candy. The child in me likes to be touched and hugged and kissed.

The child was always there, I think, but for years he was suppressed as I focused on other things. Ironically what I remember most about my childhood years are the hours I spent alone in my room reading and studying and practicing the piano downstairs in the living room. Later, older, the decade I lived in New York, I focused on graduate school, a career in the theater, a circle of friends, writing a book, and paying my bills on time. Sometimes I feel that perhaps many of those years I was too self-absorbed, caught up in my own little world, searching for everything from the right apartment to the right man. But then I thought of myself as most urban gay men in their twenties did: handsome, important, and indestructible.

Long before I moved away from Manhattan I began to shed layers of stress from my life: quitting a job I didn't like, avoiding people who made me uncomfortable, accepting that there were things I knew nothing about and might never have a chance to experience or learn. I don't consider this a defeatist attitude. It is simply my way of adapting to the world. At the same time I also began reassessing my expectations and goals, constantly checking my ideals against reality, rationalizing the difference between my intellect and behavior. And as the pressures and tensions lessened, I found underneath the grumpy, grouchy urban dweller I had become was the man my friends had been able to see all along: a nice guy just trying to find happiness.

But life is more complex. Sometimes I fear I am too many people: to my friend Debbie I am a pillar of strength, offering advice and inspiration and encouragement; to my friend Jon I am a confidant, exchanging anecdotes on everything from our latest dates to backstage Broadway gossip. To my employer I am a source of frustration, to my co-workers an advocate for better, more fair working conditions, to my parents I'm a mystery. Every person I know brings out a different facet of me. The last man I dated seriously didn't know who he wanted me to be for him: friend, companion, acquaintance or lover;

hence one of the major problems of our relationship. But I had no such confusions as to who I wanted to be for him. I wanted to be them all.

And when I realized this was not possible with him, that in fact, no matter whom I was for him, we were still not right for each other. I had walked away from the relationship and again examined my expectations, goals, ideals, intellect, and behavior. And when I had sorted things out, put things back into perspective, and decided I was ready to move on, I discovered I was still depressed. But this time I remembered the child within me. This time it was the child who saved me.

It was the child who led me outside again to explore and observe the village streets and rural roads around my new home. It was the child who took me out on bike rides, for a swim at a neighbor's pool, on trips to the beach or to visit old friends. It was the child who made me laugh and turn on the radio and sing along. It was the child who allowed me to enjoy simple things: fireflies on a balmy summer night, the smell of freshly cut grass, snow falling beneath a street lamp. And it was the child who made it possible to meet new people, inspiring a man who felt he had been burned too many times with a combination of innocence and optimism and belief that anything he wanted was obtainable.

What I guess I'm trying to say is that people find their inner strength in many ways. For some it is through jogging or exercising or meditation or visualization. For others it can be by crying, writing, screaming, eating or perhaps, as one fictional heroine displayed, simply walking through Tiffany's. For me, it is the child who offers hope. It is the child who leads me back to the park: to think, to solve, to understand, and to relax. And like the man who stood on this same land two centuries ago with a dream of a new nation, I, too, come here with dreams. Dreams of a world without disease and friends not dying, dreams of an open, accepted lifestyle, dreams of a life in love with the right man. Simple dreams of a normal, modern gay man. A man who dreams it is still possible to look at the world like a child.

THE RIGHT MAN

In the last three months I have had over thirty dates—more, I think, than perhaps the total I have had in all the years I have been dating gay men. In this short period I have dated men younger, older, and the same age as I. I have dated blonds, brunets, a redhead, and a few who have been balding. One, I remember, wore his hair in a ponytail. Another had a body so astounding it made me nervous to sit near him. And for the most part I have met these men on neutral territory, neither his place nor mine, our rendezvous occurring outside restaurants, theaters, bars, bookstores, and once, a grocery store.

And these dates have been simple activities: a drink, maybe dinner, sometimes something athletic—bowling, biking, just walking around town or hiking through a park. I have met these men through a variety of methods: a friend's introduction, a personal ad, a dating service, a social organization, and yes, even at a bar. As one of my friends says, I am on the prowl. But as I carefully explain, these dates are not arranged or intended as sexual encounters. These days, I am more interested in a long-term relationship. In fact, these dates have served other purposes for me as well: a way of getting over a prior unfulfilling relationship, a way of meeting new friends, a way of discovering and exploring the area around my home, and yes, possibly, a way of finding that special someone, the right man for me.

Who is the right man? Does he exist? In the last three months I have had a brief affair with a younger man in Philadelphia, a slightly longer one with an older gentleman who owned a farm near the Delaware River, and a much shorter one with a man whose biggest passion was belonging to a gay water polo team. Each man was intelligent and attractive; each possessed a personality that both interested and intrigued me enough to want to see him again. And each possessed the right sexual chemistry. But with each, something was also wrong or missing. On some level there wasn't a connection or need or spark between us. Each presented me with a major problem for which I could find neither a solution, an adjustment, nor an arrangement. And each one I let end in its own way, drifting politely apart through either neglect or avoidance. Each one hurt when it was over. And every time, I managed to pick myself up, go out, and find another date.

One friend of mine thinks I'm too particular. I tell him I don't think I'm particular at all, I only expect the same qualities in my dates that I enjoy in my friends. Another friend thinks I place too much emphasis on looks. He thinks I'm shallow and insincere when I tell him that the chemistry wasn't right with someone I just met. And I tell him that I expect that attraction to be a part of any relationship I undertake, though I am quick to add I have no particular type or demand any certain physical requirements. For me he can be tall or short, blond or brunet. He can be muscular or lean or smooth or hairy or even overweight. I know this as a fact; I have fallen for a variety of men. So, physically, I know the right man for me exists; I see him all the time—at the beach, at the bar, at the gym, on the street. I'm not talking about a man so beautiful and handsome and flawless that he approaches and becomes a fantasy or ideal or god. Even if I were to meet such a man, he might still not be the right one for me. All I ask is that the package be right. And the right package includes the right attraction, in both directions, for both me and him.

And as I tell my friend, chemistry implies much more than just physical aspects. It includes a combination of other qualities and traits—background, education, personality, intelligence—and encompasses not just similarities but a mixture of differences as well. And as I explain further, I don't expect to find someone perfect; the right relationship, I believe, includes a certain amount of give-and-take, complements and compromises. Finding the right man means a lot more than being at the right place at the right time with the right attitude. Theoretically, I cannot describe the right man for me. I can't really supply a list of right or wrong, or good or bad qualities.

This realization slapped me in the face one day last week when my friend Jon called me at work. Jon, a man my age and height with a similar educational background and professional and avocational interests, had recently ended a seven-year monogamous gay relationship. His ex-lover had moved out of the apartment, and now Jon was ready to start dating again. But he did not feel comfortable in a gay bar and was unaware of what he should do in order to meet the right man. So he turned to many resources I had also used: friends of friends, personal ads, a gay religious organization. But each had left him unsatisfied. Now he was ready to try a dating service. His frantic call that day was for help filling out the application form.

Here, in black and white, in words, phrases, sentences, and questions, he was asked to list the qualities of the men he would like to meet as well as to rate his own characteristics, both in temperament and looks. As he read the questions to me over the phone and we discussed each of his decisions and answers, I was struck by the absurdity of it all. How could you choose between a man who acts more from his thoughts than one who acts from his feelings? What if you wanted someone who was both imaginative and realistic, which this questionnaire didn't allow? What if, as in my case, you didn't care if he were clean shaven or had a mustache or a beard? What if the man who is perfect for you, according to this questionnaire, prefers someone who is taller? What if the only man you're right for is a deaf and dumb, hunchbacked midget? I understood my friend's dismay when I told him I thought he was a man who is ruled more by his head than by his heart; but that's what friends are for, they keep you honest and grounded. Before hanging up, I gave him some advice, the same advice, in fact, he had given me shortly after a relationship I had been both serious and committed to had faltered. "It takes time," I said. "You just have to keep trying."

So who is the right man for my friend? Who is the right one for me? What is it I want or expect or need? A therapist once told me I'm searching for a father figure. But for her, that was an easy concept to grasp. Yes, in many ways I am initially drawn to men who seem to be the fatherly type. But that's not the type of relationship I want. What I want in life is what most people are searching for: a nice home, self-satisfaction from career, and a chance to share my time with someone. And that someone I expect to be attentive and caring, loving and loyal, masculine and well-grounded with morals and ethics: a man who brings out those qualities in me and who regards me as an equal in all aspects of the relationship. Someone preferably close to my age, someone within the same generation. I am looking for someone honest and communicative and committed, not someone who'll—as one man I dated said—"give it a try and see how it turns out." And as for dating, it's not so much the activity but the person I'm sharing time with that matters.

So what exactly was wrong with all these dates? Nothing specific; they were all sincere and genuinely nice guys. My friend Barry thinks I put too much emphasis on first impressions. He constantly reassures me that it took him six months of dating his lover, Mitchell, before he fell in love. In many ways I know there is something right in what he says. And I keep reminding him that the last man I fell in love with certainly fit into that pattern. So I'm realistic enough not to expect a white knight to sweep me off my feet. Yet perhaps I'm sometimes too rational in following my instincts, never allowing a second date to happen with someone who is interested in me.

There's nothing more I want right now in my life than to be in a relationship. But it's not a crime to be single. As I tell one friend, I would rather spend my life alone than spend it with the wrong person. But I go out on dates and keep looking for Mr. Right. I don't know what it will be that will make me fall in love. All I can answer is that I keep trying and looking and I'll know what it is when it happens. And all I can hope is that I, too, am the right man for him.

ONE WAY OR ANOTHER

It was the day after Thanksgiving and I had walked across the paved brick courtyard which separates our two houses to see my friend Barry before I headed into town to do some grocery shopping. It was cold and windy outside and the snow which had fallen two days before was now solid and slippery, packed into a frosting of ice. I walked cautiously, the soles of the old sneakers I wore had long ago disappeared, and by the time I had reached is front door, Barry had seen my approach and unbolted the lock. Dressed in a purple and white stripped terry cotton bathrobe, or rather undressed and wearing a robe, he was poking apiece of kindling into the stone fireplace that heats the kitchen of his stone house when I closed the door. He turned and gave me a smile and I could tell he was surprised to see me but glad I had stopped by, his expression full of a thousand questions. Barry and I had been friends for eleven years, friends since we met each other in graduate school in New York City. Now, in the mountains of Pennsylvania, Barry was also my landlord; he and his lover, Mitchell, owned the cottage I was renting, their house next door they used as a weekend escape from the city.

Barry stamped his foot and wedged a twig under a smoking log. "I don't know why my fires never work," he said. "I do everything like you do."

We both looked into the fire and I picked up a section of the Sunday *Times* which he kept in a wicker basket near the store and tore pages from the paper, crumpled them up, and slid them under the grate in the fireplace. Soon the paper had caught fire and we both stood back and watched the flames shoot upward into the neck of the fireplace, fade a bit, and the thin strips of fatwood kindling blacken and ignite.

"It looks real," a voice behind me said and I felt a hand slide across my shoulder. I turned and said good morning to Stuart, Barry's house guest for the holiday weekend, and watched his eyes, large amber circles, dart between the fire, Barry, and myself.

"The coffee's ready," Barry said and walked to a cupboard and retrieved a cup for Stuart.

"You're up early," Stuart said to me. He took a seat on a stool and leaned an arm on the counter. He was wearing a white T-shirt and old, faded jeans, shredded at the knees, and his long black hair, iced with streaks of gray, fell across his brow like a boy's; and, though he shifted his body so that his legs straddled the stool, his eyes did not veer from me; I could feel the intensity of his examination even as I looked away from him.

Since I had met Stuart two days ago I felt that electrical spark which sometimes draws me toward a man I know nothing about. And I sensed Stuart felt the same way. But we were both in awkward positions. Stuart was one of Barry's ex-boyfriends. And I had just begun seeing someone regularly, and I knew I was not the type of guy who could have sex with one man when he was sleeping with another, and certainly not the type of person who would trick with a friend's ex-boyfriend. I leaned against the frame of the door, Stuart ran his hand through his hair and Barry poured the coffee, placing the mug on the counter beside Stuart.

"I always get up early," I said to Stuart. "It's a habit."

"But you were up late," Stuart noted, lifting the cup to his lips and blowing over the steam.

"Spying on the neighbors?" Barry laughed.

"I couldn't help noticing the car population next door doubled in the middle of the night," Stuart said.

"Ray stayed last night," I answered, studying the chest hair which crept over the collar of Stuart's T-shirt, a sight which I found unbelievable sexy.

"Is he the lawyer?" Barry asked.

"No, he's the one with the moustache," I answered.

"Did he leave already?" Stuart asked.

"He's picking up his ex-lover at the airport," I replied, knowing to give them the news they were waiting for instead of letting them interrogate me and put it out painfully in little pieces. There was an awkward moment of silence as we all shifted our positions.

"I'm warning you now, Jimmy," Barry said. "You're going to get burned."

I looked at the floor, then at the fire. Stuart ran his hand through his hair again and then, out of Barry's sight, placed it against my back, sliding it down to where it rested at the dip of my buttocks.

Months later Barry told me he knew that morning what would happen. I think I knew it then too. But I still had to give it a try with Ray. I still had to let it happen. And I let a chance with Stuart slip away, all because I'm a guy who can only go one way or the other.

JUST LOOKING

It feels like November, my boyfriend, Ray, said when he entered my apartment. Outside my kitchen window I thought it looked like spring had arrived early, the sky a solid pale blue, the sun bouncing off my car in large silver spots. Though it was mid-February, last night when I pulled the car into the driveway I had noticed the green tips of the day lilies pushing their way up through the soil. According to my boyfriend, it was windy and chilly outside this morning, though perhaps it would be somewhat warmer when we reached Washington, D.C., where, we had decided, we were driving to spend the weekend together.

The drive to Washington from Pennsylvania is somewhere around three and a half hours, and Ray had made cassette tapes from us to listen to on the drive: recordings by Sarah Brightman, Holly Near, and the original cast album of *Miss Saigon*, a hit London musical which had not yet opened on Broadway. Ray, a professor and a playwright, has a wide range of musical tastes, much wider than my own. He has patience for many things I do not, for example Charles Ives, Philip Glass, and Twentieth Century Opera. But then he doesn't like country music, which I do, and when I switch the radio to a Top 40 station, I notice him squirm in his seat and clench his teeth together, though he will not make me change the station if I am the driver. I think that is perhaps one of the things I like best about Ray, that we are not the same person and neither one of us is trying to make the other into someone else. We have our differences and we have our similarities. There is enough to connect us as friends, enough to keep us interested in one another in bed, although our relationship has not been without complications.

We met three months prior to this trip to Washington, for brunch at a Philadelphia restaurant a few days before Thanksgiving. Ray had replied to my personal ad in a Philadelphia gay newspaper. His note was short: "GWM, 30, professor, new to area. Enjoys music, theater, movies, reading. 5'10", 140 lbs, br/bl, mustache. I am usually home in the evenings." When we first spoke on the phone I learned he had recently moved to New Hope from Boston, and, like myself, was adjusting to life in a more rural environment. The major complication, I found out on our first date, was that he had left a floundering relationship and a lover back in Boston.

I once told Ray during an argument that though he was here, physically in Pennsylvania, he was still mentally in Boston. I had noticed when we were together he would thumb through Boston magazines at a bookstore, listen to a broadcast of the Boston Symphony on the radio, or mention a snowstorm might be headed in our direction because a friend of his in Boston had said there was one on the way. Often, when we were discussing a subject, Ray would begin a remark with, "back in Boston," or "at home in Boston," but I could not fault him for that, for I, too, had a propensity to start a sentence with, "When I lived in New York." So that did not irritate me. I was not even jealous of the lover he left behind in Boston, or what he someday expected to go back to. I, too, was struggling and floundering in my own way when we first met. I was at the point where I needed and wanted to connect with someone. All right, I told myself after that first date, we all carry a lot of baggage around with us. I, myself, was trying to get over a previous unsuccessful relationship, trying to forget a string of lousy dates, trying to make some new friends, and trying to make this place my home. And so we started dating each other. And as things turned out we spent almost every night together. We cooked for one another, went shopping together, helped each other with day to day tasks: banking, laundry, cleaning. In short, because we became so comfortable with one another so quickly, we bypassed a lot of the exploration that true dating and courtship involves: finding out who the other person really is. So what bothered me almost three months after we met, was not an itch or restless desire to move on to someone else. What bothered me was the issue of monogamy.

It happened like this: We were eating at a Mexican restaurant a few days before Valentine's Day. We were both in good moods, though both tired from work. There were many things left unspoken in our relationship, one, in particular, was the dangling relationship Ray had with his lover, Nick, back in Boston. I had never interrogated Ray about Nick and Ray had not offered much explanation. And yet part of our own relationship included the mutual admiration of other men. We would often comment on a man who caught our attention, defining him as something like "handsome," "sexy," "intriguing" or "stunning" or commenting on some characteristic the man displayed, like a great face, great eyes, nice arms, or nice ass. I did not find this practice as distressing as I have sometimes felt with other boyfriends. Particularly, I think, because I perceived I had Ray's sexual interest whereas with others I had felt only tenuously linked. I sensed some sort of underling, unspoken trust with Ray, that he wasn't looking for anyone else and neither was I. And so it happened in our dinner conversation that we were both remarking about a nearby young man's beauty, when I mentioned in a light-hearted manner that it was all right for Ray to "look" but not the "touch." My comment seemed to take Ray off guard and I added, a bit more forcefully, that if he were sleeping with me, he should not be sleeping with someone else. He answered by saying he didn't believe in monogamy. I felt as if I had been slapped in the face but I was smart enough to remain silent, and when we reached our cars I informed him that I needed to be by myself that night, that there were some things that I now had to do a lot of thinking about.

And the next day this is what I told him I had decided: I said I was not asking him to marry me, not asking him to say he loved me, and I never expected us to be joined at the hip to one another, after all, we had only known each other for a short time. But I did say I was certain about the statement I had made last night: if he sleeps with me, he doesn't sleep with anyone else. I asked him since we had been dating if he had slept with his lover Nick. He said yes he had, when he went back to Boston for the Christmas holidays, and then he asked why I was trying to make him feel guilty about it. I answered I would never make him feel guilty about something which we had never discussed before. But we were discussing it now, and this is what I believed and what I wanted and expected. And that if it happened again, then he should feel guilty, and he should start looking for someone else, someone who would be comfortable with that type of arrangement because I wasn't. But, I added, the real essence of our problem, as I saw it, was that we were traveling two different roads when I had thought we were on the same one. I wanted a serial monogamous relationship and he did not believe in monogamy. It wasn't entirely an issue of *only himself* being monogamous, but of *both of us* being monogamous. If he couldn't make some kind of commitment to me, why should I make a commitment to him? In my opinion there was nowhere else for us to go together.

Ray was flustered at this point. We both were. And I knew he was upset. Neither one of us wanted to give up what we had going with the other. He began to backtrack, explaining he moved to this area because he was offered a good teaching job, but it had been a harder adjustment than he had imagined. He admitted he missed Boston, then added that he had disliked Boston when he had first moved there several years ago. But his opinion had changed. And that though he didn't believe monogamy was possible for himself at this moment, he did believe people do grow and change, that I, in fact, had even written about myself changing. I didn't mention that someday we might be able to *evolve* into an open relationship, in part, because we had not yet navigated the basis of any sort of commitment. And I wasn't ready to compromise because there was nothing in my favor.

After a long silence, neither of us budging, he said, "I can't promise you a lifetime commitment. I can only make a commitment to you right now." And I knew that was all I wanted and expected at this point. A step in the right direction.

And so our weekend in Washington was part vacation, part celebration. Ray wanted to see a matinee performance of Sondheim's *Merrily We Roll Along* which was being produced by a local theater company and I, having seen enough bad theater from having worked in the theater for almost a decade, said I would drop him off and go to the mall, the mall being that huge array of buildings between the Capital and the Washington Monument. My destination was the National Gallery.

It was still windy and chilly when we arrived and we ate lunch at a restaurant overlooking the Washington Channel. Already we were starved and anxious, though the view from our table was both settling and memorable: a small harbor of docked sailboats, sunlight reflecting off the water as brilliantly as an evening dance of fireflies. After lunch Ray left for the theater and I walked the few blocks to the mall. Washington has always reminded me of some unknown, European city: low buildings, boulevards of monuments and memorials and galleries. The mall was busy that afternoon, full of tourists and cameras and joggers and dogs, the bright sunshine doing its best to dispel the cold. Inside the National Gallery it was crowded and warm, and after a few minutes I shed my coat and carried it balled beneath my arm.

I have never been a big fan of museums, though I have been to most of the major ones in both America and Europe. As a child my parents took me to as many museums as I could stand. Living in New York I was forever leading out-of-town visitors to the Museum of Modern Art or the Metropolitan. One reason why I have always felt uncomfortable with museums is that I never know what to do with my hands. I feel as if I am walking in a priceless china shop, knowing even if I had the money, I would never pick anything up or want to buy it. My favorite museums have the kind of exhibits you can touch, like moonrocks and tortoise shells. And so I thought it odd that I should choose to spend my afternoon in an art museum, but after sitting for such a long drive, it was nice to be moving, walking and looking.

I spent the afternoon wandering through the permanent collections and a few of the special exhibits: an interesting display of paintings made from woodcuts, an absorbing one on an artist named John Marin who painted landscapes, both urban and rural, in dull, dry looking tones, and an uninspiring retrospective of Twentieth Century Art on the Concourse. The tourists on view in the National Gallery, particularly the East Wing which houses the contemporary art, are often more interesting than the art itself: one, a young man wearing black jeans and a white turtleneck, fascinated me as we hovered around each other while viewing a series of French sculptures: from the rear, I was awed by the way the thin cotton fabric of his shirt stretched taut at his shoulders and then billowed out like a skirt at his narrow waist; beside me, I noted his strong profile; in front, I studied the blond bangs and large brown eyes. I lost sight of him somewhere amongst the Impressionist paintings. But I noticed that there were several other men strolling alone, something I have never thought about or done before on a Saturday afternoon in an art gallery. But here I was alone and I couldn't help notice the other men who were alone too. After years of being a single gay male living in Manhattan my eyes are trained to seek out other gay men passing, cruising, and there, that afternoon at the National Gallery, the population of gay men was as thriving as any street in Greenwich Village on a Saturday night.

After a couple of hours my eyes were tired from looking at all the men and art, and I walked outside, across the mall, and down to the theater to meet Ray. The production, he said, when he greeted me, was not inspiring, and we hopped into the car and drove to our hotel near DuPont Circle. The rest of the weekend we spent together: eating, shopping, browsing, drinking, and in bed with each other. Before our drive back to Pennsylvania the next afternoon, we stopped at a bookstore on

Connecticut Avenue. Ray waited in the car while I picked up a copy of the Sunday edition of *The New York Times*. Waiting in line to pay for the paper I noticed a dark, swarthy young man standing in front of the shelf appropriately labeled "Mysteries." He was looking at me, giving me a cruise so long you would think he was admiring one of those amazing Greek sculptures on the main floor of the Metropolitan Museum. I looked at him and I felt my heartbeat quickening; I thought he was quite handsome. But I was also absorbed with another, more important thought, as clearly as when I first recognized it the day before while at the art gallery. Wasn't it nice not to feel the need to know more about this man, that a simple look between the two of us was enough? I didn't wonder how big his arms or chest or cock were. I didn't care where he lived, or how he earned his living. I was not interested in his name, his phone number, or going home with him. The mere moment of the look was all I wanted; it was satisfying simply in and of itself.

Driving back to Pennsylvania, I was struck by the impermanence of many things: the changing landscape—new exit ramps, office buildings and motels being built along the highway; the changing seasons—already forsythia was blooming in short strips at the side of the road; the music of *Miss Saigon*—a score which will and should change many times before it reaches Broadway, as much perhaps as a show such as *Merrily We Roll Along* did. Even Degas once said a painting is never finished.

But then, somewhere around the Delaware-Pennsylvania border, I became sure of where I was driving, of what road to travel. I was headed toward my home. I was headed deeper into a relationship. But that was all I really knew, all I really know now. I don't know how far Ray and I will travel together; I don't really understand the permanence or impermanence of the heart. But that moment, as the road appeared and disappeared beneath the car in an unchanging cycle, I was content that we were together: just driving, just listening, just looking.

FRIENDS

He will say it was my fault. I will say it was his. He will say it was his idea to break up, that I was too demanding, expected too much too soon. I will say it was my idea. He made me unhappy. I couldn't trust him. His friends thought I was controlling and manipulative Mine thought he had an attitude problem.

We did share some good times. But in the end we were both overrun by our own differences and stubbornness. I wanted a monogamous relationship. He didn't. I had reached a point that in order to continue seeing him I had to have some sort of commitment. But he couldn't give it to me. And so, another attempt at a relationship has dissolved and it's time once again to rebuild my confidence; time for some self-repairing, some strengthening of the self-esteem. And so, this first weekend without him, without Ray, I'm heading out of town. I'm spending the weekend in New York City with a close friend.

I do not have any good, close friends in New Hope where I have lived for the last two years. I have never been someone who was able to make a wide circle of friends, even when I was in college, when I worked in the theater or when I lived in Manhattan. I am the type who has a small, strong, stable, and supportive core of four or five everlasting friends. Unfortunately, and sometimes fortunately, these friends live far away from me. Fortunately, I sometimes think, because I am not able to drive them completely crazy. The closest one, Jon, the one I'm visiting this weekend, lives in Manhattan, an hour and a half drive by car from my home.

Though there is a lot of geographical distance between me and my good friends, I talk to them regularly on the phone.

And I see them as often as possible. I know what's happening in their lives and they in mine. And when we get together, we do not have a lot of territory to catch up on. Time apart has not created any awkwardness for either of us. We are simply ourselves with each other. For me, that is one of the most important gifts I and my friends can and will give to one another, for sometimes on a date or in a relationship I have noticed that I can become someone who I don't know, someone I don't recognize, someone I would never, ever acknowledge as myself.

And so I am turning to my friend Jon for advice and comfort and support this weekend. He has helped me through similar situations before. With Geoff. With Clarke. With a string of lousy dates. And I have helped Jon through some of the same feelings as well. Jon knows more about my life, I think, than any boyfriend or ex-boyfriend ever will. I find it odd that I have, in my adult life, picked my friends much more carefully than my tricks, affairs, boyfriends, and lovers. It's a statement I've heard made by others many times, over and over, but one I have not necessarily agreed with.

It seems that within the last few years, for me, lovers and sexual partners have come and gone, but my friends have always remained loyal to me. A lot of things have been written already about friendships, about how it is seldom the stuff of drama or that we reflect and measure our lives against our friends. But the most important thing about friendships, I think, for a gay man, a single gay man, is that they become his surrogate family.

Friendship happens in many ways. The bonds are sometimes obvious: school, career, youth or similar backgrounds. There are links in my friendships which will never exist in any sort of relationship I could or will ever have. Perhaps that is why, in some relationships, lovers are often jealous of best friends. Two of my strong, close friends, John and Debbie, I have known since college when we all sang together in the university choral group. Another friend, Barry, I met when I first moved to New York and we were in graduate school together. Another close friend of mine, Kevin, is now dead; we met because we were on similar career paths in the theater. And in his place, now, is my best friend Jon. We became friends because of Kevin's death.

Recently, someone asked me why hadn't I ever thought about dating Jon, why hadn't we become lovers, or why don't we? It has been a thought, I must confess, that has crossed my mind many times too. And my explanation to them was that it has always been a matter of bad timing: When I was free, John had Tom. When Jon was free, I was seeing Geoff. When I was getting over Geoff, Jon was dating Lenny. When Jon was free, I had met Ray. And as Ray now ends, Jon is seeing Ken. And, I added, there was also the geographical distance between us. Neither of us wants a long distance relationship.

But now, thinking about the question again, I realize I have been asked that question many times in my life. It was asked when my oldest friend John and I were college roommates and when we lived together in New York. It was asked about me and Kevin. It was asked of me and my friends Joel and Steve and Mark. And now, trying to sort through what went wrong in a bad relationship and what is right in my friendships, I am confused why my lovers can't be more like my friends and why my friends can't be more like my lovers. I am aware that I expect my lovers to be my friends, in fact, that I want that to be an important part of my relationship. So why shouldn't I expect my friends to end up as lovers? The answer is fear, I think—fear of losing a friend if he doesn't work out as a lover. And it all has to do with sex, of course. For me, stepping over the sexual line adds another dimension to any relationship. It automatically creates certain elements and expectations in myself and of the other person. For example, I am much more possessive of a person in a sexual relationship than I am in a friendship. In a sexual relationship I expect a man's complete sexual attention, affection, and focus when we are together. And I expect to trust him when we are apart. I am not saying that he cannot look or notice or cruise or flirt with other men; everyone does that, it's part of being human and an important and fun part of being gay. What I mean is if he is sleeping with me he does not and cannot sleep with someone else. It's just a simple fact of what I want and expect and need. But a friend can sleep with as many people as he wants—unless, of course, he begins to sleep with me.

That's not the norm for a lot of gay men, I realize. For many gay men of my generation, the men who were coming out in the middle and late Seventies, sex could be an introduction and a bond to friendship. If you slept with someone once or twice and things didn't work out exactly the way you both wanted, but you both liked each other, found each other interesting, you still could end up being good friends. I, too, have a few friends I have met in this fashion. But I wonder, perhaps, if that was not simply due to the times, the prevalent attitudes of the era or maybe, because when it happened, I was younger. I do know that now, in my middle thirties, I am not interested in sex being the link or the bond in friendships. I don't want to have to deal with sexual jealousy. I have learned the hard way it's a very ugly, ugly side of me.

Someone could probably rationally question my logic, by asking, "Well, if you and Jon are such good friends before you try to become lovers, wouldn't you be friends again if such a relationship didn't work out? Aren't you devaluing the strength of your friendship? Wouldn't it survive that sort of test?" My answer is that sex is a powerful force. It has the power to influence and move and confuse. And maybe, perhaps, it's not only the fear of losing a friend because of sexual complications, but also the fact that what I need of a friend is him to be a friend.

Which is what I need this weekend. The problem this weekend is not just sex or the lack of it or the wanting of it. Sex (and a few other things) was the means I fell in love with my now ex-boyfriend Ray. And the problem is not that I fell in love. The problem is I fell in love, again, with the wrong person.

And so my weekend with Jon in New York City will be spent doing simple things with great difficulty: trying to concentrate and relax while watching movies, cooking dinner, eating ice cream, walking, shopping, and, yes, talking it all out. I will disassemble the pieces of my psyche, clean and polish the parts, and put them all back together and hope it works better this time. And I know all my problems will not be solved this weekend. For Ray and I, though we did not work out as lovers, still hope to work out as friends. But as I told another boyfriend, Geoff, a year ago as we were going our separate ways, I wanted more than anything for it to be possible for us to become friends. But first the hurt and disappointment had to disappear. And as I told Geoff when I saw him last week for the first time since we broke up, sometimes it just takes time. And you never know how long that time is going to be.

THAT SUMMER

I remember the afternoon we spent at the beach and he remarked why would anyone want to bring reading material along when there was so much to see. Look at that one, he said, tipping his head in the direction of a young man whose shoulders were broader than his hips. Dark and handsome, I thought. Sexy, not smart, he said.

That was not the only one who caught his eye. He had a fascination that summer for tall blond men. I remember I had known him long enough by then not to be jealous of his attraction to other men. I was old enough and smart enough to know that I had something of his which they, even with their masculine perfection, at that moment did not possess—his friendship of many years. I knew then, that summer, that we were never destined to be lovers, that what we were to be to one another were simply and especially, best friends.

We went to the beach together for many years. But that summer our first day on the beach he spent staring at the water, staring at the sky, staring at the constant parade of unclothed bodies. He refused to go into the water, afraid it would make his hair stand up in spikes, but he took every opportunity to walk away from where we had laid our blanket, journeying to the concession stand, the boardwalk, in the direction of a tall blond man.

I did not mind that summer, I was lost in books I remember. I was caught up in my own need to escape, my own dissatisfaction of a year of frustrating dates. And I felt sure that someone would interrupt my reading, that the act of reading itself would intrigue a man into approaching me.

Fantasy, he said, when I explained it to him. He had rented a large green and yellow striped beach umbrella and shoved it, tilted, into the sand. When he walked away I looked up and watched the wind flapping the brim. I sat underneath it reading and waiting. I remember I fell asleep and when I awoke he had returned. He was again staring at the water, staring at the sky, staring at the boys. He, too, that summer was waiting for someone. I remember he nudged me and I looked up at a man passing by. The man returned my look and I felt my heart quicken. I knew then anything and everything was still possible.

He would recall the anatomical details, of course. He would remember the bare chests and tan lines and bulging swimsuits. The body as its soul. He met the same kind of men at the beach that he hated dating in the city—shallow and narcissistic, only interested in one night stands—but there, the mere fact that they were skin against the skin of the sky, mesmerized him. One night at the bar when he had stopped dancing he stood beside me, sweating, and said—Anyone can look perfect with the proper lighting. And he went home with anyone who would ask.

This summer I went back to the beach. He was not there, of course. Nor were any of the others we met that year. I wondered if they, too, had died. I sat with another friend on a towel, not far from where we had, years ago, pitched that crazy oversized umbrella. This summer I noticed I needed to wear sunglasses; I was forever squinting. Radios, this summer, seemed to be spilling music everywhere. I could not stay at the beach for more than an hour. This summer, I noticed, I was more restless. Everyone seemed younger, more beautiful than I remembered. But I learned that though times change, a handsome man still rends the heart helpless.

And this summer I drove past that shack of a diner off the highway where we ate so many meals. The shutters had been repainted and hedges planted along the walkway. But it also seemed smaller, I know, because my memory had enlarged it over the years. But I was afraid, though, to continue toward the house, afraid that it, too, might have changed.

He would have tilted back his head and produced a sharp, rowdy laugh, saying I was silly and that it was only a house. He would have remembered the warped front door, the bald spot on the lawn beneath the hammock, and the way the soles of our bare feet turned black from walking on the sooty floor of the kitchen.

These are only remembered fragments of our summer together, examined, now, with the same curiosity as the shards of shells along the shore. There were, of course, the days it rained that summer, the days we spent hunched up in blankets playing backgammon and watching old movies on TV, and the mornings we walked through fog so dense we could only sense each other's presence. And there was the night we sat together on the empty beach, bathed by the warm ocean breeze beneath a sky of fiery constellations. Isn't it perfect? he said, not expecting anything more from me, not a touch or a kiss or even a word. And all I expected was for him to be a part of my life forever.

So this is what happened: a young man moves to a city and meets another young man. They become friends and share a house near the beach one summer. The part that is difficult is when one man dies unexpectedly. Who would believe that the images of one summer are what would be remembered if the larger portrait of life had not been stolen before completion? Time passes; little things provoke: the smell of coconut oil, sand between the sheets. "My friend" becomes an emptied phrase repeated throughout the years.

And I have not forgotten the sound of the waves that summer, rising, falling, and breaking, silver blue to the horizon, engraved in my memory like an etching on glass.

Who knew then where we were headed, my friend? Who knew then I would remember it like this?

FINDING NEW HOPE

The journey between Manhattan and New Hope, Pennsylvania is somewhere between one and two hours, the longer or shorter the length depends on whether you are traveling by car or by bus. Not far from Flemington, New Jersey, where the sky flattens out and the highway rises and dips, the ride feels something like a roller coaster in slow motion. Traveling between the beige pastures of unused farm land and the blacktops of strip-shopping centers, it is possible to feel the weight of the change taking place, as though Time itself were slowing down, lengthening, expanding out into the thin air as the light rearranges its reflections into a deep, pastoral glow. For years I debated on whether I was a city boy who enjoyed the country, or a country boy who enjoyed the city. Now, realizing I get as much of a visceral thrill at the sight of a city skyline as I do from a river bank slope of an autumn forest, I merely accept the fact that I require a balance of both urban and rural lifestyles, equal parts frustration, solitude, tension, and distraction.

I moved to New Hope in 1988 after the death of a close friend. After a decade of living in Manhattan, I left because I was tired of city life, frustrated in a job, frustrated, too, with my stagnant love-life, and scared, terribly scared, of my own mortality. I wanted nothing more than to change myself, disassemble all the components of my psyche, clean and polish them, reassemble all the pieces and begin again. But what happened the two years I lived in the country was a quick spiral into a breakdown and a recovery period of setbacks and an examination of shards, only to find that the one thing I really needed, the thing that I wanted most, was merely to have some sort of faith in the future restored. When I returned to live in Manhattan in 1990, I was not exactly reborn or rejuvenated, but ironically, as I told my friends, psychologically inspired with a cynical, yet optimistic, spirit of new hope.

My life in the country was not without other rewards. I rented a stone cottage with two bedrooms, larger than I could ever find and afford in the city, on a half-acre of land. Less than a minute from my doorstep was a forest of maples and meadows and a small pond which reflected the ruins of an abandoned aqueduct. Next door to me lived a field hand who worked on the farm across the street, a smoky, toothless man full of local wisdom who brought his homegrown vegetables to me in exchange for rides from me to take him into town or to the store or the train. I learned how to do a lot of things in the country that I would never had done if I remained in the city: how to thaw frozen pipes, how to bridle a horse, how, even, to operate one of those large industrial mowers used by landscapers. I also learned a lot about myself: that my allergies are worse in the spring, that I'm jealous and possessive of the people in my life, that I'm moody, high strung, demanding, intent and intense, all of which are not exactly flaws, just part of my stubborn personality. I spent days and days biking across some of the most breathtaking scenery of the eastern region of this country, aware that my bicycle and the simple act of motion, a lightweight machine of pedals and wheels combined with the raw, physical exertion of the human body, were important and necessary in saving my sanity. Now, trying to step back and look at the larger picture, I think the pull I feel toward the country has a lot to do with my Southern roots, that Scarlett O'Hara inspiration from the land, the power of terra firma to relieve the dull ache of homesickness.

* * *

New Hope has a large gay and lesbian community; on weekends the surrounding area of Bucks County swells with tourists exploring flea markets and antique stores. At night the parking lots of the Cartwheel and the Raven, the two gay meccas of the area, are a maze of cars stacked side by side, riders squeezing in and out of almost unbelievable tiny cracks of doors, cigarette tips flashing in the darkness like fireflies on a summer night. What I did in New Hope was not really that different from life in Manhattan; only the faces, places, and pace had changed. I went out on dates, too many dates, really, motivated from that relentless tug I feel of wanting to find my Mr. Right. I searched out an income, experimented unsuccessfully with gardening, spent a week sanding and repainting patio furniture till I was dizzy from the fumes and the pride of accomplishment—a distraction, really, designed to keep my thoughts from hovering too much around myself. For a while I was successful, but when I gave up smoking I escalated into a nervous wreck, becoming dependent instead on a variety of medications: Xanax, Halcion, Buspar, and Restoril. But that too passed, just as the man I met and fell in love with. The odd thing about living in the country was that I had trouble falling asleep no matter whether I was alone or not, the huge vacuum of emptiness of the night only magnified my loneliness and despair; a soul can only take so much solitude and self-examination until it becomes finally, ultimately, irrepressibly, mad.

Fortunately I have been blessed with wonderful friends. It was fiends who suggested I move out of the city, friends who found and rented me the cottage in the country, friends who visited and said I was looking better than they had ever seen me, friends, too, who led me around like the shell-shocked victim I had become, friends who suggested courses for therapy and healing and finally mentioned, when I had shed my neuroses like a snake's skin, that I might want to return to live in the city. I think this all has to do again with that concept of balance I feel is now so essential to maintain in my life. I am a man divided into many parts, a man moving between many worlds, many desires, many dreams and hopes; it is no surprise to me that I have as many straight friends as I do gay, one as equally important and necessary in my life as the other.

If I look for any place to put the blame, I blame it on the Libra moon.

* * *

Ah yes, autumn. The mere mention of the season conjures up images of golden foliage and abundant harvests, and as the days grow shorter and shorter and the light stretches across the horizon to burst into clouds of violet sunsets, I find I become subject to forces well beyond my control. It is no surprise to me that my favorite season is autumn; I am a child of October, born into the season of hot cider, scarecrows, and chimney-smoke air. I have found that the older I get, the less I am inclined to enjoy summer and the beach: the oppressive heat and humidity, the struggle with crowds, the fear of a suspicious freckle. I have always thought that summer divides us into those with muscles and those without, those with bodies meant to be unwrapped and displayed and those who watch, lonely and longing from the sides. It is no surprise to me to find my gay friends divided into two distinct camps as well: those having sex and those who are not. In autumn the faded flannel shirts are trotted out, the idea of sex becomes the concept of sexy, and the eyes can relax, following now the figure eights of fire-tipped leaves as they spiral to the ground.

Sometimes I believe it is simply the way they wind feels that makes me so nostalgic in autumn, or perhaps it is the early arrival of dusk, reminding me of those nights as a child when my mother would call out in the yard for me to come in and I, shrugging my shoulders, thinking, but I just got here, why must I now leave? Autumn also reminds me of time passing, growing up, changing, moving on to another year. And if there were ever an idyllic time to visit New Hope I would have to recommend autumn: the arch of flame-colored trees along the canal, deer darting cut of the mist, roadside stands selling pumpkins and white-yellow corn. Every autumn I still rendezvous in New Hope with a friend from Washington D.C. who I have now known half of my life, every year we remember things we did together as we drive along the narrow country roads in search of another adventure, the wind surging through the open windows of the car; Time unharnessed and unfastened, paradoxically moving backward and forward.

But Manhattan, too, is not without its charm in the fall. I remember stumbling late one afternoon onto Columbus Circle and seeing the shock of the yellow leaves of Central Park. It's fall, I said to myself in that millisecond of recognition, and then felt the thin membranes of my nostrils expand, seeking out the remembered smell of chilly, damp soil. Autumn in New York can be as vivid as in the country; sunlight washing the corner of a building in amber, the rhythm of the city sounding like a romantic Cole Porter song, the full moon appearing round a corner like an unexpected friend. But most of all, I think, autumn in New York means the season of new books, new movies, new theater: things to look forward to, something different just on the horizon. I suppose that's what I like best about autumn, the newness of it all juxtaposed against the cyclical turn of nature, the unexpected and expected, the equilibrium of change.

The first time I moved to Manhattan, in 1978, I had just graduated college. I lived in a small apartment in Greenwich Village, where the rent was high, but I was also young and fearless; New York City to me meant exploration and adventure. When I moved to New Hope, away from Manhattan, I never anticipated I would return to live in the city again only two years later. But the road from the city to the country is as much psychological as it is geographical, and a road that can be traveled in both directions.

Yet sometimes I feel as if I am running from my life; sometimes I feel as if I am always struggling—struggling to find the right job, a nice home, a good man, the right sides of my personality. Sometimes I think I will never understand anything at all. My apartment in Manhattan is now half a block from the street where my friend lived, the one whose death embarked me on my route of self-examination; it is impossible for me to pass buildings that do not remind me of him, impossible to escape, too, reminders of the others I have known who have passed through my life much too quickly.

    I have always wanted to move to a place where I knew it would be the last place I would move, a place where I wouldn't have to think about leaving or looking for another place, a place small enough for comfort and large enough to grow into. I still don't think I'm there. How long that journey takes, I have no way of knowing. All I know is that I'm no longer afraid of losing my balance; things just happen, you know—they always will. But sometimes it takes a different light to let you see more about yourself, or a season of change to give you hope.

BEHIND THE SCREEN

On your way to work you have a great idea on how to write a scene, the dialogue just keeps rolling around your mind in remarkable, witty lines. You are frantic to write it all down. You make it to the office, past the receptionist, past the coffee pot, past your smiling, schmoozing co-workers. You make it to your desk and turn on your computer and you have typed in a rough draft of about half of your scene when you see, out of the corner of your eye, your boss approaching your desk. You quickly shift to a blank screen on your monitor to keep him from reading your material. Your boss hands you a letter that he says has to be typed right away, pronto, as soon as possible, before anything else you do today. He thinks everything he does is important. Your boss also thinks you are not really busy, anyway, from the blank screen of your monitor. He walks away and you shift screens again and start typing. You know your boss, walking down the hall, must hear the tapping sound of your rapid keystrokes. You know he must be pleased that you have jumped so quickly into typing his letter. You, however, are finishing writing your scene. You work your way through to a comfortable stopping point, shift the screen again, and then type your boss's letter.

Your boss knows nothing about you. You are a writer who makes over half of his income from temporary word processing jobs. Your boss doesn't know what you write about. Or even that you write. He doesn't know where you live, how old you are, what your last job was or how long you were there. He is so self-focused he probably doesn't even know what sex you are. You are an entity that only types for him. No personal contact comes between him and you. He even places the letter for you to type on your desk instead of placing it in your hand. But that doesn't really bother you. You've been doing this so long all those prickly little nuances just wash right over you. You actually prefer there to be as little personal contact as possible.

You know about seven different word processing software programs well. Your assignment this week is at a large law firm which uses your favorite software; your favorite feature is shifting screens between two different documents. This week you are convinced it is the most important invention used in your daily life. It keeps your co-workers from snooping. It keeps your boss, a lawyer, from snooping. It keeps everyone thinking you are busy. You can hide what you are really typing, what you are really writing, what your life is *really* all about, right behind another screen. You know most of the people at this company have no idea what you are up to, what you are *really* doing. Yesterday you found out that even the girl in Word Processing didn't know you could shift screens so quickly between two documents.

After you finish your boss's letter he brings you a proposal to revise. You have been working on this proposal all week. Or rather, your boss has been making corrections and revisions all week. Before he leaves your desk he tells you about his daughter, nine years old, winning a dance contest at a summer camp this week. This is the fourth time you have heard this story—once when your boss told it at the water fountain this morning, another time to someone on the phone when you were in his office, the third time you overheard him telling it to another lawyer when you were on the way back from the restroom. You try to pretend you are interested in the story but when he leaves your desk you grow more annoyed. Your boss isn't even aware of how hard you work, how hard your days are. He doesn't know you are gay, doesn't know you spend your evenings delivering meals to men who are sick, doesn't know you worry every minute about your health. He doesn't know you've lost a generation of friends, boyfriends, and **lovers** to AIDS. You try to brush it out of your **mind**; you don't really *want* him to know. It would only complicate things; he would stutter or **become** embarrassed, stumbling for some half-hearted words of compassion. It's better this way. Let him think you me**r**ely type. **M**erely work for *him*.

And so you simply go back to work. You shift screens, type, print the **proposal,** and return the whole thing to your boss. And then he reappears **with** more revisions. The proposal shows up on your desk several **times** throughout the **day,** just like an uninvited **dybbuk.** Doesn't your boss realize you have other work, *real* work, your work you **have** to do? Sometimes you feel that the world is just too naive, some people are just too self-absorbed. For revenge, on the last revision, you don't even **correct** your boss's grammar.

Toward **the** end of the day, you have finished three letters and four **more** revisions **of** the proposal. You have also finished your scene. When **you** print it out and read it you think it is witty and remarkable. At **last,** you think, there is something worth living far, something that makes you feel, **well,** creative and **human** again. You still **have** about an **hour left** before **your** work **day** is over, **before** you can go home and **do more of** the work that **you want** to do, *have* to do. **To** kill some time you begin to write a piece about a **temporary** word processor who writes while at work. But then you notice your boss, out of the corner of your eye, walking down the **hall** toward your desk. You shift screens again, hiding your real work **behind** a screen, ready to type another letter, **but** instead **he** asks you for your advice.

Seen any **good movies?** he asks you. My wife **wants** to go to the movies tonight.

A first, you think. A real, **hon**est-to-goodness personal question, even if its motive is self-directed. You reach for your newspaper, wondering what type of movies he prefers. Comedies? Mysteries? Something with a little skin?

Opinions are, after all, insights to the human soul.

WHERE YOU'LL FIND ME

April, 1993. I have come to activism late in life, late in the sense that today I am closer to forty than I am to thirty; late in the reason that I have been gay for almost twenty years and am only now beginning to raise my voice in frustration over the repression of homosexuals for decades; late, too, in the sense that now, twelve years into an epidemic that has robbed me of my friends and co-workers and changed the direction of my life, I am becoming as disheartened as my peers over the continuing inactiveness of the government. I have never considered my voice as one of rage; I have always searched for some sort of rational path of understanding, even in irrational times. But it is impossible not to be caught up in the fiery issues of the day: whether gays should be allowed to serve in the military after they have already for years fought silently and valiantly and nobly within the nation's ranks; how effective AZT is in battling AIDS; whether children should be educated, positively, about homosexual behavior in school systems.

To be gay or lesbian in the Nineties is to be political whether you like it or not, whether you are in or out of the closet; our lives in this decade are suddenly charged with meaning. In recent weeks we have seen our lifestyles discussed in Congressional hearings and a survey of male sexual behavior diminish our numbers from the often quoted ten percent of the population to barely over one percent. Any gay or lesbian can tell you that it is not how large or how small our actual numbers are, but that we are treated with the same equality and respect due every member of this nation. That was one of the reasons for our March on Washington, where we descended on the nation's capital in numbers of over one million men and women and children. The real strength of our movement and our community is in the fact that we incorporate such a wide and diverse spectrum of the population, from our drag queens to our Latino lesbians to our contingents of color and bisexuals, leaving, of course, everyone involved entirely bemused by this one percent paradox. Still, as heady as all of the activity was in Washington last week, few of our battles have been won. In fact, we are only at the starting point of our war.

Our war is against ignorance and intolerance from everything against the hate crimes directed at homosexuals to the criminal neglect of people infected with the HIV virus. Few can now dispute the influence of AIDS over the last few years in politicizing the gay and lesbian agenda. But AIDS, of course, is not a gay disease. Any gay and lesbian will and can tell you that, but unfortunately in the United States the perception still remains. And any gay or lesbian, any volunteer at GMHC, God's Love We Deliver, Action AIDS, and the numerous AIDS service organizations around the city and the country can explain to you the troubles our inner cities will face from AIDS, the troubles, too, our youth in any part of the country will encounter; we can point out, too, the decimation that lies ahead in the entire continents of Africa and Asia.

Recently, while working as a writer on a documentary called *Living Proof*, based on the Carolyn Jones photography project of people who are living with the HIV virus, I watched footage of a young man—a straight, hemophiliac teenager named Henry Nichols, an Eagle Scout who contracted the HIV virus through a blood transfusion, journey to the White House to meet President Clinton and present him with a book of the "Living Proof" photographs. After his meeting with the President, Henry says on film that he hopes President Clinton will remember that you can never do enough about AIDS. Certainly Mr. Clinton has not done enough, and this is something as a new activist I must remind him of now. Three months into his first term, six months after his election, he has still not appointed an AIDS czar, a person of governmental authority to provide leadership and direction in this epidemic, a position many activists feel should have been made by his first few days in office.

Mr. Clinton, of course, has many wars: revitalizing the economy, health care reform, helping settle the strife in Bosnia and Herzegovina. But deconstruct any of them and their purpose becomes the same as ours: freedom, equality, respect. This is why our crusade must continue.

I missed the march for gay and lesbian rights that was held in 1979; missed, too, the march in 1987. But I was there last weekend in Washington, and I will be in Central Park this Sunday for the annual AIDSWalk. The word "annual," here, has a truly frightening ring to it, which is why, more than ever, we must continue to fight and march and contribute and volunteer. I will be there this weekend as a son and brother and neighbor and friend and lover, walking beside fathers and mothers and sisters and daughters. Americans must now realize gays and lesbians are a part of the national family. And I will be at the Gay Pride parade, too, in June. And next year at the Gay Games IV and the twenty-fifth anniversary of the Stonewall riots. To quote a lyric from Judy Garland's theme song, a woman whose death ironically propelled the gay and lesbian rights movement significantly forward, this is "where you'll find me." I will be where ever necessary to be counted, where ever I need to be until our war is won. AIDS is not a gay disease. And civil rights is a human issue.

STRENGTH

We were headed downtown in a cab toward a club in the East Village and my friend Rhett was talking about George's memorial service. "There was the story someone told," Rhett said, "about the trip George arranged white water rafting. He wanted to make sure the tour-package company knew who was booking the trip. 'There are six of us,' George told the travel agent. 'All men. And we all say *fab-u-lous* a lot. Get the picture?'"

The picture was always important for George—how things looked, how *he* looked. He had, after all, worked in fashion. "I was a schmuck who sold dresses," I once heard him tell a mutual friend. Another friend, however, had been astonished by the beauty of George's body; when they first met, George had answered the door clad only in a towel. I had heard from another friend that George's spirits were floundering because of the increasing number of Kaposi's sarcoma lesions on his body. What I remembered in the cab, that evening with Rhett, spinning through the ever-changing neighborhoods of Manhattan, was that George always seemed so physically strong to me; even after he began chemotherapy, his biceps looked like they measured a good eighteen inches.

And then the next day my friend Eric called to say that he had heard Mark had died. Since I had first met Mark, fifteen years ago, he had stopped smoking, drinking, and doing a host of recreational drugs; he had started macrobiotics, experimented with herbs, acupuncture, and meditation, and had settled into a long-term relationship with another musician named Mike. I did not even know Mark was sick until a few months before his death; his change of habits I had always attributed to the eccentricities of his talent. On stage Mark possessed a mischievous spirit and the rubbery face of a clown. Offstage, however, he was painfully shy, especially when I first met him when we worked together on an off-off-Broadway show. The first night we slept together he confessed he was frightened about being on stage, but what he got out of performing, he said, the strength from recognition from an audience, outweighed all the fear he confronted.

Tuesday evenings Mark and I used to drink margaritas together in the West Village, where we both lived at the time, swirling thin, short straws through the icy blue drinks while we dreamed up ideas for songs. We were in our twenties then and we had a lot in common, notably our recent arrivals in Manhattan and our need to escape our Southern, religious roots. And those were the days where the only thing we were afraid of was going home alone, the world shimmered in front of us with possibility.

Now, years later, loss comes to me in waves, death after death, shock after shock; grief and anger possess a cumulative power. This has become life in the epicenter of the epidemic of AIDS in America: a constant struggle with guilt for surviving a generation of friends, lovers, co-workers, and peers who have died at an early age. Depression, I believe, is a perpetual emotion; what strength I can find to lift myself out of it at times evaporates as easily as morning dew.

And then a week after I had heard about Mark's death, I noticed in the obituaries that Carlos had died. Carlos was an AIDS Administrator at the office where I had recently worked as a part-time temporary employee. I had only met Carlos briefly one day in the elevator, where we exchanged names and handshakes. I had noticed him often, however; he came in a couple of days each week, only for a few hours, mostly sitting at his desk, attempting to eat something. He was, at that point, unbearably thin, his hair lost, the color of his skin like the ashes of wood. What I knew about him—from office talk—was that he had lost his lover five years before, and had been diagnosed

HIV-positive for nine years. He knew nothing about me, of course, nothing other than what he could detect from my eyes. What I saw in him, though, was a man determined to keep his job, wanting order in his life, finding, I think, a sense of meaning and purpose in what he did.

The last time I saw him was a few days before his death; I was in the office restroom. From a stall I heard a feeble cry of "help" and the door swung open. Carlos, now weaker and thinner, did not have the energy to lift himself off the toilet. I went inside the stall and placed my hands beneath his elbows to help him stand. What he wanted from me was simply my strength. And what I gave him that day was nothing compared to what he already had; a strength, I believe, made perfect through weakness.

OLD THINGS

A few years ago, when I was renting a cottage in New Hope, Pennsylvania, I had a neighbor who collected old things. My neighbor, Mitchell, was the new owner of an eighteenth century stone house, and, settling into the area, he easily became addicted to the numerous flea markets, antique fairs, and auctions held in Bucks County. Every weekend Mitchell would knock on my door and ask, in his polite and excited manner, "Do you want to see what I got today?" And no matter what he showed me—from a wrought iron bench to an antique cookie jar in the shape of a clown—he did so with both awe and delight. His joy was not simply because he outbid a competitor or purchased his find at a bargain price; it stemmed from something we all hope to accomplish in our lives—to surround ourselves with things we like, things that make us feel comfortable, things from which we can draw a sense of pride. My friend was only doing something we all do at some point in our lives: He was making his new house into a home.

I, too, have my collection of old things, things which I have had for many years, things that I have bought or been given, things that to anyone else might seem useless or frivolous: a hand-painted canteen from my trip to Romania, a wood inlay box from my parents' vacation in Israel, an ashtray from Paris, a stuffed dinosaur, numerous swizzle sticks, and two etched glasses from the sorority dances I was invited to in college.

Sometimes I think it is odd that I, a gay man now in his mid-thirties, attach so much sentiment to these things, which only sit and collect dust. Perhaps it is because I have moved around a great deal in my lifetime thus far—geographically, intellectually, and emotionally—and these things have become, in some sort of strange way, my anchors, my security blankets, my safe harbor. For each old item holds a story of a particular place, person, or time in my life; they are a part of my past and a way to keep it from existing entirely in my mind: The miniature red double-decker bus I bought when I was a school boy in England, the silver goblet I was given by the cast of a play I directed in college, the amber sea shell was discovered on a Delaware beach one morning with a boyfriend.

When I lived in New Hope, I was no stranger, either, to the flea markets and antique shops of the area, though I could not help but think, as I weaved in and out of the aisles and booths that some day my old things might be lined up like this, for people to point to, pick up, look at, perhaps even dismiss. What saddened me was that these people would not know what my old things had meant to me. My most priceless possession, an inexpensive snow globe of a winter skier in a red jacket on a mountain slope, would mean nothing to these shoppers. They would not know that it was my gift to my friend Kevin after my trip to Aspen one year, to add to his collection of snow globes from the distant cities and places he had been. They would not know, either, that a year later the snow globe became mine again when Kevin died of AIDS, and while helping his family and friends empty his apartment, I was asked if there was anything among the possessions that I wanted to keep for myself. I chose the snow globe, because it was what reminded me most of my friend.

And so the snow globe now sits on a shelf in my apartment with my other old things. And there are days, when I pick it up and flip it, watching the flakes fall around the skier, that I feel what makes growing old for a gay man these days so difficult is not only the acceptance of his youth and beauty fading, not only the fear of disease and the witnessing of death, but also the fact that for most of us, there is little we will personally pass on to the generations after us. For most of us are men without children. I feel certain that I will never have a child—a biological son or daughter of my own—to explain what the snow globe means to me; so I will never be able to tell my child that my friend Kevin, at a much too young age, fought valiantly against a very awful disease no one understood. A stranger would think my snow globe was just an eccentric object I owned; I would simply be a man who collected odd little things. Perhaps that is one of the reasons why I feel so impelled to write about gay life during this epidemic; as gay men, both as individuals and as part of a community, we are still capable of leaving behind other things beside children: imprints on art, culture, history, and politics.

And so my old things today take on a new importance for me; each item now requires a reexamination of its significance—in essence, a review of the history of myself juxtaposed against how my life has changed because of AIDS. As a man who has been a member of the gay community for over twenty years, a man who knew gay life before the plague of AIDS, a man who witnessed the first horrors of the epidemic, a man who has, for the last twelve years, volunteered and helped and cared for and buried more friends than he wishes to list, this evaluation of change fueled the desire to write and report the stories of gay life I heard and experienced during these confusing years.

Change is inevitable in any life, whether one is straight or gay, black or white, an immigrant or an expatriate, male or female. And so it happened that one day I moved again, packed up all my things, and said good-bye to my neighbor Mitchell, leaving Pennsylvania and returning to live in Manhattan. And I began to write, without hesitation about the way AIDS has impacted my life, my community, and my generation: in essence, a gay man bearing witness to his uncertain times. But there are days I wonder if I will ever stop moving; other days I think about what I will some day leave behind. I cannot stop the passage of Time; cannot, too, pause the continuum of aging. But the old things never grow old for me; they are my memories, feelings, opinions, and choices—they are evidence, too, to the process of my own evolution. But most important of all, no matter where I live, no matter how my life adapts or changes, they are what make my house my home.

WHAT COMES AROUND

You are thirty-seven and eleven-twelfths. Or fifteen-sixteenths. It is the eve of your thirty-eighth birthday. You look into the mirror and try to decide who you are. You are not handsome, or so you think. You are not ugly, either, you decide. In this city, this city of drop-dead gorgeous actors and models, you are somewhere in between. Somewhere in between is what you are. You are an almost thirty-eight year-old gay man who is somewhere in between drop-dead gorgeous and troll-like ugly.

You turn and study your profile in the mirror. It is not a strong profile. But it is not weak one, either. Your hairline has receded but you are not bald. You do not have a bald spot but you no longer have a full head of teenaged hair. You no longer have beautiful brown bangs. You no longer have to push your long brown hair out of your eyes. You look at yourself again in the mirror, this time deeper at the hairline. You do not have any gray hair, either. You are a guy approaching forty without any graying hair.

You weakest spot is your chin, you decide. It is all about your chin, you think when you study your profile again. You have never liked your chin from this angle. Your chin is up but it is not defying gravity. You notice too much skin on your neck. You turn and study your chin from the other side. You decide you don't like that angle either. You face the mirror. You like this position best. The dimple in your chin is now faint. But prominent. You decide this is who you are. You are not a right or a left profile kind of person. You are a straight-forward kind of guy. The kind of guy with a faint but prominent dimple in his chin who hopes someone doesn't notice his developing turkey neck.

You are not in the habit of dwelling on your looks. Not when you have a boyfriend. Or a date. When you have a boyfriend or a date you do not study your looks so much. When you have a boyfriend or a date you are outwardly focused, not inwardly obsessed. But since it is the eve of your birthday and you have neither a boyfriend nor a date everything is out of sync. Forty is looming. You are approaching a time zone of trauma. Everything loses perspective when you realize forty looms closer. You wonder if you are capable of still finding a boyfriend or a date in a city where there are so many drop-dead gorgeous actors and models as your competition, and most of whom are now younger than you are.

It is the morning of the eve of your thirty-eighth birthday and you have no plans tonight. Jon is busy with a new boyfriend. Barry is never available. You have plans tomorrow night with Dennis but no plans tonight. You could rent a movie tonight, but you are too restless. You want to get out of your apartment. Your planets are all in the place where they are supposed to be and you do not want to be in the house tonight. You are supposed to be at your zenith. You are not forty but you are not twenty, either. You are not as attractive as you were ten years ago but you should be ten years smarter. You should use your experience to keep yourself entertained. You should know what you want to do tonight.

So what should you do? You could call a phone line, hook up with someone for sex, but you did that earlier in the week and it would feel like a desperate thing to do tonight. You do not want to be desperate. Or act desperate. You could jerk off and then decide to call the phone line, that way you wouldn't have to get off because you already did. The necessity of it would be gone and you could simply have a good time getting someone else off. You decide that is an outwardly focused idea and not something to do when you are inwardly obsessed. You decide that you should do something other than look for sex.

So what should you do? Ten-plus years' worth of wisdom tells you you should go out and look for sex.

You decide you will go to a bar. You stomach churns at the thought. Your stomach always churns and bubbles when you think about going to a bar. It is an ingrained habit. It's as if your stomach knows you will drink too much and then try to soak it all in with a quick stuffing of donuts or pizza before you go to sleep to prevent a hangover the next morning. You decide you will go out to a bar and have only one drink. Your stomach calms down but it is not convinced. One drink barely sets you at ease in a bar but your stomach rumbles with appreciation.

You rinse your face at the sink, dry it with a towel, pull your underwear off, and sit on the toilet. You pick a magazine off the floor that you picked up at a bar the last time you were out, four days ago. This magazine comes out every week. Every week there is another handsome young man on the cover, a drop-dead gorgeous model or actor getting paid for what he does best—look like a drop-dead gorgeous cover boy. If he is not handsome then he is beautiful or sexy. Sometimes the cover features a porn star. If he is not beautiful or sexy or a porn star then he has a great set of abs. Or arms. Or chest. Or something else. You are not something else or any of the above. You are almost thirty-eight years old and you are spending your morning of the eve of your last day as thirty-seven on the toilet reading a magazine you picked up in a gay bar four days ago.

You study the magazine like it was a text book. You read the advertisements. There is a party for a drag queen which you will not go to because you are not a pretty faux-blond boy or a beautiful faux woman. There is another party on a boat which you will not go to because it will make you seasick. There is a party for the launch of a new CD and another one for the launch of a new movie. You live in a city of parties that you never go to. You are not a pretty party boy. Faux-blond or otherwise.

In fact, you are not good at parties. You have never been good at parties. The one you threw in seventh grade stank. (No one made out.) The one in high school was a bomb. (Everyone made out except you.) In college you went to parties where you didn't fit in. (You didn't want to make out with a girl.) Two decades later in the city you can no longer make small talk at a party. You are not a small talk kind of guy.

You flip through the pages of the magazine till you reach the personal ads at the back. You begin to read the small type. It is so small it makes your eyes squint. This gives you a bit of a headache but you continue reading this way. You think you might find another no-small-talk kind of guy. You hope there is another no-small-talk kind of guy looking to meet the same.

What you find is what you are not. You are never the same as the guys who are looking. This happens every time you read the personals. Every time you discover you are not what someone else is searching for. You are not an in-shape Latino. You are not an Italian bubble butt bottom. You are not a hot muscle uncut horse-hung top. There is a Hispanic guy into poppers looking to hook up with other brothers. (Not you.) Another guy is looking for a slender Asian with big nipples. (No, not you, either.) A master wants to give orders to someone into SM, BD, WS, CBT, FF, TT and any kind of kink. (No, sorry, not you, either.) You wonder what kind of kink any-kind-of-kink is if the master has already listed all of the other stuff. Enemas, you decide. The master didn't list enemas, did he? You decide the kind of kink this guy is looking for is enemas and you are not the one to give it to him.

You continue reading and squinting. At least you are working out your facial muscles, you think. At least this activity is burning up some calories even though it is creating a big sense of depression and an almost-headache. You are not nine-and-a-half or more. You are not a slave who can shoot a big load. You do not want to be humiliated by someone smoking a cigar. When you reach the end of the page you realize that what you want is not in this magazine. You want a three-dimensional no-small-talk kind of guy who wants to meet another one, or at least one with a faint but prominent dimple in his chin.

You realize you have spent too much time reading this magazine. You realize that this could make you seem shallow to a potential boyfriend, studying personal ads as if they were formulas that could cure the epidemic. You wipe and flush even though there was no action back there. Your toilet is simply a great place to catch up on reading the magazines you pick up in a gay bar. You pull up your underwear. You turn on the water at the sink, rinse your face again, open the cabinet, and pull out the shaving crème.

You lather up your face. You dip the razor in the running water. You are about to shave away the last beard of your thirty-seventh year. It makes you pause in front of the mirror and study yourself again. You think about growing back your goatee. Your goatee was multi-colored. Brown around your lips, blond at the corners, black at your chin. It was not a good goatee but it was good for sex. You got plenty of cruises and plenty of sex when you had a goatee. Guys found you more approachable with a goatee. They talked to you in a bar. They bought you drinks. They took you back to their apartments. But you never saw the same guy twice. A goatee did not help you find yourself a boyfriend. A goatee was no help to you. And it hid your faint but prominent dimple. You were not a goatee sort of guy. What you wanted was not another guy with a goatee. What you wanted was a guy who would call you back.

You look into the mirror and think about being someone different. Someone not just clean shaven with a weak, dimpled chin and a receding hairline. If you were someone different you wouldn't be a no-small-talk kind of guy without a goatee and with nothing to do on the eve of his thirty-eighth birthday.

You look first at your hair. You imagine yourself with a different haircut. You could cut it shorter or shave it all off. You are not the short-short-hair type of guy. You also do not have the proper shape of a head to shave it all off. You try to imagine yourself with a bald scalp but you are haunted by a vision of when you tried to be faux-blond. Your one attempt to be a faux-blond left you looking like a copper shag carpet—your hair became a strange, reddish color and broke into a million brittle split ends. You did not even make a good faux-blond. You were miserable for days, weeks, months, before it all disappeared. You could not bring yourself to cut your hair short even when it was riddled with a million brittle split ends. You could certainly not shave it all off. You were stuck with wearing caps wherever you went. You avoided swimming in pools, not wanting your copper-colored shag carpet to turn green. Your hair is fine, you decide. You will keep it the way it is. Nice and brown and natural.

You think next about getting your ear pierced. If you had a pierced ear then maybe you would not seem so uptight. You try to imagine what you ear would look like pierced and decide it would not be a good look for you. A stud would look out of place on your ear. Like a mole or a freckle. You are not a hoop-earring sort of guy, either, though you think it might be fun to wear something that dangled. You think again about your lost hairline, the time many, many, many years ago when you grew your hair so long that it whooshed when you turned your head. This is what comes around year after year after year. Your hair changes without your help, whether you want to be bald, faux-blond, or otherwise.

This thought makes you depressed so you look at your ears again. You have good ears but not a good pierced-ear look. You think one pierced ear would set you off-balance. You are all about balance because you are a Libra. You are a thirty-seven year-old gay man watching himself turn thirty-eight before his eyes.

You look down at your chest. You think about piercing your nipple. Or nipples since you would have to have a balance there, too. This makes you laugh. You are not a nipple pierced kind of guy either. You think briefly about a tattoo. A chain link line around a non-existent bicep. You lift your arm and flex your non-existent bicep. No matter how much you pump iron your muscles do not seem to grow into muscles. The only thing that really grows is your whole body. Every year you grow a little bit older. That is what grows. This is what changes. Your body becomes heavier. It becomes harder and harder to fight gravity.

You step away from the sink and look at yourself in the full length mirror on the back of the door. You try not to laugh at yourself, even though you look like an undressed Santa Claus with your beard of shaving crème. You pull in your stomach, lift up your buttocks. Maybe you should pierce your navel, you think. That is the center of you, your middle point. This makes you laugh harder and you lose your posture. Then this makes you upset. And more depressed. You look at your stomach and decide that your pierced navel might make someone else sick. Your navel is not flat because your stomach is not flat. No matter how hard you exercise you cannot get your stomach to be flat. You do not have any abs. You have never seen your abs. You will never see your abs. You are almost thirty-eight years old and your potential set of abs are history. All you can hope for is that your waist size will never again be a number larger than your age.

You return to the mirror in front of the sink again. You start to shave. You think again about all the things you are not in this city of drop-dead gorgeous actors and models and porn stars. You could be worse off, you think. You could not be someone stuck somewhere in the middle but further down the rung. You could be someone trying to impersonate a faux-blond, you think. You could be an aging self-absorbed wanna-be faux-blond guy and someone a lot dumber than you are. You shave some more, decide that what you are is lucky you are not a wanna-be faux-blond and self-absorbed. Well, at least not a wanna-be faux-blond, you correct yourself. You would not be happy if you still wanted to be blond.

STILL DANCING

The class begins at 8 p.m.; the room looks remarkably like a miniaturized version of the cafeteria where my high school held its sock hops. I am always amazed at the people who take this class on a Saturday night, a beginner's introduction to country-western two-step dancing sponsored by the "Southerners," a social group of expatriate gays and lesbians in the New York City area. The men and women are wildly diverse tonight: ponytails, buzzcuts, tattoos, and earrings. If anything is predominant, it would have to be denim and T-shirts.

The instructor is named Lori, a tall, handsome woman who in different clothing could pass as one of Chekhov's sisters, but tonight is wearing jeans and a sleeveless plaid blouse, her blonde hair twisted into a braid that hangs down her back. She assembles everyone into the center of the room, there are about fifty of us now, and she shows us the basic step—a rhythm of shuffling the feet back and forth in a quick-quick, slow, slow pattern. We spread out and try the steps alone, but I feel so oddly exposed dancing by myself that I concentrate, perhaps too seriously, on my steps. Beside me a beefy guy with a goatee hooks his thumbs through the belt loops of his jeans and casually sashays through the steps as Lori repeats over and over, "Quick-Quick, Slow, Slow. Quick-Quick, Slow, Slow."

Next we form a large circle and Lori explains that two-step dancing follows a circular, counterclockwise motion around the room. A short black woman with huge, expressive eyes helps Lori demonstrate the dancing we will be learning, and then we are paired up into couples. My partner is a lesbian named Judy, and Lori informs us that we must make a decision within our couples as to who will lead and who will follow. (In Fred Astaire ballroom lingo that means someone must dance the boy's part and someone must dance the girl's part.) Judy says succinctly, but nicely, that she would like to lead, and though I squirm a bit, I know it is just my male chauvinistic, reactionary act; I actually want her to lead, so far every lesson I've had I have been the leader and tonight I want to practice following.

Lori gives out more pointers: where to place the hands, how to keep the steps going in different directions, how to weave around the other couples. Before you know it a Bonnie Raitt tune is pumped timidly through the loudspeakers and Judy, amazingly agile, leads me steadily in a dance around the room. Next thing I know Lori is teaching the leaders how to twirl the followers and as Judy and I work our way through the motions I have this silly thought racing through my head: this is a girl who likes girls who's dancing like a boy with a boy who likes boys dancing like a girl. When we stop I pitch my eyes toward the floor, unable to control my smiling.

I am here tonight for several reasons: trying to conquer my shyness, escape some frustrations—bills, solitude, the news of a friend who just died. My friend Jon who now lives in California told me he goes two-stepping and has a great time. "Forget cruising," he said, when he first recommended I give this a try. "This is better than disco was in the Seventies. And you get to touch someone while dancing." I am a single gay male in his mid-thirties, but I'm not here tonight to try to meet anyone; still, there are several men here who intrigue me: the sandy haired man I recognize from a television commercial, the lanky brunet who reminds me of an old boyfriend, the guy behind a table of refreshments who I will study all night—fair and hunky, dark eyes, great arms, a balding patch at his forehead.

Though I mastered the basic steps a few months ago, I still take the class to practice; I also find it's a way to break the ice with other newcomers. Lori has us change partners and I'm paired up with a guy named Gus, a man I find so good looking I probably would never speak to him under different circumstances. Dancing with him, I get this crazy, pornographic thrill when he shifts his hand from the center of my back to the base of my neck and my hand slips down his shoulder, feeling out the bulkiness of his tricep. Our eyes keep meeting and breaking apart, and I feel myself beginning to sweat, confused as to whether it's from my sudden nervousness or the physical exertion of dancing. I am almost thankful when Lori stops the dancing to teach everyone a simple line dance.

And then suddenly the hour is up, the class is over, everyone applauds and thanks Lori. But no one leaves the room: the lights are dimmed, the music brightened. The class was only an appetizer; now the main course—The Dance—begins. An awkwardness momentarily descends, everyone looking eagerly from the sidelines at the empty dance space until two guys whom I suspect are lovers break the spell and begin dancing. When I first starting coming to these dances, I hardly danced with anyone, preferring to watch from the side, trying to pick up the steps as the music changed. But one of the things I like most about these dances is the unspoken rule of Southern politeness—that if someone asks you to dance you do not say no—a rule which has pulled quite an assortment of strangers toward me, and me hesitantly out to the dance floor, cautioning my partner of my inexperience.

Tonight I dance more than I have at any of the other dances I have attended, attributed, I think, to the fact that I am more comfortable and the rhythm of the steps now feel natural to me. Two-step dancing has its hits like every other style of music, and the crowd swells to the dance floor as the taped music reels through favorites by Dolly Parton, Garth Brooks, Clint Black, Mary Chapin Carpenter, and almost anything by k.d. lang. More and more people begin to arrive—the better, more experienced dancers—and they take to the floor, whirling around the room, making all this motion as giddy as a ballroom competition. I recognize several people I have noticed or met from the other dances I have attended; in fact, I am beginning to sense a regular crowd who follow the underground circuit of bars and clubs in Manhattan where gay and lesbian two-step dancing is done on different nights of the week. Everyone I speak to here tonight seems to find this type of dancing addictive, as invigorating and popular as country music has become.

There are few things I enjoy as much as dancing, an outgrowth, I believe, of being a product of the disco generation. When I was first struggling with my sexual identity back in the Seventies, the most important thing a friend did for me was to take me to a disco, opening up a world of men who acted, believed, thought, and danced just like I did. Even when AIDS began changing the landscape, I found comfort and solace simply through dancing; by then dancing was no longer for me a cruising ground for sex; it was simply a physical pleasure, as narcotic and indulgent as going to a gym.

The hours literally dance by, every now and then the dancing breaks into a waltz or a pseudo-square dance called the Cotton Eyed Joe. When the room shifts into the Texas Cha Cha, a line dance performed to Clint Black's song "Gulf of Mexico," I am convinced it is one of most romantic and breathtaking moments I have ever witnessed, the choreography merely a simple series of fluid walks and pivots. And then a tall, handsome man asks me to dance. As he leads me to the dance floor, it occurs to me that I met him years ago at a house party on Fire Island. When he introduces himself as Tim, I am convinced it is him, but I do not say anything; I merely place my hand at his shoulder and we begin to dance. As I recall Tim had a lover back then, a man named Randall, and as we move brightly, swiftly around the room I wonder if his lover succumbed to the same fate as the friend who accompanied me to all those parties that summer. Tim tightens the grip around my waist, and as he leans in closer I can smell the sweat of him. Even if he remembered me, he leaves abruptly when the dance is over.

A little later when I glance at my watch I notice it is almost midnight, and like Cinderella I decide to leave the ball early, not wanting to break the enchantment. Gus catches me at the doorway and writes his phone number on a slip of paper for me before I leave. It makes me feel buoyant and hopeful. On the subway uptown, I wonder if all this dancing, all this Southern country stuff, is a way of finding the roots I left behind when I moved to Manhattan from Atlanta almost two decades ago. In the last few months I seem to have been searching out Southern culture in the city more and more—in restaurants, music, bookstores, even in the way I dress—I have now adopted an affinity for wearing boots.

Back home in my apartment I'm still dancing, floating through some remembered steps by myself. Quick-Quick, Slow, Slow. Quick-Quick, Slow, Slow. No, I think. It's not the roots. It's in the genes. I just love dancing. It makes me forget a lot of things.

EXCERPTS FROM A STONEWALL DIARY

Monday, June 20, 1994
    Should I begin this diary with sex? Isn't that what is at the root of our struggle for gay pride, our ability to have sex without losing our self-respect in the process? Should I begin by writing that I jerked off Monday morning before I got out of bed, or that I slept through the night with erections, aroused by dreams aggravated by alcohol and indigestion? Should I try to remember the last date I had with a guy I was interested in seeing more than once or, better yet, the name of the last man I slept with? Or should I cut to the uneasy heart of my lack of self-respect—a four-room railroad apartment that catches the afternoon heat like an oven, an air-conditioner which will not cool one square foot and blows a fuse located six floors below in the basement of a bodega (which may or may not be open for business at the time of implosion). And should I include the smell which lingers in the paint and flooring that reminds me of the mustiness of elderly men's clothing? Or should I dig deeper into my psyche and say that my real depression stems from my inability to make enough income to pay the rent, pay the utilities, pay the monthly charges on credit cards (which I abandoned long ago because I could not manage them). And do I mention that every time the phone rings it is another creditor asking for money I don't have; even Con Edison representatives threaten me—the one who called last week said, "Aren't you aware I am trying to save your life?"

Or should I write that all this has been of my own making? A string of temp jobs because I don't want to deal with the stress of a career other than of my own making? That my writing alone doesn't generate even a small portion of New York City expenses. Or should I take another tact, take a deep breath of air and write down the things that I am lucky for—should I begin this diary with a list of thanks? Should I thank God or some unknown Higher Power that I am still alive when so many others have already died from AIDS? Should I be thankful that I have not been beaten to death by homophobic bigots? Should I be grateful that I am alive and able to date, able to have sex, able to bounce through the potholes of my fork in the road with a depression that does not require drugs or hospitalization? Is that my pride? Should that be how I begin this diary?

* * *

Tonight was the Lesbian and Gay Center's eleventh annual Garden Party, an event which kicks off the beginning of gay pride week events every year. This year, because of the scheduling of the athletic competitions and events of the Gay Games and the events and celebrations of the twenty-fifth anniversary of the Stonewall Riots, pride week is a flurry of activity that is overwhelming. Every magazine and brochure lists a different, detailed schedule of events this week. This is the beginning of Gay Overload, which, to harken back to the subject of sex, sounds like an appropriate title for a porn video, although it would probably be shot in a West Hollywood apartment and not on the streets of New York.

My friend Rhett, who works at the Center, walked me into Garden Party. West 13th Street in the Village was blocked off between Seventh and Eighth Avenues, and the street was full of tenting and canopies, folding chairs, a stage, and a string of white-clothed tables, where vendors of gay organizations hand out brochures and buttons and marketing materials. I used to live on this block, fifteen years ago, before the Center purchased the former high school building, in an apartment that was broken into so often I was forced to move out of it. It's always strange to me to return to this block and see that it has become so central to gay life in the city when it was such an unmanageable portion of my first years in the city.

Today was beautiful, the way summer ought to be in Manhattan, and the weather and Rhett's chatter lightened my mood. There was a scattering of gay celebs at the event—comedian Kate Clinton and her activist-girlfriend Urvashi Vaid, transgender author and activist Kate Bornstein, Jean Marc, a reporter from the syndicated cable show *Party Talk*—and I followed Rhett inside the Center building where I autographed a copy of my book that a bookstore in upstate New York donated for the silent auction to raise funds for the Center. While wandering through the aisles of other donated items, I ran into David Feinberg. He looked pale and agitated, more than usual for David, but he was as sarcastic as ever, mentioning his editor's vacation and the fact that he has noticed that I am now writing articles for *Body Positive* magazine. Rhett and I picked up our boxed dinners and retreated to an air-conditioned room on the third floor where we talked about mundane things (Rhett's diet, my lack of one), while at the same time we admired a young man with gorgeous arms. (If this is what a diary must record, then I apologize for inserting such triviality here, such as Rhett giving me his brownie to eat and me giving him my plum.) Yet my feeling, really, of the entire night, felt like being on the brink of something historic but without it really being that way, that it didn't quite *become* as important as everyone wanted it to be. Or, perhaps, it was just that things like this event and other ones throughout Manhattan this week have been hyped up so many notches that there is a giddiness floating about town. I felt that way when Rhett and I parted and I went downstairs and watched the evening's entertainment—Kate Clinton, a southern band called Ya'll, a choir of gay gospel singers. The evening was a magical New York one, the lights from the stage illuminating the undersides of the leaves overhanging the street and clusters of men and women draping their arms around shoulder and waists.

I only saw two old boyfriends at the event tonight, not speaking to either one because there was nothing for us to say to each other, really, and once Rhett had left me to do his schmoozing job, I felt, once again, like an outsider watching something he could not really connect to. It was then that I realized I was alone and my legs were tired, but I walked the thirtyplus blocks up Seventh Avenue and over to my apartment on Ninth Avenue, stopping for a glass of wine at Cleo's, a local gay bar a block from where I live, hoping, in the crowded night, to find some kind of connection with someone who felt as I did.

It did not happen and I went home alone.

Tuesday, June 21, 1994

Yes, today was about sex, too. I left work early to meet my friend Jonathan at the Penn Hotel in midtown, ground zero of the Gay Games activity. Rhett, Jonathan's ex-boyfriend, was competing in the bodybuilding competition and the preliminaries were this afternoon at the hotel (also the site of registration for volunteers and participants in Games). Everywhere in the hotel the eye was challenged, one good-looking jock after another, the volunteers as pumped-up as the competitors.

It's so odd to me how much gay lives now revolve around athletic activities, when as a boy it was something that I felt so excluded from and inept at participating in. Even today, sex has been marketed into an athletic activity—video after video seem to have guys meeting up in locker rooms, boyish bodies now amazing muscular. My own sexual fascination with well-built men seems a logical progression to me; even though I was no good at sports, I was drawn to the pumped-up superheroes of comic books, imagining that one of them could rescue me from my ordinary suburban life. For years I have tried to build up my body, but I've never been able to shed my boyish, undefined frame or flabby skin tone, particularly around my waist. And, in recent years, I haven't been able to afford a gym membership and, though I've come to accept that I will never possess the kind of body that I and other gay men think is sexy, it still makes me feel as if I were an inadequate specimen of a modern gay man, and thus, so at odds with this community promotion of "gay pride."

The crowd inside the ballroom where the bodybuilding preliminaries was held was as intimidating as the competitors flexing on the temporary stage which was set up in one corner of the room. When Jonathan and I entered, the middleweights were still on stage and I recognized Teddy Kladitis, a bodybuilder with KS and a catheter implanted in his chest, from the publicity he had been doing to help promote the Games. Jonathan and I spotted Kermit Cole in the room, too, the director of the film I worked on, *Living Proof,* and together the three of us found a row of seats behind a fortysomething-year-old man with a gray goatee and two thin young men seated next to him. (I thought they made an interesting intergenerational group, but as time passed in the room, I would discover that the younger men were not even acquainted with the older one.)

Rhett's weight class arrived on stage (bantam weights) and I was surprised that I was not comparing physiques but body make-up—some guys were heavily oiled and they all seemed to have a fake tan complexion, complete with darker wrinkle lines instead of muscle striations. That's not to say there was nothing to "look" at. I zeroed in immediately on competitor number 47 who had a gorgeous face, military good looks, sharply cut black hair, and the best body in the class (and his tan looked natural). My eyes also happened to stray to the competitor next to him, and I was amazed by the shape and size of the equipment his swimsuit attempted to support, and I pointed this out to Jonathan. We laughed like school girls ogling good-looking boys, which led me to ask him that if God could grant us only a beautiful face or a beautiful body which one would he want to have?

"A face," he answered. "And you"

I nod and said, "A face, too."

"That's good," he added, "because that's what we have and we're lucky to have it."

Rhett's routine was very good, an orchestral version of the Act Two overture from the opera, *Madame Butterfly*, and though he didn't place in his category (he was eliminated from the finals), when he met us in the audience I commended him on his chutzpah—I could never stand in bathing suit in front of a room of strangers.

Number 47 and the young man with the big basket both made the finals and, before we left, I imagined them developing a friendship like beauty queen contestants. A few sexual positions ran across my mind while we watched the heavier (and bigger) competitors on stage. When a black bodybuilder collapsed on stage (from dehydration), Rhett went to make sure he was okay, and then the four of us—Jonathan, Kermit, Rhett, and myself—went for sushi near Herald Square.

Back at my apartment my neighbor, Jon, explained that he has been invited to see Barbra Streisand's concert at Madison Square Garden. He had been invited with a group of people that included Liza Minnelli and Billy Stritch. Jon's a playwright and a lyricist and he runs in circles of celebrities and producers and directors who want him to work on their projects. (He's always working on something that is doing a workshop, or a demo, or a reading.) Jon's money problem is not quite as bad as my own (he's much more frugal and thriftier than I am) and, after he left, I tried not to let my own poverty and personal disappointments overwhelm me. (I became a much less Streisand fan these last few months when I saw how much money she was charging for tickets to her live concert and felt she was becoming too elitist and exclusive a performer.)

As I write up these events of my day now, I am desperate for a drink or some kind of release from my internal aggravations. I'm reading *The Folding Star* by Allan Hollinghurst, in order to write a non-bylined review for *Publishers Weekly*. It depresses me because it is so good—richly written prose with a complex plot and characters—and I think I will never be able to accomplish something like this. It's also about sex, a man's obsessive desire for a young man. It makes me wonder if everything in life breaks down to sex, and not into homosexual and heterosexual divisions, but into those getting it and those not getting it. The haves and have-nots. Maybe that is what God or that ever elusive Higher Power should grant us. The ability to have sex without emotional involvement (something I have *never* been able to accomplish). My mind drifts back through the day to see if I've left anything out. I end up abandoning the reading and the writing and look through a drawer of pornography I keep to escape from myself.

And so the night and the day ended with sex. Or, rather, with sexual fantasies.

Wednesday, June 22, 1995

Pride arrived today fleetingly like a trick, stayed for an orgasm, and faded into a contentment until that, too, was washed away and replaced by a need to experience it again.

It started with a phone call from Bob, an entertainment publicist I used to work with. Bob is a tall, good-looking man who looks so similar to a guy I used to date in Pennsylvania that I immediately graft him with a sexual and emotional history that doesn't belong to him. Bob called and said he was reading my book of short stories, which felt like a tease to me, and I flirted back with him, until he seemed surprised by the volleying and changed the subject to say he was calling to see if I wanted to see Ian McKellen's one-man show tonight, *A Knight Out*, which was playing at the Lyceum Theater on Broadway (and part of the Cultural Festival activities of the Gay Games). I told him I only needed a single ticket, everyone I could immediately think of had plans for this evening and it was too late for me to call around to find a date. (I had my pride to think about, after all—Wouldn't anyone I could call now know I was available myself and not doing anything that evening?) I spent the rest of the day writing a book review and then reading deeper into *The Folding Star* until it was time to leave for the theater.

One thing that I felt certain I would have to confront at the theater was my solitude and I brought *The Folding Star* to read at my seat before the show began to escape it. I was surprised that Bob had left me a ticket for a box seat and my self-consciousness was eased by the location and the box gave me a view of the audience and stage that I always seem to seek out on my own—a view that could allow me to be both a participant and a voyeur of an event. The audience was slow to arrive at their seats, and, once there, it was clear that ninety-eight percent were gay men. (I was also somewhat relieved to see quite a few bald spots from my vantage point; it made me aware that I was not the only aging gay man still living and residing in New York City.)

McKellen's show was a compilation of monologues, anecdotes, and readings, and he was met with a wild applause when he arrived on stage. I had seen him years before in *Acting Shakespeare* and knew what to expect; he's a hammy actor but full of both bravado and honesty. He began the night by describing the joy and beauty of the Lyceum Theater, comparing it to the best of the British houses. He then turned to describing the class system of the audience—the middle class of the mezzanine seats, the upper class of the orchestra seats, the peasants of the balconies. The spotlight dipped and targeted the areas as he described them. He didn't leave out the boxes, either, describing us as the royalty or "queens" present for the performance, and, just as the spotlight highlighted my position in the theater, McKellen identified the location as reserved for those "obscure princesses." McKellen's spiel created both laughter and applause and I was able to laugh and clap along with it as well, though once the routine was over I couldn't help but feel that my loneliness had been uncovered for the rest of the audience to momentarily notice. But I was lucky that I did not have to dwell on it; the performance was full of enchanting moments: the recitation of Michael's coming out letter to his parents from *Tales of the City*; author Armistead Mauphin's cameo on stage with McKellen; playwright Martin Sherman's account of the Stonewall riots; and another cameo with actor B.D. Wong, where McKellen re-enacted a kiss with the actor from film version of *And the Band Played On*.

The evening left me with a feeling of pride which seemed to evaporate on the walk back to my apartment, the way the heightened expectation of ejaculation is replaced by an aftermath of incredulity over what has just transpired. I stopped in at Cleo's before heading back to my apartment, drinking myself into a dizzy state of complexity: Sex, pride, writing, honesty, stories, men, orgasms swirling around in my head until my self-consciousness made me retreat to my apartment, alone.

Thursday, June 23, 1994

It is hard not to be overwhelmed by it all: the island of Manhattan now sports close to fifty gay bars, and more than one hundred-fifty gay organizations regularly meet at the Lesbian and Gay Center or at other venues around town; there are gay sports organizations, gay theater companies, gay religious organizations, gay business organizations. It is hard to know where I fit into all of *this* Gay Overload. Only to see that I am such a small picture of it all and feel at times like an island unto myself, even though I am out, I am gay, have gay friends, go to gay plays and restaurants, read and write gay literature, try to spend my income on doing gay things and supporting the gay community.

It wasn't always like this. That is what I should remember and what, I know, is at the gist of gay pride. In June of 1969, I was thirteen years old, just coming into my sexual awakening. I knew nothing of the Stonewall Riots; in my hometown in North Georgia there were no reports of New York City police officers and agents from the Alcoholic Beverage Control Board raiding the Stonewall Inn for alleged violations of alcohol controls but essentially to harass the gay patrons. I knew nothing of my own sexuality either that year, other than the dim desire to worship comic book heroes, and Tarzan and Hercules movies; I hadn't even discovered musical comedies yet. But I was aware of Judy Garland's death, one of the events which has often been debated as fueling the emotional pitch of the Stonewall riots, and her death struck me noticeably hard. My eighth grade year had been full of taunts from other students—I wore white socks to school, which were ridiculed as queer by my classmates and I crossed my legs in a girly fashion, which was definitely seen as something queer by my peers—and I had spent a considerable amount of time rectifying and correcting my image to blend in with my schoolmates. And *The Wizard of Oz* had led me to believe that there existed some place more enchanting and magical than the suburban neighborhood where I was growing up; it had led me to believe that it was okay to be different, that the pungent feeling of incompleteness could be solved.

Eight years later, I arrived too late during the summer of 1978 to watch the gay pride parade in Manhattan. A year later I walked across town with my friend Kevin to watch the parade down Fifth Avenue; it had never occurred to me that men would dance through the streets in sequin dresses and skimpy bathing suits or that women would go topless while riding motorcycles—and it was both an empowering and confusing experience for me—as much as I admired their pride and chutzpah at parading like this in public, I did not see myself within their celebratory ranks. It would be something that would continue to confuse me, year after year after year.

* * *

My friend John arrived from Washington, D.C. at 7:30 p.m. tonight, anxious and sweaty. Before this extravagant week of pride events began, I told John that we needed to make a plan of the activities we were interested in doing, so that we would not flounder over what to do next or moan about what party we might have missed. We had both agreed to volunteer to help with the Gay Games—we had served as marshals the year before at the March on Washington and wanted to repeat the enjoyable experience—and it didn't require any extra money or tickets for us to participate in this way. After John had settled into the apartment, washed his face, and explained his train trip, we walked downtown to the Penn Hotel to pick up his credentials for the event we were volunteering: we are helping with the marathon race on Saturday morning.

While we were waiting in line to buy tickets for closing ceremonies of the Games on Saturday at Yankee Stadium (John's treat since he accepts the fact that I am rock-bottom poor), I noticed a volunteer get a phone call and his complexion turn pale as he listened to someone on the other end of the line. I knew at once that the guy had been offered last-minute tickets to the Streisand concert (across the street at Madison Square Garden), and when he puts the caller on hold and talks to another co-worker with a flushed, anxious expression, the co-worker breaks into a smiles and waves him away without a concern. The story ends happily with the guy running out of the room without looking back.

John and I walked back uptown and ate at Cafe Elsie, a small gay restaurant around the corner from my apartment, and we talked about one of John's co-workers who may or may not be making sexual advances at John. (Everyone is always making sexual advances at John; I've seen porn stars cruise him on the street, so it doesn't surprise me at all to hear that it could be happening in his office.) After dinner, we walked uptown to Roseland where there was a country western dance competition taking place.

We watched the end of the competition and the winners dance around the floor, and then John and I danced two songs. When we stopped for drinks, John spotted someone else from Washington and he was back on the floor, dancing some more. John never fails to arouse a complex set of emotions within me that I can never seem to escape, a combination of worry, love, romance, jealousy, nostalgia, and friendship. Watching him dance around the floor that evening, I recognized that I also felt possessive of him, and I decided to leave the dance and go home. I stopped in first at Cleo's for a drink, then went upstairs to my apartment and got involved in a phone sex line with a guy on Long Island who wanted to imagine that we were in a three-way. When the L.I. guy revealed that he desired the third partner to be a nine-year old boy, I disconnected the line, not at all proud to be drawn into that kind of scenario. In bed, I tried to fall asleep but was restless, and considered if I had enough time to jerk off before John was safely inside the apartment. I tried to sleep instead, and fell into a strange dream about a guy I saw on the street in the neighborhood who I wanted to date and I was using his apartment to throw a party. Sometime around 3 a.m., John buzzed me from downstairs, and I let him inside the building. It was still not an easy route to sleep or relaxation. Once again I was thinking about sex; why it was so easy for John and seemed to be an insurmountable obstacle for myself, even in my dreams.

Friday, June 24, 1994

Perhaps I should stop moaning, stop complaining, dig down deeper and find the root of something which creates a sense of satisfaction or contentment for me, a foundation for pride, after all, gay or otherwise. There is my writing; I get a great sense of accomplishment from that—it is a source of pride and honesty for me. But I should start, of course, with my friends, and that is what today was, in fact—a gathering of friends.

My friends and I share a lot of common interests—theater, music, books—and share a sense of personal history as well—college years, new boys in Manhattan, the loss of friends from AIDS. I would like to say that being gay didn't factor into all of this but if I were I would have to say we were all gay-accepting. For the truth of it is, being gay has given me a quality and level of friendships I might never have experienced otherwise.

After breakfast, John and I walked to Central Park and sat in Sheep Meadow, which was full of gay boys sunning themselves on towels, even though the weather was very humid. Once we got tired of throwing a Frisbee, we took the subway downtown and saw the movie *Wolf,* which co-starred a friend of Jon's. Jon had mentioned that during filming of the movie that his friend, playing a book editor, had brought a copy of my book,

Dancing on the Moon, to use in the set of his office (though I didn't notice it in the film.)

Later, a bunch of us met for dinner at Virgil's in Times Square—Wade, John, Jon, myself. Wade, John's friend from Washington, D.C., is over six-feet tall and something of a dreamboat (in my opinion). He was nervous about scoring some drugs that evening to use at a dance the following night— the one which was being held on the U.S.S. Intrepid, a military warship docked at 42nd Street and the Hudson River Piers. Wade left us before the check arrived in order to make his drug rendezvous and the rest of us wandered out into Times Square and over to the Marriott Marquis, where we discovered that we were not interested in watching drag queens arriving for a ball. Instead, we decided to cab it down to Chelsea and walk the Eighth Avenue "homo mile" that stretches from 23rd Street to 14th Street.

In Chelsea, the sidewalks were crowded and it was impossible for us to walk three abreast, so I let Jon and John walk ahead of me, preferring to watch the cruises and glances they get as we headed downtown. This strip of Chelsea is replacing Christopher Street and Sheridan Square as the heart of gay New York—there are gay-owned and gay-frequented bars and restaurants and clothing stores and health clubs on both sides of the street. The heavy humidity of the day was finally dissipating into a light mist of rain, and the dampness layered the air with a chill. Before we reached 14th Street, I was ready to return home, and, when we reached the entrance to the 14th Street subway stop, all of us struggled over continuing our walk downtown into the Village or returning uptown to my apartment. John wanted to continue on, and I would have let him do it on his own, but even Jon, who is usually the one of us who is so quick to poop out, was eager to continue on, so I followed them once again, across the crosswalk, and over to Greenwich Avenue. The mist continued, but the traffic, street lights, and shop lights gave the wet surfaces a glassy, though colorful, smear. We stopped in at Uncle Charlie's, a bar on Greenwich Avenue, because John thought one of the guys he met the night before at the country western dance might be there, but just when I was warm, we headed back out into the misty night, deciding to walk over to Sheridan Square and site of the Stonewall bar.

Christopher Street was astonishingly crowded; in my three different decades in the city—the late Seventies, the Eighties, and now the early Nineties—I have never known it to be this crowded except on Gay Pride Days. If the mood were not so cruisy and festive, it would feel as if we were tourists who have made a pilgrimage to some kind of holy, revered shrine. In a way, I suppose, this has to be the most revered spot in the world for gay men and lesbians and this was the reason why we ended up there that night. We stopped outside the Stonewall bar long enough to watch a cluster of young men have their picture taken as a group. John wanted to go inside the bar, but I reminded him he had been there many times before. When we lived together on Bleecker Street, this site used to be a Bowl and Board and a bagel store next door. I remembered my first year in the city—I was twenty-two years old and had learned about the riots and the history of the place, and I recall being drawn here as one is to a historical war shrine or cathedral in Europe, thinking, as if by some sort of strange magic, it would reveal a kind of inexplicable psychic energy for me.

The police had set up barricades in several places in Sheridan Square—lines of string tied from one to the next formed strange patterns of east-west pedestrian traffic. It successfully herded us as though we were cattle across Seventh Avenue and we continued down Christopher Street in the direction of the Hudson River. The crowds of men and women were thicker now, and the patterns of groups and individuals weaved into and out and against one another as if they were tumbled by turns of a toy kaleidoscope. By now the chill had left me because of the strange and surreal moment we had wandered into, even though the mist continued to change into a light rain and the wind blew harder against our clothes. What was the most overwhelming thing, however, was that the night was fueled by the energy of our group and those with us. We were here, bonded, together, witnessing, even though there was nothing really to be seen except us and them. This moment lasted until we reached the West Side Highway, when the prospect of continuing on by foot seemed daunting. We hailed a cab and returned uptown.

At home, Jon disappeared next door, John left a phone message for Wade, and I stood in front of my bathroom mirror, wondering if I should keep the goatee I have had for almost four months or shave it off.

I decided I would keep it until the end of the week.

Saturday, June 25, 1994

I would have thought more about sex today if I hadn't been so tired. (Perhaps that is the clue to this obsessiveness—to mentally and physically tire myself until I just subsist with action and not thought.)

We woke at 4:30 this morning, or, rather, I woke up at 4:30 this morning covered with a clammy sweat and a clouded head which showering and a cup of coffee did not clear. John waited to shower until the last possible moment and then we caught a cab to 72nd Street and the Park where we hooked up with the other volunteers for the marathon race. We walked over to the booth where the registrants and volunteers were to sign in and we were given extra-large blue T-shirts which, on the front and back, MARSHALL was spelled out in large block letters. I slipped mine over the shirt I was wearing but John asked several officious volunteers if there was a smaller size, who waved him away as if it were a silly request. (John prefers his shirts form-fitting, has always preferred his clothing to be too small and too tight in order to show off his physique.)

Our post was back at 72nd Street and Fifth Avenue and, though the sun was now up, when we reached our position, it was humid and overcast; a heavy mist hung over the park. The twenty-six mile course of the marathon started at Tavern on the Green, wound through the lower loop of the Park, then headed east on 72nd Street to the FDR Drive, down to Battery Park, where runners circled back to the FDR Drive, up to 72nd

Street and York, and back to Central Park for a final loop. Our job was to make sure runners exited the Park correctly to 72nd Street, and then, about two hours later, make sure they enter the Park correctly for their final lap.

Around 6:30, the first two runners appeared at our point. The rest came in fours, then in larger clumps. John and I became cheerleaders, yelling and clapping for them, "Looking good!" "You can do it!" I sounded like someone I don't know, or very seldom recognized. Every now and then some kind of event propels "musical comedy Jimmy" to take over my body and become a sort of smiling, good-time guy. (And this was one of those moments).

By 7, all the runners were out of the Park and all John and I had to do was wait two hours for their return. A city policeman on duty for the race and stationed at our posts asked John how many runners were participating (about 600) and fell into a discussion with John about whether that was as many as they anticipated. (I, of course, thought the cop was a cutie and a catch—he was in a tight uniform, not too tall, and had a beefy, college jock sort of appearance. Not only was my "musical comedy" personality unable to attract the guy's attention away from John, but it disappeared as soon as the sun heated things up and fried the humidity against my forehead so that I turned into a cranky old man who should have stayed inside.) Instead, I talked to the *Advocate* photographer (also a cutie) covering the event, until John and I walked over to a bench and waited until it was time to move back into action.

By 10 a.m., all of the runners were back in the Park and John and I walked across the lawn to the finish line and watched the finalists being sprayed with jets of water. Then it was a cab back downtown and up the rigorous five flights to my apartment, praying that the air-conditioner would continue to work the rest of the day.

* * *

After our afternoon naps, our amazing journey to Yankee Stadium began. On the subway line, we rode cars which were full of gay men and lesbians. I stood between John and some unbelievable hunk that I fantasized must have arrived from a dairy farm in the mid-west just to participate in the city during these days, or better yet, from somewhere near the mountains of Sweden. There were a few "straight" riders on the train, and it was clear to them where they were seated or standing that they were now in a minority on the train, and it was interesting to see the realization of this filter into their consciousness.

At the stadium, the Closing Ceremonies of the Games began with a boring parade of athletes (from where we were sitting they looked like small clusters of color and I would have rather have stayed on the subway and watched the riders). But it was astonishing to grasp that everyone who had assembled in Yankee Stadium—and there were thousands and thousands of us—had at some time felt that they were different and isolated while growing up, the usual route to recognizing one is homosexual. Rumors circulated through the crowd that Streisand or Madonna would sing at some point during the ceremonies, a rumor that never came true, but the performers—Cyndi Lauper, Barbara Cook, and Patti LaBelle, among them—were not at all a disappointment. Everyone was so eager to be in a happy and gay mood (including me). And we were.

Sunday, June 26, 1994

Another early morning. We struggled with exhaustion, showers, coffee. I considered canceling our plans, just watching the parade, but by 9 a.m. we were at the "March with a Buddy" temporary office on East 45th Street. After watching more than a dozen gay pride parades in the city pass me by, I decided it was time this year to march in one; the biggest problem I faced this year, as in past years, was finding an organization I wanted to march with. Priority Pharmacy, a pharmacy that helps gay men with AIDS, was sponsoring a "March with a Buddy" program for Stonewall 25, which allowed volunteers to carry a placard of an enlarged photo of a person who was not able to march (due to illness or death). It seemed to me the most compassionate and worthwhile thing I could do, considering that I did not desire to be trapped with 2500 other people carrying an immense rainbow flag that weighed 7000 pounds, which was the centerpiece of an exhaustive campaign during this year's celebration.

At the Priority registration site my name was not on their list of volunteers, but John's name was, and, upon the suggestion of a volunteer, was asked to wait about fifteen more minutes and I would be given one of the placards of a no-show for the parade. A few moments later I was handed a placard with a photo of "Angel," a Hispanic man from New Jersey, and given an extra-large T-shirt that read "March with a Buddy." John, of course, had no intention of wearing his T-shirt (he had on a skin tight tank top on and was not changing his look), and we walked over to the location on First Avenue where our group was to assemble. It was a beautiful morning, the sky a flat blue with a few puffs of clouds, the air light and free from the humidity of the earlier part of the week. Shortly before the parade began (at 11 am), Jonathan, his friend Arnie, and Rhett also joined us in the line to march. The five of us talked about the guys we had seen this morning, the lack of tiaras and leathermen in the crowd, and the rumor of the renegade parade which ACT UP was planning along the customary parade route of Fifth Avenue.

And so the little group of us eventually marched up First Avenue, a small part of seven hundred other men, women, parents, family, friends, and volunteers who were marching for a larger purpose, the recognition of those unable to participate in today's parade and the need to distinguish our continued presence and roles in society. And the hundreds of us were only a smaller part of an even larger assembly of gay men and lesbians and their families and friends who were marching to acknowledge the twenty-fifth year of the moment gay men and women spoke up publicly for their right to exist, a right that today's march past the United Nations building, sought to address internationally to the rest of the world.

This was what it what it was like to march that day in June, 1994: It was sunny, it was full of friends, it was full of a cause. We were happy and proud. And it was clear to me as we passed by those watching us on the sidewalk that our group was making a statement. When the parade turned westward toward the rallying point in Central Park, I found myself near the blue wooden police barricades and the crowds of spectators. No one was looking individually at me or John or any of our group; instead, I noticed that their eyes were drawn to the entire crowd of us and to our signs held high. And as I looked across at them—the spectators—at the sea of faces and caps and eyes—I noticed their smiles and their sorrow; we were collecting as much applause as we were tears—a young woman applauding us was standing next to a man who had to bury his face his hands to hide his quivering lips.

Reports said that as many as one million people marched that afternoon in the parade. There were no clashes between police and the marchers this year; the official First Avenue parade politely paused to let the renegade parade, which had assembled after all, pass calmly through the entrance into the Park. The parades culminated in a rally on the dusty Great Lawn, where Liza Minnelli and others performed. John and I stayed as long as we could, till we left our group behind so that he could catch an afternoon train back to Washington.

By 6 p.m., I was again alone in my apartment, drifting in and out of sleep. I was too tired to think about going to the dance on the pier, too tired to even make back down five flights to the street to watch the paraders heading downtown for other events. I spoke with Joel, another gay friend from college on the phone that night, and explained and described the events of the day to him. When I hung up the phone, I felt an emptiness arrive and replace the exhaustion and I found a porno tape I had not watched in more than ten years and put it into my VCR.

And so my celebration of pride ended as the week began—with thoughts of sex. I clutched and groped and pulled at myself, remembering the days when I was growing up in Georgia when I might have been ashamed at what I wanted to do, while watching men have sex on a screen a few inches from my eyes. Somewhere before I reached an orgasm, I remembered that self-perception is at the root of any kind of basis of pride. Yes, I should be thankful that I have not been beaten to death by homophobic bigots. Yes, I should be thankful to God or some unknown Higher Power that I am still alive when so many others have died from AIDS. Life could be much harder for me that it really is. So that is how I will end this diary. I was glad I could live to see the hype. I was glad I found a reason to march. I was glad to say I was there for Stonewall 25.

FUNNY GUY

David B. Feinberg was a very funny guy. But I do not have a funny story about him. Our friendship was not based on his perpetual sense of humor or my often lack of one. Instead, it was founded on our mutual desire to be writers—*gay* writers grappling with and writing about the changes of life we had experience because of the epidemic of AIDS, gay men who, incidentally, knew what gay life was like *before* the epidemic.

I first met David in 1987 when I joined the Gay Writers Workshop, a group of about five or six writers who met once a month in members' apartments throughout the metropolitan New York City area. David had been a member for some time, and though we had no leader to our group—we considered ourselves peers—we all looked to David to be our leader. Most of us had been minimally published, and David, by that time, had just begun writing his humor columns for *Mandate* magazine.

The writers in our group were a diverse lot. One guy was writing a gay version of *Romeo and Juliet*, another was concentrating on poetry, another was developing the saga of a drag queen who attended law school. It was clear right from the start, however, that David and I were writing about the same subject—gay life during the plague years—but our approach was wildly dissimilar—his fiction was dark, humorous, and witty, and focused around being HIV-positive, as he was in real life; my short stories were realistic, minimalistic, and compassionate, as I tried to understand my role as a carepartner for a friend who was struggling with many of the issues David, himself, would later deal with.

Not long after I joined the group, David had his first novel, *Eighty-Sixed*, accepted by Viking. Each month when our workshop met David would update the other members on the publishing process, flashing the proofs of the jacket cover of his book around the room or waving the author's questionnaire he had received from the publicity department to fill out, adding little joking asides about the experience. He didn't do this to brag, really, though many of us were ruffled a bit by it, each of us was continually sending our writings out and facing rejections. David believed, I think, that each one of us would one day go through this same process ourselves, which is why he was so eager to share his experience of it. A few months later, after I gave him a collection of my short stories that I had finished—half of which dealt with the impact of AIDS on the gay community—he surprised me and sent them along to his editor at Viking to consider—perhaps one of the most generous things one writer can do for another.

As it happened, that collection was not published, though it did serve as my introduction to Ed Iwanicki, the man who would become the editor of a later collection of my short stories that was published and who continued to edit David's subsequent books. Real life, however, suspended a lot of my desire and momentum to be a writer—my friend died and I moved away from Manhattan and went through what I have often called my "minor major nervous meltdown" period. David, however, continued his "Life in Hell"—a highway of memorials, demonstrations, and doctors' visits. And he continued writing about every aspect of it. Eventually I returned to the city, emotionally stronger, and moved into an apartment in the Theater District, a few blocks down from where David lived on Ninth Avenue, an area he had affectionately dubbed as "Hell's Kitchenette."

Occasionally I would run into David on the street and he would go into a riff about his anal warts or something equally as shocking. David was never squeamish about disclosure of anything, and I would often stand in front of him thinking that if I was shocked about hearing about anal warts on Ninth

Avenue then what would my mother think about this? Or better yet, what would *David's* mother think about it? After all, his family was often his fondest, quickest, and easiest source of comic anguish—as was mine, one of the many things I felt which connected us emotionally. A few minutes later, David would tell me he was having a party on such and such date and to be sure to come. And a few days later an invitation or a postcard would arrive in the mail reminding me of it. I have never been much of a party person, but I would go to David's parties because I liked David, curious about how many people he could fit into the sliver of his apartment, curious, as well, as to what sort of crowd his other friends were. I had, by then, heard and read many, many stories about them.

David's apartment, in those days, was painted a light shade of lavender, with a darker colored trim, and on the wall by his bed was an enormous collage of photographs and drawings of men that David admired—the "hot ones" as they were called— culled from a variety of publications such as *Advocate Men*, *Torso*, the *International Male* catalog or the advertisements for the Chelsea Gym that would often appear in *The Village Voice*. It was as easy to be drawn to this wall of beautiful faces and bodies as it was to David and his real world, but I could never stay long at his parties, shyness and a need for fresh air would pull me back out onto the street. As I would walk back to my apartment, I would often dwell on the differences between David and myself—the photographs I had clipped of men that interested me, for instance, *my* hot ones, were hidden in a drawer beside my bed, never to be displayed in public, never, even, shared privately with another man.

It was in the fall of 1993, I think, that I noticed that things were really beginning to change for David. I ran into him at the bus stop—he was headed downtown to his new apartment in Chelsea, the one that a boyfriend had hand-painted a wall trim near the ceiling that David despised—and I could tell he had dropped weight. Not long after that I decided that I would start going to ACT UP meetings on Monday nights because I felt I needed to find a more angrier and political approach to my writing. What I found, instead, was a way to find David.

And so it happened that on Monday nights I would wander into ACT UP and look for David, say hello, briefly gossip, and sometimes sit beside him, listening to him mumble asides as he scribbled notes on the photocopied agenda, his free arm draped around my shoulder or touching my thigh to make a point. I don't think I really ever officially joined ACT UP; I had wandered in and out of meetings for years and shown up for a few of the bigger actions and rallies, and when I started going again I never felt as if I were rejoining the group. Instead, I felt I was joining David.

ACT UP, Monday nights at The Lesbian and Gay Center in the West Village, was somewhere where I knew I could find David, even if it just meant spotting him across the room. This was the place where I could check up on him without really seeming to check up on him. I suppose this voyeuristic distance is just another part of my WASPy upbringing, that polite reserve of wanting to know but not wanting to ask, the Southern writer whose view of the canvas is of a broad perspective as opposed to the Northern activist whose life is specific and lived on the edge and at the front lines. David, of course, went on to denounce ACT UP in the last month of his life; in an infamous speech delivered to the organization on the night he was released from the hospital for the last time, he chided them for wasting time bickering amongst themselves and "indulging in its obsession with the Catholic church."

In addition to being a funny guy, David was also a consummate critic. One of his favorite pastimes was to pick up the phone and play "trash the reading" or "trash the movie" or "trash the play"—a game, I will also admit, he was much more superb at than I. I often feared, even, that one day I might fall victim to his satirical attacks. One night, for instance, at a benefit screening for a documentary I wrote called *Living Proof*, based on the Carolyn Jones photography project about people who are successfully living with their HIV diagnosis and in which David had a five-second appearance, David waved me over through the crowd at the theater and asked me to sit beside him. When the lights came up at the end of the movie, I tried to push my way into the aisle, fearful of being caught in a "trash the movie" scenario in which I did not want to participate. But I couldn't get away, caught in the crowd, and I stood with my back toward David, not wanting, at that moment, to know his opinion. The movie, after all, was upbeat and positive about living with HIV, and David, I knew from our conversation earlier that evening, was struggling with issues of his own dying and death. In the lobby, before the movie had started, he had confided to me that he was worried about living to see his next book—*Queer and Loathing*—published, and I knew he wasn't exactly feeling in a positive or upbeat mood about anything that evening. He must have sensed my worry, however, sensed *my* sensitivity, because he clasped my shoulder and said, "It even made me feel good," and then, in that dry, nasal tone of his, as if to deflect his own good mood, added, "For a moment."

I once defended David to a reporter by saying that sometimes it takes a sense of humor to understand a sense of humor. At his darkest, David could also be potentially offensive—he seldom held anything back when it was on his mind. Personally, I often felt so inadequate around him—I have never considered myself a funny guy; at best, my sense of humor is either situational or very dry. I was not always tuned into David's satirical wavelength, but I could always rationalize the genesis of his humor. David was always *on*, as if he were isolated in a soundbooth and being broadcast across something like AIDS Public Radio. Sometimes, however, when he would go into one of his riffs, I would stop him with a "What? What?"—not totally comprehending what he was saying (or hearing—David was also a superb mumbler). Oftentimes, I would question him purposely, or bequeath him one of my unknowing blank stares, my own sort of private joke with him: Nothing is more funny to me than making a comic *have* to explain his own joke, one that David *enjoyed* having to do in my company. And I enjoyed playing his straight man.

David's humor, both in person and in print, was frank and ferocious. Critics often cited him for his lack of self-pity. He was one of the first, if not the first, to write humorously about AIDS, paving the way, in essence, for other writers to write comically about life in the epidemic, particularly the string of comic plays about AIDS that appeared in the early Nineties by Paul Rudnick, Christopher Durang, Terrence McNally, and Tony Kushner. Though David once said to a reporter that B.J. Rosenthal, his randy and troubled fictional alter-ego in *Eighty-Sixed* and *Spontaneous Combustion*, was "more well-endowed" than himself, he was nonetheless quite close to the same skin as David. One of the hardest things for a writer who writes creatively about AIDS is to be able to separate the fiction from the facts of his experiences, and which is why David's last book, *Queer and Loathing*, a collection of his non-fiction articles about living with HIV, is perhaps his most insightful, intimate, and controversial book because David did not steer away from any of his own truths, adventures, and opinions. David was also an extraordinary journalist, often using a first-person narrative technique that would not only describe an event, but one which could capture an absurdly comic portrait of himself within it.

Is humor an acceptable way for an activist to write about AIDS? Certainly, it is one of the most viable and accessible ways to stress and reveal the troubling truths of the epidemic, at least in my opinion, but it was also a point which polarized David against many other gay men, gay writers, gay editors, and gay publications. Edmund White, himself HIV-positive and co-author of a collection of AIDS fiction titled *The Darker Proof*, wrote in an essay entitled "Esthetics and Loss" in *Artforum* in 1987, "If art is to confront AIDS more honestly than the media has done, it must begin in tact, avoid humor and end in anger."

Avoid humor? The thought of it could send David into spasms of laughter. David, incensed by White's logic, went on to campaign for more humor in AIDS writing, expressing himself eloquently on the subject in *The Advocate* and at the

1992 OutWrite conference of gay and lesbian writers and editors in Boston, as well as on numerous panels. "I'm not trivializing AIDS," he told an interviewer in 1992. "I've seen too many people die. It's hard to write about AIDS. If I wrote about it straight, I couldn't face it. In a lot of ways, this is therapy for me. I had a lot of anger and depression in me when I learned I was HIV-positive. Some of the anger I channeled into ACT UP, the rest I sublimated into writing. Part of why I do it in a humorous way is to make it manageable for me. Humor is a way of taking control—or trying to. If you laugh at a situation, it's no longer in control of you. You're in charge. For a minute, anyway."

One of the ironies of this anecdote was supplied by Edmund White, himself. In *Muses from Chaos and Ash: AIDS, Artists, and Art*, published in 1993, White remarked, "I'd really like to write a big novel, probably similar in form to David Feinberg's *Eighty-Sixed*. That's probably been the most successful of all the AIDS novels." This was the same author who had earlier suggested that it was inappropriate to combine AIDS and humor and who went on further in this interview to compliment David's book as "quite funny" and "full of all the characteristic verve and excitement of gay life of that period."

Even at the end David continued to be funny; and he continued to write. In the hospital the last two months of his life he filled a composition book with sketches, lists, and anecdotes of his often trying and humiliating medical experiences. If there was any particular technique that David originated or perfected in his writing, I would have to say it was his lists, which he incorporated into both *Eighty-Sixed* and *Spontaneous Combustion*, but which became the barometers of David's emotional and physical health in *Queer and Loathing*. As David's health deteriorated, his humor, of course, became darker and darker.

I have, of course, many other personal memories of David—the way he gathered his friends together to see a movie on Christmas Eve, listening to his riffs about Bob Satuloff or the *Native* erroneously reporting the demise of his best friend John Weir, Ryan White's remark about how he was an "innocent victim" and David's succinct reply, "Right, the rest of us *deserve* to die," the photos he would take of the audience at his bookstore readings, watching him barely breathing as he watched his stage play being read before an audience of friends, the provocative postcards he would send me of bare-bottomed gym boys.

These are, of course, only *my* memories of David; others, I am sure, have much more riotous and vivid recollections of him. I was not part of his inner circle and he was not a part of mine, but our orbits crossed nonetheless in this expansive and crazy metropolis because of the epidemic. And, oddly, I have to say, the epidemic created a stronger friendship between us. Each of us could have taken the other to task for the way we wrote about the disease, but there was something between us, a desire to see an end to this plague and a realistic need to report its continuing uncertainties that kept our respect in check with one another.

So I will write it again because I really mean it. David B. Feinberg was a very funny guy. He was also a great and original writer. His sense of humor prevailed even as it was tested by the ravages of a virus that invaded, disrupted, and humiliated his body. Unfortunately, I must also remember him as another friend lost in the epidemic. David died November 2, 1994 at the age of thirty-seven.

IT

There is not a day I do not think about it. There is not a moment that I am unaware of its presence. I am reminded of it in a headline in the newspapers, an announcement on the radio, a special report on television. It is in the sports reports, the lifestyle pages, the entertainment reviews, in the health, international, and political articles. I notice when it is missing from an obituary.

It has been in several feature films, Broadway plays, documentaries, and made-for-television movies. It has inspired pop songs, paintings, ballets, and orchestral symphonies. Books have been written about it. So have short stories, poetry, novels, and essays. Some people, however, believe it is as strange as science fiction.

But scientists *are* fighting it. So are doctors, researchers, nurses, interns, buddies, fundraisers, and volunteers. My friends Keith and Hugh are fighting it. So are Maria's eight-month-old daughter Jeannie, Patrick's older brother Rob, Renee's husband Marco, and Luther's grandmother Penny.

There are hotlines and switchboards for it, special magazines published about it, special newsletters circulated suggesting treatments for it. There are support groups, hospices, and special wards for it. There are personal ads that mention it, and special dating services for people who have it. There is a blood test to detect it, and another one to make sure that the first one wasn't incorrect. Soon you will be able for test for it in your home.

There is a government-appointed czar for it, a ribbon for it, a new postage stamp issued because of it, and a memorial quilt for the people who have died from it. There are also symptoms for it and reactions from drugs that attempt to treat it

There are walkathons and danceathons to raise money for funds to fight it. There are special performances and benefits to raise more monies to provide services to people who have it and are fighting for their health. Non-profit organizations have been founded because of it. There are international conferences, candlelight vigils, a day without art, and a night without lights because of it. There are, however, no days and nights without it. It is a crisis and a war; it is a *global* epidemic.

It has caused many forms of discrimination. It has created government scandals in France and Germany. Thousands of lawsuits have resulted from it. Immigrants have been denied entry because of it. Insurance premiums have been raised and canceled because of it. Some places will not allow you to marry if you have it.

There are people who have had it for many years and are still capable of living full, asymptomatic lives. These people give us hope and inspiration, but don't let this fool you. That is not always the case. In 1993, one death resulted from it every 15 seconds. In this country the first 100,000 cases were diagnosed in the first nine years. The next 100,000 in eighteen months. From 1981 to 1993 it struck 339,250 Americans; 204,390 of them were killed. In 1994 it was the number one killer in America of men between the ages of 25 and 44. By the year 2000, 13 million women worldwide are expected to be infected by it.

For years this plague has been plagued by rumors, theories, and suppositions. It is not a retribution from God. It is not a curse unleashed from opening King Tut's tomb. It cannot be transmitted by mosquitoes or toilet seats. And it is not a gay disease.

It has killed actors, dancers, ice skaters, pianists, football players, and U.S. Congressmen. It has killed lawyers, designers, nurses, computer technicians, and six-year-old girls. It has killed my co-workers Peter, Warren, Bill, and Robert. It has killed my friends Kevin, Mark, Sam, Jerry, and David. It has killed Michael's lover, Darren's girlfriend, and Marcia's son-in-law. It has killed reporters, editors, secretaries, and proofreaders. It has killed truck drivers, waitresses, factory workers, and messenger boys. It has killed both white collar professionals and blue collar workers. Babies are born with it. And babies die from it. It can kill any race, either sex, and at every age.

If you don't know what it is then you better wake up. If you are not worried, you should be. It can be found in the blood, saliva, semen, and teardrops. It has changed the political, social, and medical fabric of this country. It is part of our history but this history is not over. There are demonstrations because of the high cost of treating it, demonstrations because of politicians' weakness to fund research for it, demonstrations because religions ignore it, demonstrations because no one seems to be educating anyone *about* it. Its transmission can, however, be *prevented*. Condoms can help prevent it. So can clean needles. Guidelines have been issued for prevention, though many local governments, schools, businesses, and churches *still* pay no attention to them.

If you are sick of hearing about it—you shouldn't be. *You* could be sick from it. So get used to living with it. These are only a few of the things about it. There will be many more. There is no vaccine for it. There is no cure for it. And this is *not* science fiction.

It is a *virus*. It is *still* a virus. It still *kills*. And it is a part of *our* world.

It is *here*.

TREATS

Only in hindsight do I recall the watch, and my memory has now restored its first impression to the moment we were seated and holding hands. It was there on his wrist the night we first met, large, gold, heavy, and expensive-looking. It was the kind of watch I knew I would never be able to afford for myself, and so I had admired it only from a distance and without a comment, as if it were something I had fleetingly noticed while passing a department store window.

I don't remember my opening line or his opening remark, though I do recall that the weather was hot—an unbearably humid late-summer evening. I had not come to the bar to meet a trick but to escape my overheated apartment. I was poor that year, poorer than most of the other ones, and even if I had been able to afford an air-conditioner in my apartment, I would never have been able to pay the electrical bill it would create. I had gathered enough coins before leaving my apartment to present to the bartender for a glass of wine and a small tip. When I took my drink to the downstairs room where the air was the coolest, I noticed him standing against the wall. He was dressed in a button-down shirt, chinos, and docksiders, a much more elegant costume than that of my old, misshapen polo shirt and jeans.

Later, in his bathroom, I studied the row of bottles of cologne that lined a shelf of his cabinet and I opened a few to see if I could match the scent of him which remained on me. I had never bought cologne for myself; it was an indulgence that arrived to me as gifts and something I turned to only for special occasions.

It must have showered while we were inside the bar, because when we walked toward his car, the street was a smeary reflection of lights and neon signs. I thought it a luxury that he drove a car in the city where I walked to my every destination. When we stopped in front of a black Porsche, I was flabbergasted that he had not parked such an expensive car in a garage where it would be safe. He said it was not his usual car—he had traded cars for a week because a friend had wanted to test drive his Lexus. I had never ridden in a Porsche before and I know I must have stood there with a crazy look on my face, dumbfounded by the concept of friends trading expensive cars in the same way they might swap neckties to better match a jacket.

After sex, we watched TV and ate scoops of rich, chocolate ice cream out of tiny espresso cups. I did not regard this as an odd, late-night habit of an eccentric stranger, only another reason to stay and escape the heat.

The apartment had a river-view, fifteen stories above the ground, and it was a like a large black curtain full of starry lights. I don't recall what his furniture looked like that night or shape of the rooms we walked through, only that my old sneakers floated from the river to the bed as if they were standing on the deck of a yacht.

It did not occur to me that night that I could be regarded merely as another luxury in his life or that I might be considered an older man's younger toy by someone who had seen us together at the bar. I was also not aware that he was not a man of substance until much later; my first impression was of his extravagant detail.

The watch reappeared later that night. We were in bed and it was the only thing he was still wearing. I found it odd that he had not taken it off, but continued to wear it while we had sex, and it occurred to me that he might think it was something I could steal, since I had admitted to him at the bar that I did not share even a fraction of his wealth. When I stopped and asked him why he still wore the watch, he said he must not have realized that it was still on his wrist, and he unbuckled the clasp to remove it from his arm. Before he laid it on the table beside the bed, he handed it to me and asked if I wanted to try it on. I slipped it on my wrist and held it up to catch the light which filtered into the darkened room. The metal felt cold and expensive against my skin and it was clearly an uncomfortable fit on my arm, a fact I overlooked because I was hypnotized by the image of myself as a wealthy man. In retrospect, I realize now I was seduced by the luxuries of the night and not by the man who brought them to me, something I continued to overlook when I needed them again.

ART HISTORY 101

"Would you date the type of guy who would draw something like this?" I nervously laughed and asked my boyfriend Adam, a forty-six year-old businessman from Connecticut. We were standing in an alcove of the spiral rotunda gallery of the Guggenheim Museum, trying to decipher a quartet of somber paintings by Ross Bleckner, darkly hued canvases crammed with luminescent urns, trophies, and candelabras connected to ghostly planetary and geometric shapes, designs which have been described as metaphors for the AIDS epidemic.

"Depends on how cute he was," Adam answered quickly, without much forethought, which summed up to me the strongest metaphor of our own relationship. Three years before I had published a collection of short stories based on the lives of friends whom I had lost to AIDS, and which I had given Adam a copy of a few weeks after we met, and which he seemed, at times, to have forgotten that I had even written. It often made me feel as if my past never existed, but then I'd always felt that Adam was more attracted to my looks than to any other attribute I possess.

It was a misty gray Saturday afternoon in February, 1995, when Adam and I wandered through the Guggenheim's mid-career retrospective of Bleckner. The Guggenheim, designed by architect Frank Lloyd Wright, is Manhattan's novelty museum, a continuous upward spiral ramp like an inverted corkscrew, with paintings evenly hung on the walls above the sloping floors. The Bleckner exhibit began about mid-way up the ramp with a series of paintings which were nothing but different colored stripes. Earlier, I had read something about these unimaginable paintings as being inspired from the way the artist interpreted light. Standing before them that afternoon, they seemed impassive to me, till I reached a red, black, and white one which had the words "Remember Me" spelled out across the surface in a three-dimensional trompe l'oeil design. All at once it made me remember a friend—a writer who had died more than five years before from AIDS, but whose life when he had lived in New York City had consisted of outings such as this—running to whatever au courant exhibit or gallery or movie or play one needed to go to in order to keep up—in order to be an up-to-date, fashionable urbanite.

Much has been written, of course, of Bleckner's own fashionable life—a second or double life so different from his often dour art. Bleckner has a high society profile—friend of David Gefffen, Barry Diller, and escort to Bianca Jagger, who, as I had read in an account in *The New York Times*, came with the artist to the opening night reception of this exhibit at the Guggenheim, a party which was thrown for the artist by *Vanity Fair* magazine and Hugo Boss (who incidentally designed the suit Bleckner wore that evening). Though he may not have been born with a silver spoon in his mouth, Bleckner, from his bio, was also never a starving artist. The son of a well-to-do Long Island parts manufacturer, Bleckner's father bought the artist the downtown Manhattan building where, now in his mid-forties, he still lives and works. Bleckner also owns a much publicized house in the Hamptons, Truman Capote's former one, and he currently serves as President of the board of directors of CRIA—the Community Research Initiative on AIDS—a role which to the public eye seems to function more as a society fundraiser than as an AIDS administrator.

As Adam and I continued up the Guggenheim's spiral, weaving around other heavy-coated tourists, into the artist's more lugubrious, memorial-conscious paintings, the connection between Bleckner and myself—or how I saw my writing somehow mirroring his art—Adam missed entirely, which did not, in the least bit, surprise me. I credit one of the reasons why I had had such a bumpy start in my relationship with Adam with the fact that we are both highly self-absorbed individuals. I have my own agenda for how I live—from what I wear to what I write about, to what I expect and want and will compromise with in a lover. Adam, I think, lives on a faster and more expensive track than my own, and at times it feels to me as if I am dating a clone of Malcolm Forbes. Adam, for instance, seldom shows an interest in things outside of his own life except when it relates to money, and with us, nothing beyond anything primarily sexual. That's not to say he isn't a generous and giving man both in and out of bed. He is—when, however, it suits his own purpose. For Adam, himself, lives a double life—one foot out of the closet, the other firmly hidden inside. He works as the manager of a stock brokerage firm in Connecticut, drawing an income that would take me about twelve different lifetimes and triple as many careers as a writer of gay fiction to earn. Adam is closeted about his sexuality at his office—no one even suspects that he could be gay, and he only recently revealed to some of his co-workers that he has been separated for some time from his wife of fourteen years. His wife, also, doesn't know the truth about why Adam is in the process of divorcing her—he's as closeted with her and their two kids as he is in the office.

But Adam also maintains a separate gay life, separate from the one he shares with me on weekends and dates, and which became, at one point, the greatest source of frustration for me within our burgeoning pseudo-relationship. When I first met Adam he had only been separated from his wife for shortly over a year—he was enthralled, then (and still is), with the varied homosexual landscape of Manhattan—the many permutations of sexual activity which are continually offered up around town for an inquisitive and "out there" (to use Adam's own words) gay man. Since leaving his wife, Adam has lived in a posh Upper East Side tower apartment with a view of the East River. Adam's a happy hour habitué of that A-list gay bar, The Townhouse, just around the corner from Bloomingdale's, and his favorite pastime, I have come to believe, is to see how many guys he can pick up, and the different assortment of types of men he finds himself attracted to—though I know for a fact, he is particularly drawn to the young, All-American boy-next-door type, but he has also informed me that he isn't at all discriminating over looks or body types when it comes to one-night stands.

At first, when Adam and I started seeing one another, none of this really bothered me; I wasn't looking for a relationship then myself (and I didn't feel that Adam was capable of giving me the kind of relationship that I wanted anyway). Yet the longer Adam and I dated one another, however, especially as we passed that six-month marker, and the more I found myself falling for Adam, the more I became upset with his perpetual quest to meet and bed other men, a product, magnified, I believe, from the liberation he feels from the end of his marriage. "You're not perfect," he said to me the day I confronted him with this issue. "I don't love you"—pretty, wounding words, really, that no one wants to hear no matter how fragile their relationship may seem. Still, I wasn't ready to give up what I was feeling for Adam, and, after a period of falling out of sorts, Adam and I resumed dating one another with the stipulation that he kept the details of his affairs, dates, tricks, and potential other boyfriends (or whatever he calls them) to himself. I had no desire to know of my competition, although I often found our conversations perpetually punctured with clues: "I have a business dinner on Thursday," he once said to me, "and I'll be home too late to call you." Even a housewife in Connecticut could figure out that line.

And so Adam's *triple* life sometimes reminds me of my own double life—my constant search in recent weeks for another date so I won't take dating Adam too seriously until he's ready for some sort of commitment. In the last month I've had something close to twenty blind dates—the product of being set up by a few friends, answering personal ads, and punching buttons on the phone lines. All these other dates, while I'm feeling serious about someone, goes against everything I believe in, of course—I've always seen myself as the one-guy sort-of-guy, and one bad blind date after another led me only, of course, to re-evaluate the needs and desire of my own life and relationships. I have been consciously an open gay man now for close to twenty of my thirty-nine years; I have had boyfriends, friends, fuck buddies, tricks, and anonymous encounters—I've gone to discos, clubs, bars, baths, beaches, meat racks, glory holes, sex orgies, and even had international phone sex. And I've lost, thus far, over these twenty some-odd years, dozens of friends, lovers, boyfriends, peers, and co-workers. And what I've been left with is a looming and ever-present sense of survivor's guilt. What I want right now in my life is not so much a respite from the politically correct gay life, nor even a hiatus from gay life, but instead a serious committed relationship within it—a no holds barred monogamy sort of thing, really.

I'd been in this position many times before. It wasn't an issue of expecting my boyfriend to be monogamous, but both of us being monogamous. Why should I want and expect and make a commitment to someone, if they are not treating me the same way?

Monogamy, so it seems, is a controversial issue within the gay community. Every one of my closest friends advised me to get out of my relationship with Adam when I mentioned that he was messing around with other men. We were, after all, living in the age of sexually transmitted diseases and viruses, they all reminded me, and if I was sleeping with someone who was continually sleeping with someone else, wasn't I continually putting myself at risk? But monogamy, I have also learned from the great gay debates, is also not something I should *want* or *expect* as a gay man—pretty much an impossible goal in any gay relationship—and I know this not just from myself and my own previous relationship examples, but from the stories I hear from friends and friends-of-friends. Regardless of all the stories in the gay press about how much monogamy is in these days, especially in gay relationships, especially because of AIDS and the transmission of HIV—don't believe it. It's another urban myth, as refutable as the fact that all gay men today practice safe sex. Yet I do expect a relationship to have some sort of fidelity and trust embedded within it before it evolves into an open one. If not, what is its purpose? Isn't a relationship supposed to make you feel good? Isn't one of its purposes to provide a source of comfort and joy? Who needs to be aggravated all the time because your boyfriend is too busy to see you because he is out looking for a better boyfriend?

Don't let anyone mislead you. Sex is tantamount in urban gay life—which is why I noticed, roaming through Bleckner's canvases that day, the cruisy crowd of gay men on view in the museum. After years of being a single gay male living in Manhattan my eyes are trained to seek out other gay men passing, cruising, pausing to look at one another and there, that afternoon in the Guggenheim, the population of gay men was as thriving as any street in Greenwich Village on a Saturday night. It is no wonder, then, that the tourists on view were more interesting than the art itself; in fact, I found much of Bleckner's work vague and mysterious. For a painter who is gay, Bleckner's paintings are highly asexual. A gay presence, style, and sensibility is absent from even his densest and most lush paintings. What gay man, after all, could hold his head up proudly and say he painted *stripes*? Nonetheless, Bleckner has been able to successfully capture the melancholy that haunts the gay American panorama of the last two decades.

Adam, however, is unamused at this bleak view of life, and, by the time we reach the spiral's tip, he seems almost belligerent to that fact. The trip to the Guggenheim was at my suggestion; after fifteen years of living in the city I had never visited this museum, and the prospect of the outing clearly intrigued Adam, as well, when I mentioned it. One of our first dates was a Saturday afternoon auction at Sotheby's where Adam bid on several prints by Sultan, Katz, and Lichtenstein and which now hang in his new river-view apartment. But Adam is clearly drawn to a more Sixties pop-art style of painting than Bleckner's bleak and blurry vision. Adam does note, however, a distinct sort of pretentiousness in some of Bleckner's work, and I agree with him on certain cases, especially the paintings hanging in the top floor of the Tower—the dull gray stripes of the "Unknown Quantities of Light" series and the throbbing images of "Yellow Hearts," "Hands," and "Faces."

As we wind our way back down the rotunda ramp, ready to leave the exhibit, we notice we have somehow missed viewing the Tower 5 gallery and we head in its direction. Entering, I note the somber trophy like urn of "Memorial" that is hanging by the entrance. Once inside this gallery I am immediately aware that this room is an attempt to create an AIDS memorial. Among the paintings exhibited here are "Light and Dark World," with its urn and lily-covered pond, "Recover," with its floating hand blotched by a maroon lesion grasping a beam of light, and "One Day Fever," with its ghostly pair of legs ascending to some unforeseen heaven.

Adam, however, has had enough, and instead of concentrating on the paintings he begins telling me about his son's grades in high school. Jake, Adam's fourteen-year-old son, is now in ninth grade, but is not earning high enough marks to get into Stanford or Harvard, where Adam wants him to go. As Adam begins telling me that he earns too much money for Jake to be given a scholarship, I am drawn to an ethereal painting that covers almost the entire back wall of the gallery. The painting, called "Falling Birds," has a rich deep blue background with a series of pale blue birds in various stages of falling flight. If there is a masterpiece amongst these collected works in the Guggenheim, this would be my choice. It is both transfixing and startling—something beautiful in its tragedy and tragic in its beauty.

Is the power of art drawn from how it reflects or refracts your life? If that is so, there is no doubt that Bleckner's paintings summon up my own emotional baggage. Is the success of art, then, a collaborative process between artist and viewer? I know little about the art of art except what or how it impresses or moves me emotionally. Emotional involvement, in fact, I have often found a necessary guideline within my own writing. A few days before Adam and I went to the Guggenheim, a man I had been clandestinely dating read a copy of my book. Finishing it, he commented on the romantic view of gay life presented within in it, something that he did not entirely find realistic to himself. "I didn't move to Manhattan for romance," he said to me as he attempted to discuss some of the subjects I had covered in my writing. This guy had arrived to the city not long after I did, in the late Seventies, and what he came for was clearly not love or romance, but sex. But he had survived the epidemic thus far, just as I had, and found himself that day, however, wanting the same thing that I had wanted all along—a long-term relationship.

I suppose, then, that's how I've come to define my life—the tragic romantic in search of unconditional love—something that I know, as a realist, however, that I will also never attain from anyone, and especially not from Adam. It's impossible not to realize, as you age beyond your thirtysomething years, that human love is inevitably imperfect and uncertain. Adam, after all, fooled around on his wife with other men during the years of their marriage—so wouldn't it make sense that he would do the same in any type of relationship we were destined to have together ourselves? But it is also clearer to me now at this age and in this decade, often after reviewing my own sexual and emotional history, that it is difficult for me to have such a casual view toward sex, that loving and being loved are the purposes of my sexuality, not, as many gay men believe or *want to believe*, the pursuit of sex. So it's no surprise to me as I turned away from this Bleckner painting of tragic and beautiful flight and back to Adam and his concerns of his son, that I felt a wistfulness overcome me as we left the room. Bleckner's work is about longing, not happiness, about loneliness and alienation. It's no wonder that I have often felt lonelier dating and falling in love with someone than I ever felt when I wasn't seeing anyone. Could that be because I define my life through how others see me, instead of how I view it myself?

We stop in the museum shop downstairs and look at souvenirs, Adam fascinated by a book on floor plans of Manhattan apartment buildings. Lately, I've become so conscious of the things I buy when I am with Adam, fearful of attaching too much sentiment to them if things do not work out between us, that they will only cause me too much sadness and heartache to keep. But a snow globe of the Guggenheim Museum catches my attention and I'm instantly impelled to add it to my collection of others I have found from around the world. As I lift it up and shake it a thought moves into my mind—how lucky it is to just meet someone you want to date more than once—how difficult even that is to accomplish if you're gay and my age and living in a city such as Manhattan.

I decide to buy the snow globe, and as I do I notice Adam looking at me from the back of the gift shop. On the sidewalk, walking across the east side toward Adam's apartment, it is my turn to steal glances at him as we reach corners or stoplights or as the conversation warrants. Adam's face, I find in this cool wintry afternoon light, is more handsome to me now than the evening seven months ago when I first met him after I decided to go to the Townhouse for a drink after seeing a movie alone—a face that possesses its own history, I have also come to understand.

It would be easy for me now to list Adam's faults, to convince myself out of this relationship, for I know more about him than his face would ordinarily show me if I were a stranger. But I'm also a guy who doesn't give up easily. Nor does Adam. The three times I have broken things off between us he has pushed them back together. And the fact is, I fell for Adam for the way he, too, first looked to me: well-groomed, well-dressed, with a penchant for Barney's suits and button-down shirts, He is my height but has a more stocky build, which I both admire and enjoy. In all, I find him a handsome but not too threateningly-so kind of man. I have always felt that he looked like the type of guy a guy could settle down with, if settling down was what they were both after. And so that, I guess, searching for the reflections of us together in the glass store windows that we pass on this misty Manhattan Saturday, is something that I must continually learn and relearn—that the dynamics of a relationship flow out of the history and interaction of *both* of its players, and like art, is continually shaped by the vision of its beholder.

DICKS

I'll begin with Bill Tyler because he was the first man who wanted to put his dick in my ass that I let do it. He was broad-shouldered, balding, closer to forty when I was closer to twenty, and had lips like Ricky Nelson. His dick was wide and chubby and looked like it should have a nickname. I think I got him inside of me for all of a few seconds before the pain overwhelmed me and I made him take it out. It never occurred to me that this was something I might have to practice at. Bill told me it didn't matter, but I knew it did. I caught him at the end of one long relationship and before the start of another.

I lied. Bill wasn't the first. The first man who actually wanted to put his dick into my ass and that I half-let do it was a Brazilian man I met at a bar in Greenwich Village. It was near closing time on a Saturday night (which meant it was really *very* early Sunday morning) and we had cruised each other all night but wasted our time trying to interest other guys. The Brazilian had a lean, bronzed body, dark wiry hair at his armpits and groin, and a dick like a serpent—long and slender with a slightly wider head. Somehow I knew he would be gone as soon as he came, which is why he didn't get inside for very long and I tend to forget I even met him.

Hank once told a friend of mine that I was the best sex he ever had. His dick is lost to me now, but I do remember his body—short, stocky, covered with fur—the kind of body I would find myself easily drawn to over and over. I somehow believed that if I was passionate and involving in bed with Hank that he would be passionate and involving out of bed. I was twenty-nine the year I first slept with him. I repeated this mistake many times.

Glenn had a dick the size and shape of a beer can. We dated a few times but when I went over to his apartment, he wouldn't take his T-shirt off during sex because he didn't want me to see the rash that covered his chest. He was the first guy I slept with that I ever suspected might be HIV-positive. Neither of us stayed interested in one another long enough for me to find out if that was the case.

Teddy told me up front that he was positive. I met him in the rain at the AIDS walk. He had a long, lean physique, a dark full beard, and a voice as deep and majestic as an old English actor. I took him back to my apartment to dry out and wanted desperately for him to show me his dick but he wouldn't. We played around in our underwear a couple of times. My imagination about the size and shape of his dick can still make me hard.

Max had no problems showing me his dick or telling me he was positive. I met him at a bar on the Upper East Side of Manhattan. He was close to fifty when I met him and in incredible shape—a fat free body corded with veins and muscle. His dick was bigger than Michelangelo's David but not quite the powertool belonging to Jeff Stryker. He wanted one night and that's what he got.

Jeff's most unusual feature was his whole genital package. His dick and balls looked larger because of vitiligo, a skin condition of pink and brown patches. It swirled like a palomino around his shaft and discolored his left ball. He courted me from California, flying in on the red-eye and calling me to meet him at his hotel near Times Square. The novelty of his cock and balls wore off quickly when he opened his mouth. He didn't know how to sublimate his personality to his body's natural work of art.

Adam was more proud of his dick than any of his other body parts. He once paid a photographer fifty bucks to take a picture of it. In my history of cock it was nothing spectacular, though I had it more times than I've had any other (except for my own).

It was a fleshy pink tube with no sign of a circumcision scar. It's most unusual feature was that when it was hard it was really no larger than it was soft. Unfortunately, I gave up rent-stabilized Manhattan real estate to keep it around. I suppose that now makes me the bigger dick.

LESSONS

There was a time in my life when I became a virgin again. It was during a period when a lot of things were going wrong, or, rather, a lot of people were disappearing without saying good-bye, and those who weren't disappearing were afraid that they would be disappearing soon themselves, and so, instead of waiting to see if I was going to vanish as well, I sequestered myself. I drew those willowy pink chenille curtains of mine closed, locked those over-painted louvered window gates up tighter than a chastity belt and decided to hide in the dark away from it all until it was safe to go back out in the sunlight again. It never really got safe again. Things never really got better but I learned how to adjust; I learned to peek through the slats, and to wear sunglasses and hats and whatever other protective gear I could get my body into when I went outside. Then one day I found myself no longer fretting about my self-imposed exile and back out in the sun again—in Sheep Meadow in Central Park carelessly sunbathing with my shirt off, without even putting on sunblock—and falling in love with a married man who was trying to fall out of love with his wife.

It was a complicated relationship for us both right from the start. Even though those gates of mine had been closed so long the locks were rusty, I was still standing outside my closet. He, alas, was hidden within his. But none of this hampered what happened between us in bed. In fact, that's how the relationship blossomed. Soon enough we began experimenting and I discovered that his greatest desire was for me to teach him how to become a bottom, or, in more technical terms, how to become "the passive partner who receives the penetration of a male's penis." And I became more than a willing coach, never one to shy away from the kind of muscular, beefcake ass he possessed. I spent hours getting that sphincter of his to relax, lubing up a small butt plug until he was comfortable with holding it inside his ass, then progressing to a slender dildo, then gradually moving up to a larger one, then a wider one, until one day we reached the point when he was ready to take my cock up his ass. I remember thinking at the time that if someone had given me that sort of time and attention, I would have no desire to find another boyfriend. I'd want to get married.

I should have realized this was too fun to last. Once my boyfriend had mastered my cock, it wasn't long before he wanted instead to play top to my bottom. The only problem was, he wasn't interested in giving me the same time and attention I had given him, nor was he interested in giving up being a bottom, either. Like I said, it was a complicated relationship—I was out and he was in and he wanted to be in and out with other guys. I never had the chance to switch from top to bottom with him, because we were too quickly switching between other partners and fighting too much about our positions. But he wasn't the only guy I had dated who, well, wanted to flip me over.

I should probably admit now that to many men I seem like the ideal bottom—boyish-looking and short, I don't even weigh in at 150 pounds—which is why I get such a delicious personal pleasure out of turning the tables and demanding that I be a top with all of these hunky macho guys who expect me to roll over and play bottom for them. But the truth is, even though I looked boyish and my boyfriend wasn't really my boyfriend anymore, by this time I wasn't really boyish any longer. I suppose this is a roundabout way of saying that I wasn't getting any younger. And, as community folklore has it, after so much time goes by, those closed gates soon look like a boarded-up wall; if you want to open the window, you have to start over again and knock out a hole to see the sun. So here I was a virgin again after all these years of isolation and waiting for the right guy to knock my window open.

And the real truth: I was a single and unattached aging gay man yearning for love. What I wanted was to find a better man than the kind I usually met, and one of the methods I thought might help me in my personal quest would be to, well, make myself more versatile in the bedroom department. Knock my own gate down before someone else hit a brick wall.

Not long after I reached that insight I began perusing the personals to meet my dream man, a habit I had gravitated to for years and years and years, whenever I felt the dating pool had grown too shallow. I picked up newspapers and magazines at the bars, the community center, the bookstore, the newsstand—wherever I could find ones that carried men-for-men personals. At home I would sit at my desk with a red felt-tip pen poised in my hand, ready to circle the most desirable ones. No matter how many personals I circled and notated in the "Romance Only" or "Let's Date" sections, I always seemed to gravitate to the "Raunch and Kink" or "Sex Only" sections, fascinated by the obsessive nature of so many gay men and at the same time frustrated that so many guys were looking for such specific requirements, and knowing, really, that my nature would most likely preclude any visits to the kinkier sides of gay life. The only thing I had ever desired of a perfect sexual encounter was to give as much pleasure to my partner as I wanted him to provide me. And that didn't necessarily include smelly jockstraps or foot worship, though it also didn't rule them out.

And so one particularly lonely and forlorn day, this ad caught my eye:

BUTT PLAY 101
Let me teach you how to enjoy your ass and asshole. I will show you how to experience ultimate pleasure from the space between your legs

.

I must confess now that I had never answered a sexual ad before. Yes, I read them and mulled them over, but I only circled and called the romantic, dream date ones. As for sex, because I'd always found enough action at the bars or the clubs or on the street—or from the dating ads—I hadn't ever needed to turn to the "Sex Only" personals as an outlet. My goal was to find a worthwhile long-term relationship or at least someone who would stick around after the third date, not someone who only wanted to stick his sticky fingers up my butt to get his rocks off. Nonetheless, I circled the ad, partly nostalgic over my lost boyfriend and partly curious about whether I should really consider a new method to snare a new one. A few days later, when I was leaving voice mail messages for all of my potential dream dates, I decided, *Oh, well, what the hell, let's respond to the butt player as well.*

None of my Perfect Husbands responded, but the butt player did. Our short, introductory phone conversation went something like this:

"So you're into butt play?" he asked.

"Not really," I replied.

"You ever had anything up your ass before?" he asked.

"Not in a while."

"I've helped a lot of beginners," he said.

"I'm not exactly a beginner," I stated, "just starting over."

"Boyfriend?" he asked.

"Not anymore."

"I can see you Sunday at nine," he said. His voice was cheerless and perfunctory, making it seem as if I had called to make a doctor's appointment for a shot of penicillin. Yet it was exactly this sexless, clinical exchange that made it so easy for me to accept his offer.

"Okay," I answered. We talked a few minutes more. He told me his address and that his name was Joey. He admitted that he was in his early fifties and had gray and black salt-and-pepper hair. As I hung up, I reminded myself that this was a learning experience—he was going to teach me to be a bottom, or at least teach me to be a *better* bottom. Henry Higgins wasn't exactly the perfect man for Eliza Doolittle when they met, either, you know.

* * *

I arrived at Joey's apartment nervous and tipsy and more than fifteen minutes late, which (even on gay median time) is more than a rude way to begin an association. I had indulged in a glass of wine at the bar on the corner of Joey's street, a trendy little smoke-filled, artsy-fartsy place with skinny women in black dresses and guys in dark T-shirts and gold hoop earrings. As I gulped down the last third of my drink, I had reminded myself that this wasn't a date. This guy didn't advertise in the "Looking for Love" section, and I wasn't expecting Joey to be my Mr. Goodbar. He was only Mr. Chips, after all, and I could leave him as soon as he taught me, uh, well, how to enjoy the pleasure of a man's penetration.

"Want something to drink?" he asked as he ushered me into his apartment. My distress must have clearly shown on my face at that moment. Joey was more like sixty than fifty, and his salt-and-pepper hair was an unshaven beard. Otherwise, he was bald as a cue ball, with a puffy face that looked like a sandbag that had been punched and hadn't regained its shape. He was slightly shorter than me but more than three hundred pounds overweight, a fact he hadn't mentioned on the phone. He was dressed in the kind of light, blousy outfit that, when worn by street people, makes you immediately cross to the other side of the street. If he had not lived in one of those high-tech, luxury apartments that always seem to end up photographed in *Metropolitan Home* or the Thursday section of the *Times*, I would have turned around and left, because this potential dreamboat more closely resembled my worst nightmare.

I should probably add that the Sunday night I arrived at Joey's apartment, it was a warm, misty late spring evening that seemed to possess more humidity and mugginess than actual raindrops or heat. I stood in his doorway holding a moist umbrella, my split ends growing into an afro. I felt old and troll-like myself at that moment; I was conscious I was standing on a clean beige carpet, worried that I had brought with me all the urban dirt and soot and grime I had carefully tried to avoid out on the street. Joey's apartment was clearly more showplace than home. The smell from flowers in a crystal vase on a table near where I stood wafted up to my nose as I shook myself out of my damp jacket. The vestibule where I stood frozen like a rescued stray dog opened up into a living room entirely decorated in beige—a sofa and matching wing chairs were upholstered in a neutral, beige fabric; prints of blank beige-colored squares framed by beige wood were hung on a beige-painted wall; a shiny beige lamp rested on a shiny beige end table.

"Any wine?" I asked Joey as he led me to the sofa. I took a seat cautiously, resting my derriere lightly on the edge of a cushion as if I were going to leap out of the room at any instant, because I was embarrassed at shedding particles of dust into the immaculate surroundings. Beside me, a beige coffee table jutted out close to my knees, empty except for several *Playbills* arranged in the shape of a fan.

"Red or white?" he asked.

"Whatever's open," I answered.

During our entire greeting and exchange, Joey was beaming as if a Christmas gift had just walked through the door. I sat waiting for him to return, feeling like I had played this game a million times and was too old and tired to try it again tonight with an ancient schlumper.

"I loved this show," I said, trying to deflect my discomfort when Joey returned with a glass of wine that looked more beige than white. I reached over and plucked a *Playbill* out of the arrangement, the fan quickly disintegrating into an unorganized mess. As I lamely tried to straighten it up, the thought occurred to me: murderers don't like show tunes—do they? And wasn't Joey too old to be a murderer anyway? Isn't it usually the wealthy sixty-year-old man who is found with his throat slashed the next morning? Joey seemed unperturbed by the mess I had made on his coffee table. In fact, he seemed to be amused by my nervous stumbling about; when I looked up I noticed he was smiling, his mouth widening to reveal a set of conspicuously fake beige teeth.

"The dancing was terrific," he said, "but the music was abysmal." He waved his hand in the air on his last word, as if shooing away a fly, but then he started telling me about a theatrical wig maker he knew who worked backstage and as the gossip flew from his mouth, his hand waved back and forth like a flag flapping in the wind on Independence Day.

I didn't really mind all the talk about the theater; I was grateful for any distraction from the matter at hand. We sat and kibitzed about a lighting designer stepping out of his boundaries to become a director and a composer known for his S&M tendencies. In fact, we talked so long about the theater that I completely forgot the reason why I was there in the first place. Joey was becoming a friend, not a potential teacher, and his fuzzy potato head no longer looked as if it belonged to a derelict. I could see the honesty in his face even if I couldn't imagine him successfully pleasuring my ass. But then Joey abruptly ended the conversation, leaning over and saying, "Well, shall we get started?" Suddenly his wrists were no longer limp; one hand was firmly placed against my shoulder, the other reaching around to remove my empty glass from the coffee table.

"Uh, sure," I answered, not really certain I wanted to go through with it.

"You can leave your clothes on the chair," he said, as a doctor might before leaving a patient alone in an examining room. In fact, Joey did leave me alone in the room while he carried away the empty glass, but he returned by the time I had managed to rise from the couch and fumble with the buttons on my shirt. Joey walked to a set of louvered doors that I had thought was a closet, but opened, they revealed a full-size bed built into a small nook that must have once been a laundry room. Along the bottom of the bed was a row of drawers built into the frame and Joey opened the middle drawer and began pulling out an assortment of items: a pair of latex gloves, a box of condoms, an industrial-sized bottle of lubricant, four or five different-sized dildos, none of which, I felt certain, I could possibly accommodate, a box of baby wipes and a plastic mat, which he unfolded and placed on top of the beige bedspread. I was deliberately taking my time with my clothes, folding and refolding them as he moved swiftly about his little alcove. Finally, he turned and looked at me standing sheepishly in my underwear and T-shirt.

"I sterilize all the dildos in the dishwasher," he said, as if that were my most crucial concern about sticking a giant object up my ass.

"The dishwasher?" I responded, flabbergasted by a mental image of a row of dildos sitting straight up in a car wash. The next thing I knew I was standing behind him staring at the paraphernalia spread out on the bed, all of it for the sole purpose of entertaining my ass. Things had never seemed this complicated when I played the same game with my ex-boyfriend. But that was the difference, wasn't it? I reminded myself. It had been a game with my boyfriend. This was a lesson.

"And I always use condoms on the dildos," he said, patting the plastic mat. "Take your shorts off and sit up here." Joey seemed to realize as he said this that there was hardly room for me to sit on the bed because of all his equipment, and he started rearranging things to make a space for me, or, worse, for *us*. I realized the moment I dropped my briefs that I should have thought twice before agreeing to all of this. Was I that desperate to learn how to enjoy my ass? Shouldn't I have really concentrated on finding a boyfriend *first*? I looked down at my cock and noticed it appeared smaller and more frightened than I had seen it in years.

"Have you had many responses to your ad?" I asked when I was seated on the edge of the bed, shifting myself onto the mat. Somehow Joey was already completely undressed and I was amazed to see that his body looked no different than when he had been wearing his billowy outfit: it was as lumpy and wavy as beige fabric that had been sat on all day. The only difference between his body and his clothing was the gold Hebrew symbol dangling from a chain around his neck now visible against the sparse, gray fluff of his chest. And his erection, of course: his small, slender dick popped straight out at me like a breadstick misplaced in an Easter basket.

"Nope," he said. "You're my first. I just placed the ad last week."

Great, I thought, *a virgin again. And a guinea pig.*

* * *

But it was then that the lesson began. Or life unfolded. Isn't that what teaching is all about? The passing of knowledge gained not so much on one subject but after the cumulative experiences of many years.

"When I first met my lover I was strictly a top," Joey said. I was on my back with my legs bent and my knees pulled to my chest. "I wasn't interested in somebody sticking something inside me, because all I wanted to do was to stick something myself, you know? Then, after we were together for about four years, we started changing roles. He didn't always want to be the bottom so I experimented with it some and decided I liked it, and we changed roles. He was the top and I was the bottom. That lasted for a few more years and then he decided he wanted to be the bottom again. That's when we started getting all this stuff," he said, waving his hand at his assortment of dildos.

"I think that's more than I can handle," I said, twisting my body to look at the smallest dildo, which in my estimation was about twelve inches long and eight inches wide.

"You think so? We'll see."

Joey had positioned himself at the end of the bed, a plump round period to my wavy exclamation point. He lifted one of my legs and rested it against his shoulder. The next thing I knew, his wet gloved finger was in my rectum and I could feel him twiddling my prostate gland. I leaned up to watch his hand inside me, expecting him to say at any point, "Scalpel," or "Sutures," but instead he said, "You're very tight."

I nodded, wishing there were some music playing or somebody kissing me or a video being shown or, better yet, that I had another glass of beige wine in my hand. Instead, all

I heard was Joey beginning to breathe harder, like someone with asthma. I lay back down, the mat crinkling as my skin pressed against it. I closed my eyes and tried to imagine myself a thousand miles away, but instead heard the *slumpf, slumpf, slumpf* of Joey pumping more lubricant out of a bottle and into his hand and then into my ass.

"It's the small ones that are the hardest, you know," he said.

I leaned my head up again and looked at him in surprise. "It's the truth. It's all about stretching. The walls don't stretch that much with the tiny ones. The big ones force you to relax in order to accommodate them. Give me a big, fat dick any day. It's so much easier to manage and it's a lot more fun." He started laughing, a high-pitched hiccup that started in the back of his throat and ended with the quivering of his shoulders and saggy chest.

It was such an odd moment from someone I had heretofore regarded as a clinical, professional worker. "It's all about relaxing, you know," he said, still chuckling. "Once you learn how to relax those muscles down there you can take a football."

The thought of a football up my ass was definitely unappealing, and I pumped a swipe of lube from the bottle and wrapped the oily palm of my hand around my cock, trying to force myself to become harder. Above me, I heard Joey gasp.

"What's wrong?" I asked.

"Ahh, why did you do that?" he asked.

"Do what?" I asked, shocked.

"I wanted to suck your dick. Now I can't take it in my mouth. And you have such a beautiful dick."

"Ohhh," I said, sorry, really sorry, that he hadn't acted quicker. "Thank you," I added, feeling like the moronic pupil who has disappointed the teacher.

Next, he took a slender dildo I hadn't noticed before, the kind I had once used on my ex-boyfriend, lubed it up, and inserted it into my ass. It went in easily, though I could feel the walls of my ass caving into the dildo instead of it stretching them further. "You've been practicing," he said.

"Not really. Those Kegel exercises don't work for me."

"Oh sure they do," he said. "You're just uptight. What're you so nervous about?"

Life, I thought. I'm nervous because I'm still alive after all these years. The only thing that worked out for me was that I didn't die when everyone else did.

"Open your eyes," he said and lightly slapped my chest.

I could feel the residue of lube where his hand had grazed my skin.

"I'm not going to hurt you," he said. "I won't do anything you don't want me to do. You can trust me. After a few lessons, you'll be able to take King Dong over there."

"King Dong?"

"The super-deluxe double-headed one," he said, nodding at the giant dildo with a cock head on each end. "My boyfriend and I used to play with that one a lot. There was a time when we were both bottoms. Come to think of it, there was a time when everyone in the city was a bottom. It sure was difficult to find a top some nights."

I gave him a smile and leaned back and started pumping my cock again. I felt myself growing thicker and he took the slender dildo out of my ass and lubed up a wider and longer one. Before I knew it, it was inside my ass, and I was rock hard, pumping my cock and arching my back away from the mat. And then I suddenly felt a decade younger, and a memory washed over me of a man I had dated on Fire Island. Joey bent my legs and rubbed my thighs just as the man had. He kept the dildo far up inside me and cupped my balls and rubbed them with his slippery hands. Then he reached up and twisted my left nipple.

"The first time I was fucked, my boyfriend was so impatient that he made me bleed," Joey said. "I turned him into a great lover, though. Then he left me. Then he came back. Said he couldn't find anyone better in bed. Oh, he could find others to have sex with, don't get me wrong. But none of them had my touch. It worked for both of us though. He made me feel so beautiful."

Joey was breathing hard through his mouth by now, and he moaned and moved one hand to my cock and stroked it as he returned to lightly pushing the dildo in and out of my ass. "That okay?" he asked.

I nodded back at him.

"I miss him," Joey said. "He died about three years ago."

He stopped pushing the dildo in and out of me and pulled himself up out of his hunched over position. "That doesn't bother you, does it? Everything we're doing is safe."

I nodded again that it was all right to continue. I was aware that we hadn't kissed each other, aware that not a single drop of body fluid had been exchanged between us. No tears. No sweat. As I looked at Joey's face as he worked over my ass and cock, alternating one hand between stroking his cock and my own, I realized he had survived, as I had, but his road might have been more difficult than my own. I sensed that the puffiness bloating his face was not entirely due to the ravages of aging but likely came from medication or the overuse of alcohol.

But I also realized he was enjoying his task. Obviously, he had taken out the ad because he enjoyed sticking something up a guy's butt, enjoyed giving a guy pleasure this way; perhaps this was his fantasy, his fetish, the scene he wanted to play—older teacher instructing the younger pupil. The thought of it made me smile and the delight surged through me like a jolt of electricity. I felt my body finally become sensitive to his touch. My first shot came with a wave of release, replaced almost immediately by a flood of tension and pressure and then a second shot into Joey's waiting palm.

Before he had a chance to remove the dildo from my ass or wipe my come from his hand, I reached up and gave his cock a few quick pumps with my slick, hollowed fist. He came instantly, his come spurting over my wrist and onto the mat with a plop, plop, plop. He laughed as he caught his breath. "Thank you," he said.

Thank you, I repeated in my mind, embarrassed that he had thanked me for letting him fuck me with a dildo and quickly jerking him off. As I dried myself off with the baby wipes and paper towels, it occurred to me that teaching was such a selfless act. In that way it bore a striking resemblance to being in love—wanting to do something for someone else without the expectation or need of anything being returned. You don't expect someone to thank you. Lovers can be the best teachers. And teachers can be the best lovers, too. But I was aware that my encounter with Joey had not been without a certain level of self-absorption and self-need. His. And mine. Joey had knocked a window out in my wall for me. And I liked to think I might have brought in a little sunlight for him.

When I was dressed and standing at the door in my still damp jacket, Joey held his hand out for me to shake. Instead of taking it, I leaned over and kissed him on his fuzzy cheek. He smiled and held the door open for me. As I stepped outside, I realized that I had revealed little of myself other than the intimacy of my body. I hadn't even told him about *my* ex-boyfriend. But it was already too late; I felt myself headed back into my shuttered, private little world. Before he closed the door behind me, I turned back and said, "Thank you. It was fun."

And then I was back out on the street again, slapping my tennis shoes against the puddles of water like a teenager, eager to be a teacher again.

GLASSES

The job starts it, of course, not the job but the lack of a job, or, rather, the lack of a career, not that I have a lack of a career—I know what I want to do, it's just that I can't make a living doing it because I have to work at a job and not a career but the problem is not everyone believes that my career is a career, after all, not even a job, really, because when you deconstruct the problem, I mean, who reads gay fiction, you know, everyone says now it's a limited market and now it's shrinking not growing, but that's not what makes me fill the glass—not the state of the art or, rather, the lack of the art, the lack of the state of gay literature, it's the fact that I don't have the time to work at it anyway and try to make it better, or, at least, my output of it better, and even when I can find the time, squeezing a half-hour here, ten minutes there, I can't find the energy to do it anymore because all I want to do is escape from it because it's become so hard to do now because I am always studying it or searching for a different story to tell and then when I work it all out in my head there's the time and the energy obstacles again and then I come home from the job-that-is-not-my career and all I want to do is relax and get away from the idea of that job-that-is-not-my-career and that's when I pour the first glass even when I know I should be at least be reading something even if I am not writing anything so as soon as I take the sip from the glass and feel a tiny little explosion of relaxation in my brain that's when I try to go through the mail, to at least feel like I am accomplishing something, but the bills pull me down and I end up looking through one of the new catalogs or brochures for vacations and items I can't afford which, of course, is the basis of one of the other problems, the problem that leads me to refill the glass again and sip some more even as the dizziness lets me dream that I can escape and take a vacation which will get me out of this lousy four-wall box of an apartment that has no view even though the view is not what is the lousiest thing about this apartment, what's the lousiest is that the hot water doesn't work when I need it to, the windows don't lock, the electricity goes out even though this apartment is more money than the apartment I lived in before this one but at least in that apartment I didn't have to blame anyone for the crap except myself because it was a cheap, lousy apartment instead of an expensive, lousy box imitating an apartment that I always have to work and work and work to pay the rent for every month because nothing in this life is easy anymore, you know, not even finding a trick is easy but that's not because I'm not trying, it's because I've burned out on that too, not really tricking, but on trying to make conversation to initiate the trick, because it all seems so futile, you know, not the tricking because if I wanted to I could get someone and I could do it, sex is never difficult to find in this city, it's just that I've done all that before for years and years and years and now I want something else, something different, a relationship, but even the quest for that has left me bone dry because I am trying so hard to make it work with that married-man-who can't-make-a-commitment who started me on all this heavy sipping in the first place because we do it together, or, rather, I do it with him because he likes to do it on the nights when we're together, to help him fall asleep, or so he says, and I do it to be with him and not alone in my lousy, expensive apartment, but what happens, of course, is he begins to show his honesty while he is sipping, because the saying is true, after all, a drunken man's words are a sober man's thoughts, and he begins to unravel the problems which he has with our relationship while I sip from my glass, and, you know, in all honesty, after all these years, it isn't the idea that he wants to date other guys that really pisses me off so much it is his dishonesty of trying to cover it up for such a long time, you know, because I knew he was doing it long before he admitted it, of course, but the wounding part is not so much his desire to see other guys—okay, I've accepted that we have an open relationship—what really pisses me off are the put-downs about my weight, my hairline, and lack of money and the fact that he doesn't think I have a real job and a real career because I can't even pay a month's rent, but I have to tell you, after all these years of hearing him say this over and over like a broken record I could care shit about the other guys, let them deal with him, but the problem is now that I can't pull myself away from him because at least we are having sex and at least I am not alone in that tiny-box-imitating-an-apartment, and at least he supplies enough booze for me to drink and escape him, too, you know, even though I was using him to escape my cheap, lousy apartment and my job-that-is-not-a-career and the fact that I want to drink more than I want to write because what has happened is that I am so tired of pretending I want to be somewhere else when what I really want is to just get a decent night's sleep and not to have to admit to anyone that I now have this problem on top of all the other problems, at least asleep I don't have to pretend I want to escape that, too, you know.

THE POT

The truth is I didn't steal the pot. My roommate, John, left it behind when he moved out of the Manhattan apartment we shared to return to Washington to take care of his mom. It was a particularly rough time for me as well. It was the late 1980s and I was taking care of a friend who was dying from AIDS, spending most of my evenings sleeping at my friend's apartment in case he needed help in the middle of the night. The pot was full of hundreds of pennies, which is the reason why John left it behind; he didn't have the energy to empty it out and had no idea what to do with all those pennies. After my friend died, I spent an evening rolling the pennies into paper wrappers and the next day deposited them in my checking account. Not much later, I moved out of town myself. Over the following ten years the pot moved with me from country to city, state to state, and apartment to apartment. I only recently rediscovered the pot, which now sits empty on the windowsill of my small Clinton apartment, when I had to move it to install an air-conditioner.

It's not a beautiful pot. It's certainly not at all valuable or an heirloom or an antique or has any other value except an emotional one, which is the reason why I have never thrown it away. Technically, it could hold about two quarts of water and its shape is more like a sports trophy than a vase—wider at the base than at the neck and with two winglike handles near the top lip. It should have been cast out of silver or pewter instead of its rich looking dark red clay. But the clay color is what reminds me most of Georgia, the state where I was born and the place where I first met John when we attended college together. Around the mouth of the pot, just above the winglike handles, four bands are painted: a thick black one framed by two thin white lines at the bottom and one at the top. But it is the design below the handles that captures the attention first: a white and green fossil-like impression of fern leaves that spread out from the cream-colored outline of four petals of a flower, the center stamen nothing but a beautiful, light blue dollop of paint. On top of all this is a sugary glaze coating, reminiscent of the kind usually dripped over the sides of a pound cake, but which makes the clay surface of the pot slick to the touch instead of rough.

Given the strange shape of the pot, I have used it to hold a number of things over the years: sunglasses, stamps, business cards, envelopes, keys. One year, when I rented a cottage in Pennsylvania, it served as a perfect ornament atop a black cast-iron potbellied stove. After I moved back into Manhattan, its most frequent function has been as a humidifier during the winter months, its deep cavity filled with water as it sat atop a progression of radiators in overheated tenement apartments.

The thing that I distinctly remember it holding was John's smoking paraphernalia when we lived together off-campus while attending Emory University. After class, John would retreat to his room, turn on his stereo, and reach into the pot for his small, black ceramic pipe and matches and the stash of marijuana he kept in a clear plastic bag rolled into the shape of a tube. Lying on his bed he would unravel the plastic bag, pinch out a portion of the marijuana, and sprinkle it into the mesh wire clavicle of the pipe. He'd get the twigs and seeds burning with the scratch of a match and several short, quick breaths. Then he'd lean back against the wall and take a deep toke. Occasionally, I might join him; smoking pot was the boldest thing I think I ever did in college—I had not come out as a gay man, but I was seduced as much by John's lithe, dark-eyed presence as I was by the lure of the music of our generation which he played on the stereo as he smoked: the disco arias of Donna Summer, the harmonies of Abba and the Bee Gees, and my favorite song to listen to stoned, Chuck Mangione's "The Land of Make Believe."

After college I didn't see the pot again for several years. I moved to New York to start graduate school and lived in an expensive apartment in the West Village until I found a cheaper one. John stayed behind in Atlanta and found work as a ballroom dance instructor and went through a brief relationship with another dance teacher. When the relationship ended, John realized he had an itch to see what New York City was all about. So he called me and we shared another apartment, this one a six floor walk-up on Bleecker Street with a shower stall you had to step up into and crouch while using, praying that there might be enough water pressure to send a drizzle out of the nozzle and dribbling to the floor.

I didn't regard the pot that much in those days when we lived together in the heart of the Village. John's bedroom was more like a walk-in closet than a bedroom; he was only able to fit in it the queen-sized bed which he had brought up from Atlanta, so we socialized in my larger bedroom or on the couch we wedged into the living room. John was always withdrawing his pipe and stash in his room, the clay pot tucked away from view beneath the frame of his bed, and carrying his equipment to wherever I happened to be seated in the apartment. He would light up and explain his day to me, the frustrations which he felt from being a data encoder at a marketing firm, and the even more frustrations he felt from trying to find a boyfriend.

I never understood John's frustrations with men, however. Walking down the street together, I was always aware of the stares that he was capable of drawing. Since college John had transformed his coltish physique into one of a budding bodybuilder. What set him apart from all those other clones, I always believed, was an unbelievably small waist which he had inherited from one of his Italian forefathers, a waist that remained thin, thin, thin, even as his shoulders and arms flared to muscular proportions. John was always, even in his skinnier incarnation, a more flamboyant presence than myself, prone to skin-tight styles: spandex shirts that ended before their armpits or waists began and shorts that seemed more suggestive than protective.

And so it wasn't long before John met another boyfriend, or, rather, boyfriend after boyfriend after boyfriend. John and his pumped-up physique were quite a social success in Manhattan. And it was a heady time to be young and beautiful: Charles Ludlum plays, the Saint, and the Chelsea Gym were all part of the city's gay landscape. It wasn't long before he moved out with a hunky blond guy to share a renovated one-bedroom apartment in Chelsea. I wasn't fond of John's new boyfriend—I somehow sensed he looked down on me because I had neither a flat stomach nor big arms—and I was jealous of the attention John was giving him. But another friend from Emory, an actress with a beautiful soprano voice who wanted to land a part in a Broadway musical, was sleeping on our sofa at that time and she moved into John's room. Soon, her chain-smoking girlfriend from Atlanta arrived to share the expenses. Trouble developed, however, when the girlfriend avoided paying rent and adopted a small dog which she house-trained to urinate on a patch of newspapers because the trips up and down the six flights of stairs winded her too easily. My life on Bleecker Street became miserable; I had dropped out of graduate school and was stressed out from a high-pressure public relations job and my own frustrations over men. And the truth was the daily loss of John's friendship had left a void in my life.

John's relationship with his new boyfriend fared no better than mine did with my female roommates. Three weeks after they began to live together, John's boyfriend moved out, announcing his departure, in fact, on the evening of John's thirtieth birthday. John went through several roommates before he called me and asked me to share his Chelsea apartment. It was smaller and more expensive than my Village home, but John's companionship was something I could never turn down. The truth was I was in love with John, had been in love with him since college. But the attraction I felt wasn't simply a lustful one in which sex had to be an ultimate and necessary goal.

John was the guy who brought me out, or, rather, recognized things about me before I recognized them myself. He was my first gay friend. He took me to my first gay bar, eagerly holding my hand as I looked around a club full of mirrors and swirling lights. Our attraction to one another in college was grounded perhaps on something as chemical as lust, but as our friendship grew I couldn't imagine my life without him. And it always seemed to me that John was somehow, in some kind of fashion, returning that same affection.

Not long after we began to live together again in that one-bedroom Chelsea apartment things began to change for John, or, rather, John began to make things change. He decided to enroll in graduate school, and over the next three years, he took evening classes to earn an MBA degree in marketing. Gradually, the pot smoking was no longer a daily necessity, and the red-clay pot found its way to the floor and began to collect pennies. I had several opportunities to move out and live with other guys during these years: some as roommates, others as potential relationships. But the truth was I could not leave John behind, not even as another friend fell sick. John was the best thing that I had going during those untenable times.

I had never had a best friend before I met John in college, and as John's life intersected with mine more and more, the more history we accumulated with one another, he became to seem more like family than friend. Over the years, he has been someone I've wanted to spend holidays and vacations with, the one I call on Thanksgiving and Christmas if he's not close by. After he moved to Washington to tend to his mother I'd visit him when I could afford the trip. Everything, then, came to seem memorable when shared with him, from marshaling together for the March on Washington to taking a boat ride around Manhattan.

And this was how, on a trip to visit me after his mother had died, that John noticed the pot in my apartment. There it was, just as it had been on his last trip, sitting on top of a radiator in my bedroom. John had changed again in that time. His hair was now clipped short into a military buzz cut, and, even though his body was as finely chiseled as it always was, he had developed an affection for clothes with a more subdued preppy look. But in the intervening years he had also matured from his youthful, self-absorbed personality into a more outwardly focused adult. He didn't accuse me of stealing the pot, but I could tell by his confused expression as he first detected the pot and tried to pull all of the pieces of his memory of it together, that he didn't understand how or why it had ended up in my tiny Manhattan apartment. I knew he must have forgotten how he had abandoned it; his mother's illness had proven to be a long, protracted struggle for more than eight years. He must have remembered, though, that he didn't give me the pot, and I offered no explanation about how I had salvaged it and its contents. "I always wondered what happened to that," he said, in a manner that a brother might say about discovering an old shirt in his younger brother's closet. "It's nice to know there's something of me still here," he added, which revealed, of course, the deeper bond of our friendship. And that was when I knew he had no intention of asking for the pot back. But it was also the moment that I recognized that it would always be John's pot and not my own, no matter how long it stayed in my possession.

It's odd how the mind distorts the memory over time. I'd always remembered John's pot in his bedroom of our college apartment and had assumed John had gotten it from one of his trips as a boy to Israel or Thailand or some such place. John was raised in the family of a military man, and his childhood was spent as mine was, a boyhood over the course of several homes. Not long ago John moved to San Diego to live near his twin brother. In a recent e-mail I sent to him checking up on his holiday plans, I also asked where he got the pot.

It turned out that John never had the pot in college; he used a shiny, lacquered box to store his smoking paraphernalia, and now that he has reminded me of that, there it is once again, fresh and vivid in my memory. The pot he got in Mexico, the year after he had graduated from Emory, the same year I had arrived in Manhattan and was struggling with maintaining an expensive Village apartment and floundering in graduate school. The owner of the ballroom dance studio where John and his then-boyfriend taught was Mexican and had arranged a trip for the students and instructors to Puerto Vallarta. John's recollection of the trip, comprised of rich students and attractive instructors of varying ages and sexes, was that everything was conducted on the up and up, though things had the potential of becoming wild when the tequila started flowing. The final night there was a dance exhibition and competition in the hotel ballroom and the pots were passed out as thank you gifts to members of the staff. John's recollection of the trip fails to include any memories of his boyfriend, however, though as I recall the history of his life that I know, it was not much longer before their affair ended, and John headed north to Manhattan.

My memory has also dulled our first meeting in college. It could have been at a choral rehearsal or in the lobby of the student union waiting to audition for a campus play. But I do remember what drew us closer was that sometime in the spring of that first year at Emory John's father died of a heart attack and John was gone for a week or so. One day after he had returned, while we were rehearsing for a musical in which we were both cast as dancing waiters, we sat beside one another during a break on the steps outside of the student center. Even then, not really knowing him, I yearned and ached to be closer. "I'm sorry about your dad," I said, looking over at him, hoping to find some sort of connection.

And with that John opened up to me. John has always maintained that we would have become friends earlier if I had not been so aloof. Aloof is not how I recall myself of this period, of course. If anything, I was naive, reticent, and a little too intimidated by life to be so curious about it.

And so, even as my aging memory now distorts events and details, I still find that the simple truth of it remains behind: a friendship as concrete and beautiful as a glazed red clay ceramic pot. Someone else might dig deeper and look for flaws and cracks and fissures or contemplate how the pot and the friendship might have become cracked or broken or lost over time. The only thing that I would add is that after all this time I never imagine the pot as empty, years of sentiment, after all, have been more than enough to keep it overflowing.

WRITERS

A guy I once met for sex called me up and asked me out on a date. We had originally met on a phone line and I had gone over to his apartment under the pretense that I wanted a massage and he wanted to give someone a massage. The evening of our date I met him at a restaurant he had suggested in the East Village. He showed up in a black turtleneck, black slacks, and a tweed jacket, and he had slicked back his long black hair. He looked very much like a famous writer, though I knew from our earlier encounter that he was a psychologist taking courses to become a licensed masseuse. Over dinner, he asked me questions about how to become a writer. He was a soft-spoken man and full of many questions about writing. The lighting in the restaurant made him look more attractive than he really was. At the time of our date, I was flattered that he was picking my brain for advice; it made me feel like I was an important writer myself. After dinner, we split the bill and, on the sidewalk outside the restaurant, he mentioned that he was tired and was heading across town to his apartment. I knew the date was over and somehow I felt as if I had failed a test—as if I had not been a good enough writer for him to want to take home and make love to. Only walking home, alone, did my anger overwhelm me. This was not the first time I had been psychologically raped.

I was once involved with a successful stockbroker who thought because I had written a novel he could do the same. Over the course of a summer, he wrote and typed at his computer, often during the hours we spent together. I did not mind this because it gave me a chance to write and type as well, but it bothered me that someone could think that he could just sit down and write a novel without studying how a book is constructed. After the stockbroker had finished a slender first draft of his novel, he took out an ad for a ghostwriter to fill in his blanks. He did not ask me to be his ghostwriter. Instead, he used my post office box in his ad and, for a few weeks, I carried large bundles of envelopes from the post office to his apartment. These were responses to his advertisement. He would often use the time we shared together to sift through the resumes and writing samples I had brought to him. When he had weeded the responses down to a few dozen potential applicants, he asked me to look through them and pick the ones I felt were the best writers. I could have balked at this or suggested that I be paid for this kind of work, but I didn't do either one because something in me hoped that the man would one day invest in me the amount of energy he was directing at his novel project. But I did put my foot down when he started bragging about how he would settle for nothing less than a million dollar advance before his newly hired ghostwriter had completed his manuscript. And, to his credit, my boyfriend-the-writer did change his tune. He began talking about how his unpublished novel would make a terrific movie.

 A few years before I was involved with that man, I happened to be invited by a friend to a party that was given at a townhouse. The party was during the holidays so the townhouse was beautifully decorated and there was plenty to eat and drink. The couple who were throwing the party was two men who were no longer in their fifties. One of them wore a blond wig and the other one did not have to. During the course of the evening, the one wearing the wig sat next to me on a couch and told me that I should write his life story. This has happened to me several times, because there are some people who think that their lives are so much more fascinating than anything else a writer could want to write about. As it happened, this man did have a fascinating story—he had once been a performer in the Jewel Box Revue, a drag show that once toured the country. But I politely told him that I was not the right person to write his story for him. At the time, I could not see beyond anything that was happening within my own life and that was what I felt I needed to look at first.

Which leads me to a man I dated while I was in my early thirties, which was a few years after that party. I met this man through a dating service and he was a schoolteacher and taught English composition to high school students at a private school on the Upper East Side. He was blond, bright blue-eyed, Irish, and had immigrated to New York illegally. He had gotten his green card when an off-off-Broadway theater company needed someone with an authentic Irish accent. He was also a great drinker and a great lover and sometime during the end of the first month we saw each other—when things were reaching a more emotional level between us—he ordered me not to write anything about him or our relationship. It was not a joke and he was sober when he said this. I told him I thought this was an ironic statement coming from a man who taught young students to be open about their lives in their writing. And, at the time of his command, I thought of everything in my life as a potential story, from the aspirin I carried in my knapsack to the medication I picked up for a dying friend. I could not promise the Irish writing teacher that I would not write about him or our affair and we mutually ended what could have led to a beautiful Hollywood ending or, at least, a decent off-off-Broadway play.

Once, during a phone interview, another writer asked me if I would ever write a story without a gay character. I explained to him that even if that was possible, my non-gay protagonist would still possess a gay consciousness because it was an inherent part of me which could not be removed, in the same way a black writer is always black or an Asian writer is always Asian, whether or not their characters are. Which leads me to remember now the boyfriend who once offered to "straighten" out my gay characters for me because he felt that I should make more money off of my writing. He was not a writer, himself, though he had grand aspirations of becoming famous, in the way he felt a good writer should be. What he didn't understand was that I wasn't writing for money or fame but because I felt there was something necessary that I wanted to say. He also did not understand that for me the lure of storytelling was the same lure a doctor might possess in wanting to save a patient's life.

I once turned down a date with a writer I found attractive because he approached me after he had finished affairs with Guggenheim-awarded poet and a Pulitzer-prize winning novelist. I did not turn him down because I felt my writing was any less worthy than those other two writers. I turned him down because within the context of his invitation for sex, he also put down the quality of my apartment, the quality of my lifestyle, and the fact that I was not willing to sell myself out for the big bucks as a writer. What caused me the most misery about this whole invitation, however, was that this attractive writer was HIV-positive. I felt my refusal would be seen in that context and not for its true reason. This dilemma also reminded me of another HIV-positive writer I did not have sex with. I turned this other writer down because he was already a friend when the invitation arrived and I try to adhere to my self-imposed policy of not sleeping with someone who is already my friend, particularly one who is also a writer.

I count among my friends many writers. Some of them are more financially successful than others, and some are more creative than the financially successive ones. A general rule of behavior I expect them all to adhere to in my company is not to talk endlessly about their own writing because I do not talk that way about my own. Some writers talk about their writing in the same way that some theater people talk about the theater. It is a one-note conversation that never ends and even non-writing and non-theater people find this boring. That's not to say that that my writer-friends and I don't talk about our writing or our projects with each other, we do, but they are discussed to find our strengths and flaws or to seek advice on ways to make the writing better.

A friend once told me an idea he had for a science fiction story about a gay man who becomes pregnant and flees the country when he is pursued by government authorities. My friend thought that this might be a good story for me to write. Some writers are able to use their fantasies to inch them toward creation, but I've never been able to approach writing in that matter, and I have never seen myself as a science fiction writer. As it happened, I turned to writing as a sort of therapy, to organize the jumble of thoughts swirling randomly in my head. So I became the sort of writer who had to wait until a lot of things happened to him before he could find the story he wanted to write. I always felt that this opted me out of the boy-genius category that seems so prevalent among writers who also happen to be gay, even though it was something that I had fantasized being at an early age—a young man pregnant with ideas.

A PERSONAL HISTORY OF THE EPIDEMIC

I have been actively writing about AIDS for fourteen years now, both in fiction and non-fiction, poetry and prose, grappling with issues and themes and searching for some sort of understanding to how the plague has shaped our lives. The landscape of my personal life, particularly my years in New York City, is littered with ghosts of friends, clients, colleagues, boyfriends, and lovers who have died from AIDS. I clearly remember the day in Central Park, a summer morning in 1981, waiting to meet my friend Kevin and reading an item in *The New York Times* about a rare cancer being found in gay men. That morning is engrained in my consciousness as vividly as the day I heard that Kennedy had been shot. My immediate reaction was one of confusion and skepticism, but I was also aware of being caught up in an historical moment, yet uncertain how the future would play itself out.

That feeling of being caught up in history is at the genesis of my writing my first novel, *Where the Rainbow Ends*, the story of a young Southern expatriate, Robbie Taylor, who, like myself, arrives optimistically in Manhattan in the late 1970s and meets a new circle of friends. Though the novel tackles many themes, among them the importance of family and friends to gay men and lesbians, the plot of the book follows the chronology of the first decade of the AIDS epidemic. Robbie's journey through these years finds him confronting many historical and personal markers of the plague: being tested for HIV, the unveiling of the AIDS Quilt, attending local ACT UP meetings and national demonstrations.

Where the Rainbow Ends is also an outgrowth of the national discussions of family values which were present during the Presidential campaigns of 1992. Like the Biblical character of Job, Robbie assembles one family, loses it, and assembles another. My own personal years in the epidemic have followed a similar pattern; through the friends that I have lost, I have found other, new friends.

During the six years I spent writing the novel, however, I witnessed the epidemic change its disposition; when I had finished writing the first draft of my manuscript, somewhere around 1996, it was clear to me that the perception of HIV infection was not as bleak as when I had started the manuscript, thanks, in part, to the advancements of science and medicine and the introduction of prescriptive cocktails and protease inhibitors. As journalists and gay writers began proclaiming the demise of the plague, I considered shelving the novel instead of rewriting it, worried that it did not reflect the prevailing optimistic notion that AIDS was being considered a manageable disease. But a friend, another writer, convinced me otherwise, telling me that I should not stop writing about AIDS, even if I had to approach my manuscript as an historical novel. These, he said, were stories that had to be told and retold, to prove that there had been men who have lived and loved and been lost at a too early age.

Things have surely improved since those early years when friends became ill and before AIDS and HIV could be named. But I must confess, even now, so many years later, I am still haunted by the first few friends who became sick. Their memories still come back to me as I walk back and forth through the city between jobs and appointments. I still remember the loft on 28th Street where Kevin lived, still remember Mike working out at the musty Body Center on Sixth Avenue before the gym was transformed into the high-tech one it is now. I still remember the night David assembled a group of us at the Ziegfeld to watch a badly reviewed Warren Beatty movie.

My anxiety during those years has now been replaced with a melancholy sorrow dulled even further by the passage of time. But often, while riding in a stuffy elevator filled with people in heavy winter coats and jammed in close together, I can still recall the first visit I made to a friend in the hospital and feeling the hot breaths of my fear bouncing against the face mask I wore and being forced back down my throat.

Not long ago a friend reminded me that the epidemic was not really over. He is HIV-positive and still fighting the same daily battle for health that he has been fighting since he found out his diagnosis twelve years before. AIDS is never over, he said, for any of us who have survived the loss of losing someone to this irrational infection. Like the characters I had created in my stories and my novel, my friend's personal history also incorporated the historical markers of the epidemic. He had bought tickets to that first fund-raiser at the circus at Madison Square Garden; he had delivered hot meals to homebound men in Hell's Kitchen; he had done the AIDS Walk in the rain; and he had demonstrated at the NIH.

My own personal history within the years of the epidemic is no different than any other man of my generation who has lived at ground zero and survived to tell the tales. I have volunteered, cared for, and buried more friends than I wish to admit. Another friend once commented to me before he died, that gay life had come of age in dealing with this suffering; that gay men had been changed forever, and that change should be what I must now address in my writing. My life today is certainly nothing like I expected it to be when I arrived in Manhattan all those years ago.

There are many reasons why I have never stopped writing about AIDS. AIDS summons up the greatest themes in literature, among them sex and death and faith, themes that are universal and prominent in every life. Anyone who has lost a loved one from death, untimely or by nature, can read about AIDS and understand the emotions it forces into place, anyone who has acted as a carepartner for someone who has been ill will understand the compassion necessary in tending the sick, anyone facing death from a life-threatening illness should be able to find strength and companionship in AIDS writing, anyone interested in uncovering the heart of the human soul should read writing about AIDS.

But more than any other reason my writing about AIDS is fueled by a combination of grief and guilt. I am an HIV-negative gay man who has survived the epidemic thus far. Is there a reason why I have been spared when so many others have died? Have I endured simply because of luck or fate? I still write about AIDS not just because I have survived but because it is part of my history. AIDS has changed me even though HIV has not infected me. It has, nonetheless, impacted my world. It has made me the person I am today. I write about AIDS because I am still alive.

MAGIC CARPET RIDE

I was steeped in memory before I arrived in San Francisco, having spent the weekend catching up with two college roommates who now lived in Los Angeles, reminiscing about our shared dinners of overcooked broccoli and our extra-curricular theatrics of overacted stage roles more than twenty years before. But I had started my trip sodden with personal recollection; Los Angeles and San Francisco were two stops on a book tour for a novel I had written which focused on gay life in the 1970s and 1980s and I was worried about being trapped too much in self-absorbed concentration.

But I hadn't been to San Francisco in over thirteen years and since that last visit my life had changed dramatically; since then, AIDS had redirected my career as much as it had leveled and reshaped the bay area's gay community. On this trip, however, I only expected to find San Francisco as a first-time tourist would: I was even anticipating visits to every traveler's would-be destinations of Chinatown and Fisherman's Wharf.

The notion of being swept back into time began when I unpacked in my room at the bed and breakfast inn I had chosen. At one end a bay window overlooked an intersection of streets and outside I could watch the random patterns of traffic and trolleys at the corners of Castro and Market. Watching the swaggering gait and cruising glances of leather jacketed gay men who passed beneath the window seemed no different, really, than those I had witnessed of their gay male counterparts over a decade before. San Francisco gay men, unlike their buffed Los Angeles counterparts, had not discarded that Seventies macho clone look of facial hair and swarthy appeal. Inside the inn, my room seemed to be stuck in a similar time warp. Three of the walls were painted white, but the fourth was colored a deep chocolate brown. Above a wicker desk, a framed poster of a vase of flowers hung, faded by years of light streaming in between two hanging baskets of plants. Beside the bed stood a large, custom-made mirrored armoire and cabinet. Track-lighting and navy blue-and-maroon linens reminded me of period details I might expect to find within an Armistead Maupin novel.

I expected to shake this heady pitch into reflection the following day when, buoyed by the surprising spring-like weather on the cusp of the winter solstice, I unexpectedly decided to see the city by bike.

"You're lucky you caught me here," the young operator of the bicycle shop said when I reached the Embarcadero and inquired about a rental. "I don't keep regular hours in the winter."

The young man must have been as surprised by the warmer-than-usual weather as I had been—he had shown up to work in summer clothes—a thin, white T-shirt which barely ended where his dark knee-length shorts began, a knotted strand of a leather string worn around his neck. He shook my hand and introduced himself as Victor and explained the terms and conditions of the rental as if I had only asked my brother to borrow his bike to make a quick trip to the store. He possessed that kind of *Twilight Zone* calm, and his spiky dyed-blond hair and ice blue eyes cast the spell of being someone familiar yet standing outside of time—like a catalog version of someone's cool drinking buddy or hip college pal. I stood before him eager but unaware of the continued retrospection he would soon unknowingly unlock.

My destination that day was the Golden Gate Bridge, but my trip across the city went through as many years as it did neighborhoods and streets. I biked to Fisherman's Wharf and Fort Mason, through the Presidio and down Lombard to Russian Hill, walking alongside the bike when the incline was more than I could peddle. Everywhere I went that day I encountered details of my personal past. On Polk Street, a large jade plant potted in a ceramic pot outside a restaurant reminded me of a plant I had kept in my first Manhattan apartment. On Jackson, a flower decal on the frame of a motorcycle was exactly the kind we used to paste onto notebooks in junior high school in the 1960s.

But a trip through San Francisco, I also discovered that day, is a trip through America's pop cultural past, memory explodes into recognition in every inch of the city. The city easily evokes trends of other eras, from the beatniks to the hippies to the yuppies. On Filmore Street in Pacific Heights, an elegantly restored navy blue and white 1950s Bel Air was parked at the curb in a city where it's not unusual to find several working versions of the original VW Bug passing you on the street. Renovated houses with gingerbread lattice and stained glass windows are exactly what you would expect to find in San Francisco, and they are right there, on Filmore and Hayes and Pierce. And so are the tie-dyed boutiques and psychedelic sandwich signs outside restaurants in the Haight. Even at the Tower Records outlet in Soma, the saleswoman behind the counter seemed to have been hired because she looked like an aged Joni Mitchell. By the time I decided to find my way to the Golden Gate Bridge, it seemed absolutely uncontrived that the young man with bushy black hair working outside his home on Fell Street should be listening to Steppenwolf's "Magic Carpet Ride."

At the bridge I succumbed to finally being a tourist, buying a T-shirt for my boyfriend at the gift shop, then eating a hot dog while propped up against the bike. Beyond me the city was a picture-perfect orb and a memory of sights. Hours later, when I had made my way back to the Embarcadero to return the bike, Victor was sitting outside his shop, shooting the breeze with a stubbly-bearded man wearing a red knit cap over his shoulder-length dreadlocks, an amalgamation of many fads.

I must have realized then that I was exhausted time traveler with a wild-eyed stare and jeans soggy with sweat that rode baggy around my hips, for Victor stood as I approached him as if he expected to catch me in a faint.

"Extraordinary day," I said as he took the bike from me.

I'm sure he had no idea what crazy revelations had been floating through my mind all afternoon, but he nodded and looked out and up at the buildings cut-out against the still solid blue sky. "Like riding on a bird," he answered.

As I started to leave he smiled and said "Peace," then flashed me the universal sign of two fingers widened into a V. It seemed the perfect and natural way to end a day of nostalgia in San Francisco.

"Peace," I answered back and then walked toward the traffic light, inching my way slowly back into the present.

BUDDIES

There was a time a few years ago when my life was less than idyllic. I had just moved back to Manhattan and was rock-bottom poor. Everything seemed to cost much more than what I had in my wallet or could earn in a week at the job where I worked as a publicist. I was depressed because I felt I did not have enough time to write down all the stories that were swirling around in my head. And I was desperate to find a boyfriend; I saw this as one easy way that I could bring a ray of light into all that was unhappy and unfocused in my life. I fantasized that if I found a boyfriend I could give up my job. Together my new boyfriend and I could open up a bookstore or run our own off-off Broadway theater company, or we could move in together and I could leave behind the fifth-floor walk-up apartment that did not even have enough electricity on some days for me to boot up my computer and write. And I reasoned that if I had a boyfriend, I would no longer feel that desire to write. Instead I could be content playing the happy homemaker. I could shop for groceries and plan dinner parties and worry about mildew settling into the bathroom carpet. And I could channel my energies into making my boyfriend happy.

But as it happened I was making my way through a string of blind dates and quick-sex tricks. I complained to my friends that I had trouble meeting a man who wanted a relationship with me for more than a few hours. Even though I could not afford to date anyone I asked every friend I had if they could set me up with someone who might be serious about getting involved in something long-term. I met a few guys this way but no one lasted any longer than the ones I could find on my own in a bar or on a phone line. So I complained more and more until one day a coworker dropped a piece of paper on my desk with a name and phone number.

"Call him," Chris said. "He wants to meet you."

* * *

His name was Dennis, or so I shall call him, and he was a fortysomething Republican lobbyist who lived in Washington, D.C., and came to New York frequently on business trips. Chris had worked for Dennis as a student intern and they still kept in touch, meeting for drinks at one of the Madison Avenue hotels where Dennis stayed when he was in town. Chris had told me that Dennis was in a long-term relationship that was drying up and he was looking to meet someone new. I didn't have any expectations when Dennis and I spoke on the phone and arranged to meet for drinks a few days later. I didn't possess enough confidence in either my appearance or personality to imagine that I could be the potential wedge to finally break up two warring lovers.

Dennis was short, barely five-feet-four in his socks, and a good four inches shorter than myself. He had a beautiful body; his boyhood dream had been that he'd become a professional bodybuilder and he had used this passion to create an impressive physique of oversized muscles on his short frame. Dennis had grown up on Philadelphia's Main Line and was sent off to military school and an Ivy League college. He seemed, as Chris had painted him, an ideal candidate for a husband hunter such as me—a well-bred, athletic, preppy, and professional catch.

We met in one of those mirror-lined hotel bars in the West 50s—the kind frequented by straight, married men in town for conventions or meetings and on the prowl for babes and New York experiences. Dennis and I chatted a bit after our introductions, to make sure neither of us was too off-the-rocker for the other, and then he invited me upstairs to his room.

In the room, we undressed separately and awkwardly; there seemed to be only a little passion generated between us. Dennis was somewhat embarrassed to reveal such a smooth, pumped-up physique and I was even more self-conscious to reveal my hairy, boyish one. Sex was very vanilla that night. Dennis didn't want us to kiss on the lips and after a few minutes of clutching and groping, we ended up jerking each other off. Five minutes later I was politely escorted out of the room, and the door closed behind me. Dennis was no different from the other guys I was meeting. I stood out in the hall waiting for the elevator to arrive, feeling cheap and disgusted about our hasty transaction—not that Dennis had paid for it, or that I hadn't been paid for it before, but that it seemed so impersonal and not at all what I had wanted or needed. After all, we had been set up by a friend. This was supposed to be a date, not a trick. We hadn't even had dinner or finished a drink together. And since it wasn't the hottest or most fulfilling sexual encounter I had ever had—or had even had *that week*—I wasn't too upset with the likelihood that I would never see Dennis again.

So I was surprised, truly surprised, when Dennis called me ten days later and asked if he could come over to my apartment between meetings while he was in the city. I agreed, but cordially warned him not to expect things in my home to be, well, on the level of a Main Line estate, a D.C. duplex, or even a renovated Times Square hotel.

What he liked about my apartment—I found out some time later—was the seediness of it: the lack of ventilation between the rooms, the cracked linoleum floors, the flickering electric current, the bed frame that sagged at the end because one of the support boards had broken and I had not been able to afford to repair it. Dennis loved my poverty because he could instill my life with a bohemian glow I did not wish to acknowledge. Instead, I saw myself as a writer struggling to make it in Manhattan by living in an overpriced tenement apartment. I never had enough money to afford even the lunchtime special at the corner Chinese restaurant.

I was, of course, embarrassed by my poverty and surroundings, embarrassed that Dennis had to call me from the corner so that I could go down five flights to open the front door of my building for him. I was embarrassed for someone to find that I had stopped cleaning my apartment because I felt my time could be better spent doing anything else. And I was embarrassed to lead him into my overheated bedroom; an air-conditioner was a luxury I couldn't even consider.

It was a blistering early summer afternoon when Dennis first walked into my apartment. The temperature had reached over one hundred degrees that day and the air, inside and out, was thick with humidity. Dennis wore what I would soon come to call his uniform: a dark business suit, white shirt, red power tie, black suspenders, and black patent-leather wing-tipped shoes from Brooks Brothers. In the bedroom, the sounds of taxi horns and squealing truck brakes from the impatient traffic on Ninth Avenue drifting through my open window made it impossible for us to begin a conversation. So we undressed as we had done the first time at his hotel room, separately and on opposite ends of my bed. But before our clothes had hit the floor—or, rather, before mine had hit the floor and Dennis's had been folded and gently placed on the only chair I owned—our bodies were covered with a thin film of perspiration. By the time we had finished, the sheets were drenched with sweat and crumpled as if they'd survived a tumble over Niagara Falls, and Dennis, so eager and aggressive during this second encounter, shook his muscles out as if he had just run a marathon.

Marathon running was, in fact, what now kept Dennis in such great shape, along with a two-hours-a-day three-times-a-week gym regimen. If it weren't for the gray in his full head of short, black hair, he might have been mistaken for a young man in his late twenties; his skin was tight and devoid of body fat and wrinkles. But there was something asymmetrical about him that all his exercise had not perfected, a little slope at the shoulders, one eyebrow lower than the other, and a cock which curved to the left like the base of the McDonald's arches and captured the cedary fragrance of his groin.

    Dennis left that afternoon with an air of contentment I still had not achieved from our encounters. I was angry at myself for falling into such an easy sexual trap, and in the back of my mind an alarm was going off: Don't waste your time on him if he isn't lover material. I did not have any further expectations of a relationship from Dennis and so I was surprised, once again, when he called and asked to see me a few days later.

* * *

There was no fixed pattern to Dennis's comings and goings. Sometimes I'd see him twice a week, sometimes not for a month or two. A typical afternoon get-together would find me rushing home from work to unlock the front door for him and escort him upstairs. Dennis would arrive equipped with a cold six-pack and a box of condoms, and he would chug and talk while I put out the lube and towels and found a few dirty magazines or porno tapes in case we wanted them. Unlike some of my other gay friends, I felt that fuck buddying was a less than ideal relationship; intimacy and romance have always been bigger turn-ons for me. Those few minutes' worth of conversation with Dennis at my kitchen table before we headed back to my bedroom were an important aspect of what kept me interested in him. Little details of who he was casually surfaced without my having to force any direct questions on him—enough information, in fact, to convince me that Dennis was not the ideal catch I had imagined him to be and I might best content myself with our sexual explorations and nothing more. For one thing, we differed in our degree of openness about being gay. Dennis wasn't out at work, wasn't even out to his parents or the circle of straight friends he maintained in Washington. He loved for me to use this fact in our sex play; for a while we went through a phase where I verbally taunted him for being a Closeted-White-Republican-Faggot while I spanked him and he pleaded for tolerance. One thing that worked about our relationship was that we were willing to sexually experiment with each other in ways that we had not attempted with other men.

But our conversations were also how I found out that Dennis's long-term relationship had finally dissolved and he was casually involved with a new boyfriend in Washington, though the details of his affair were often slim or mentioned offhandedly. Instead, Dennis loved to tell me all about his recent vacations; New York was often a pause on the way home from Burma or Peru or Tahiti, and he would arrive with tales of the sexual situations in which he found himself in these foreign locales, from his trips to bathhouses to hiring the local "talent." These stories convinced me that Dennis was sexually experienced in ways I had only imagined for myself. Not all of our discussions revolved around sex, however; now and then I would mention something I had written or published or try to explain to Dennis why writing a novel was such slow going, or why I had given up a permanent job and become a temporary office worker so that I could have the mental freedom to write. But I never talked to him about my most recent dates or my ongoing search for a lover, which must have been why it came as such a surprise to him when I confessed one winter afternoon that I had started dating someone seriously and that maybe we should take a hiatus from our activities.

"Who is this guy and what does he mean to you?" he asked me, alarmed, his face drawn tight. I had waited till he was dressing to leave to explain that this would be our last get-together.

"A boyfriend," I answered.

"A serious boyfriend?"

"Maybe," I said. "Maybe not."

"You don't need to get yourself into a half-assed relationship. You deserve better than that."

I was surprised by his tone of voice; a touch of intimacy had crept in where there was never one before. "Unfortunately no one is offering me that," I said.

There was a moment of silence between us as Dennis buttoned his pants and drew the suspenders over his shoulders. My apartment was cold that day, and we'd had to stay close to each other beneath the comforter to stay warm. Already there was a history of more than six months between us. He rubbed his hands briskly together to keep them warm and I thought, for a brief moment, that he might try to offer his own open relationships as a model for mine. But he didn't pursue that path. With the same tone of concern, he said, "You should complain to your landlord about the lack of heat in this place."

"I'll add it to my list of grievances."

"Do you want me to call him? I could probably pull some strings."

"He has to turn it on eventually," I said. "It's the law. Every year he gets a little later."

"You should let me help you."

"I can take care of myself."

He looked around my bedroom, then pitched his head back and looked at the ceiling. I thought he was going to make a bitter, condescending remark about the place—the lopsided floor and the cracks that traveled up the wall to where he rested his eyes. Instead he asked, "How long have you been seeing him?"

"Almost three months."

"So there's no point in getting serious so soon," he said. "You've got plenty of time before you have to make that decision. I'll call you next week when I'm in town."

* * *

We didn't stop seeing each other. My more serious boyfriend didn't stick around for a relationship. And I didn't confess this to Dennis. In the meantime Dennis had moved on to another new boyfriend and was soon juggling dates with two guys in Washington. On one level I resented the fact that Dennis and I never left my apartment together, never went out for dinner, never did the things that couples do together—go to the movies or to the theater, even though I couldn't afford to do any of those things with him—but on another level I was happy that our sexual sessions now ended with postcoital conversations and cuddling, even though this growing level of intimacy confused me. Something told me that I should not want to push Dennis into any other role than the one he had found in my life—while we were good sexual partners we might not be so good as boyfriends or lovers—and I should be happy with the status quo we had somehow arrived at and not attempt to define or change it.

And then one day during our third year of seeing each other—after we had both passed through many other sexual and romantic partners—Dennis lay in my bed complaining about a new guy he was dating named Brad, who was afraid of showing him any emotional commitment. Dennis said Brad wouldn't spend the night at his apartment. He was upset that Brad had disappeared on a business trip to Texas for eight days and hadn't bothered to call Dennis at all. I was able to realize the irony of this from many angles—an unfaithful lover complaining about an uncommitted one—and I asked Dennis if Brad was aware of our relationship.

"He knows I see a friend in New York," Dennis said.

"But we're not really just friends," I answered. "We've never seen each other outside of this room, except the night we first met at your hotel. I could tell Brad that you're afraid of emotional commitment, too. We've never even spent the night together. I don't think I've ever seen you for more than two hours at a time."

Dennis had found his way out of bed and was unfolding his pants from the back of the chair. I saw that he wanted to say something but was holding his thoughts back. "But then we're not boyfriends either, are we?" I said, letting him off the hook. "So that kind of behavior makes all of this behavior acceptable."

It was not the next time, or the time after that, but it was soon thereafter that Dennis asked me to meet him at his hotel room after a business dinner engagement had ended. "You can stay the night, too, if you want," he said.

The notion that Dennis might have thought about our relationship outside of my bedroom surprised me. "We'll see how it goes," I said, knowing that Dennis was an early riser and that he might change his mind once I got to his hotel room. Or that I might chicken out and not even show up.

At the hotel, Dennis and I lay in bed watching television after we had finished with sex. Sometime after midnight, when he was groggy, he rolled over and turned the lights out. I was wide awake beside him in bed, unable to sleep, aware that what we were doing was changing the meaning of us.

"Am I as good as your other lovers?" he asked. He had snuggled himself into my embrace, our arms floating around each other, his breath hitting the cleft of my neck in warm pulses.

I hated this comparative game, surprised that a man would put his ego to such a test. The truth, of course, was that I was much too much of a coward to hear how deeply someone else could feel for another person, particularly if the other person wasn't me. I had long ago erased my curiosity of what Dennis's life was like outside of our rendezvous—I felt I had fully accepted our being only sex partners and it would only have been painful for me to know more. The weight of his arms had pinned my own arms against my body and his hands had found mine where they rested near my stomach. He twisted our fingers together and kissed the back of my neck. I knew from the childish tone of his question that he wanted my affirmation.

"Yes," I lied, not mentioning that at that moment he was my *only* lover.

"Am I as big as they are?" he asked, again, a bit too sincerely for comfort.

"Bigger," I lied again, for Dennis was only of modest endowment, and no guy, regardless of his size, likes to hear that someone is more gifted than they are in that department—so I told him what he wanted to hear. That was what a lover should do, shouldn't he? *Any* lover, be he trick or timeless. And this was a role we were now playing. We were pretending to be lovers.

"Do they do anything I don't?" he asked next.

"What do you mean?"

"Treat you differently?"

"I think we're a little different together than what I've done with others."

He didn't pursue my path of reasoning. This was bedtime talk—talk that was supposed to be comforting and soothing, to make the worries and stress of a day disappear. "Is it working for you?" he asked.

"Yes," I answered honestly. "It's always nice to be with you."

"You should come visit me in Washington," he said.

This was another surprise. In the dark I was sure he could see the inside of my mind working. "I can't afford a trip right now," I answered.

"I can give you some money, if you want," he said. When he realized what he had offered me, though, he backtracked a bit. He pulled us closer together, rubbed his chin against my shoulder. "You can borrow it if you want. Pay me back when you can."

When I didn't answer him, he continued. "I just want to take some of the sleaziness out of this for a bit."

"But it's not just sleazy," I answered defensively. "I think you know that."

"Then there's no reason for you not to come to Washington."

"Maybe when it's warmer," I said. "I always think better when it's warm."

* * *

I never visited Dennis in Washington. We never took a trip together. Dennis never sent me flowers, never celebrated my birthday. And I never gave him a present, never wished him Happy Valentine's Day or Merry Christmas.

And more years passed between us, as if in some fairy tale. I was published but never conquered my poverty. Dennis went to Vietnam, Italy, Ecuador, and the Galapagos Islands. Chris, the friend who had set up our introductions, drifted into a forgotten memory. And then I met a man about whom I *did* become serious. For a while I didn't know how to explain Dennis's presence in my life to this guy, and then after another while I realized that things were likely to fall apart with him if I did. In bed Dennis would ask for details of my new lover and sometimes I would be vague and other times I wouldn't be. It was easy for me to describe a vacation to California with my boyfriend—the restaurants we went to in Los Angeles and the resort where we stayed in Palm Springs—but it took more effort to admit that I knew I was more serious about my boyfriend than he was about me. He was still seeing other men, still on the prowl for another boyfriend—a good friend had actually witnessed him picking someone up in a bar. I'd love to say that Dennis was supportive, that he helped me work things out, see things clearly about the different kinds of relationships gay men can have, but he wasn't that kind of talky, intuitive man, not that kind of friend or boyfriend, nor that kind of lover. Instead, Dennis became a diverting constant for me: entertaining, reflective, always coming back into town. And as it was, I had to do many foolish things to learn the error of my ways in that more serious and one-sided relationship, from snooping through appointments in my boyfriend's daybook to monitoring his movement in Internet chat rooms, things which out of context now seem appalling to admit. And I let that kind of behavior of mine stretch out longer than it should have. But there's a lot of truth in the saying that no one can change your life except yourself. And nothing is a better teacher than time and experience.

Four years later, this difficult, complicated, and now too serious relationship finally came to an end. It was early September, a Friday night, and I'd had a disagreement with my aberrant boyfriend because I felt he was shutting me out of his life and growing distant. In the end, sex had little to do with our final break; our communications had grown stale and strained. We could not share our experiences, either together or apart, and the only thing we could agree on was that it was time to end things completely between us. Leaving my boyfriend's apartment, I had walked from the Upper East Side across town feeling both burned and burned-out. I had fallen in love and now I was out of love. When I got home an hour or so later there was a message from Dennis saying he was in town for the night before he caught a plane to Rio the next morning, and if I wanted to, I could visit him at his hotel that evening. My body was aching with disappointment and rejection and an odd sense of relief, and the last thing I wanted to do was attend to someone else's sexual needs. I felt like I didn't have a sexual pore in my body. But I also didn't want to be alone.

On the walk back across town to Dennis's hotel it occurred to me that ours was the longest relationship I could lay claim to thus far in my life, outside of my family and friends. We had been buddies by then for more than eight years. I tried to let the cool Manhattan evening work its romantic charm on me—the flashing lights of Times Square, the yellow blur of taxis on the street, the great starry ceiling of Grand Central. I wanted to convince myself that I loved Dennis, that my love for Dennis might replace the love I had just lost. But I knew that couldn't happen. Dennis was not to be that man. I had learned how to divorce emotional content from our sexual relationship, but I had not yet learned if such a thing could be easily restored.

And it wasn't something I really wanted to try with Dennis. I could see now how he had pushed and challenged and changed our relationship simply by being a steady, yet evolving presence over time, and how I had at times selfishly held myself back because I was scared of feeling something deeper for him. At his hotel room, Dennis knew me well enough to know that I was not in my best spirits. "Do you want to talk about it?" he asked, when I settled onto the bed beside his luggage. He was taking clothes out of his suitcase, folding and unfolding items with the precision and deliberation he always used.

"No," I answered. "Not really." I was done with trying to make something into something that it was not. Dennis knew instinctively that I was not shutting him out, that in time, if I needed to, I would open up and talk with him. He tossed me a brochure he found from the inner sleeve of his suitcase and said, "That's where I'm headed."

The brochure was of a luxury resort and full of photos of candlelit dining rooms, hotel suites with king-sized beds and bathrooms with marble sinks and oversized tubs. For a moment I imagined walking into such a place with Dennis and discovering it for the first time, as I had done with a history of boyfriends but never with Dennis. I knew Dennis would not be traveling alone on this trip; he seldom did now, even if it meant inviting one of his well-to-do ex-boyfriends to accompany him, but with this particular trip he had been elusive about any details up till now, and I knew I was better off not asking for any more. Still, I felt an odd moment of jealousy overwhelm me, and to fight off my despair I looked up at Dennis and asked, nonchalantly, "Want to take a bath together?"

It was something in all the years we had been seeing each other that we had never done together—we had occasionally showered together, using it as a prelude to or a cleanup from sex, but we had never soaked together in a tub nor used the tub as a toy, though we had often talked about wanting to do so.

Dennis smiled and said, "The tub is awfully small here. That means we'll have to be sort of intimate with each other."

I nodded and smiled and found the energy to get off the bed and run the water in the small bathtub of his hotel room. It was hardly as luxurious as the destination in Rio where he was headed, and his tiny, cramped New York City hotel bathroom had not a shred of romance to it. I was able to muffle a nearby closet light so that we would not have to bathe in the full brightness of the bathroom and found an FM classical music station on the radio. We sat in the tub in various awkward positions with cramped knees or splayed legs, our laughter bouncing against the white tiles of the room as we tried to adjust to accommodate each other. Dennis massaged my back; I washed his hair. Both of us had erections by the time the water turned cold, so we dried off and padded across the carpet and continued in bed. That night is still one of the most vivid memories I retain of Dennis; an unexpected buoyancy heightened everything—our skin, the air, the fabric, the music floating through the room. I saw the fact that Dennis and I could go on and on like this for as long as we needed each other. Dennis was capable of suspending my life; he could make me forget, even if only momentarily, many things: unhappiness with lovers, friends who had died, money and success that eluded me. And, after all this time between us, he could keep me aroused.

I stayed with Dennis that night and we slept embracing each other as if we were lovers. Before he left for the airport the next morning, we kissed each other lightly on the lips before we disappeared back into our other lives. I realized I had something enduring with him that I'd had with no other lover. I was his buddy—the guy he saw for sex in the city—and needed nothing else from him at all. I knew I would see him again, though I didn't know when and wasn't worried about how soon. "Love ya," he said before he left me for something else that morning.

I know he didn't mean it, at least not in the way I had been looking to find it for so many years, but it was nice to hear the phrase, nonetheless, especially from him. "Love ya," I answered back. I thought it had a nice sound to it, so I tried it again, even though he was now out of earshot. "Love ya," I repeated. "Hope to see ya soon."

REMNANTS

I cannot forget that we traded clothes since I have worn the shorts several times since then. It was our last summer together and we were both gaining weight. I had bought a pair of khaki shorts too big for myself and his shorts were so tight they were making him uncomfortable. One afternoon at his summer house, we traded shorts before going out to the beach. It was one of the last times that things were perfect between us. He looked good in my shorts and I looked better in his.

That was not the first or the last time I would wear his clothes. The first year we dated one another I needed a jacket to wear to a job interview. I was a freelance writer and he was trying to steer me toward a corporate world where a job also had benefits. I did not have much money that year and he had plenty to spare. He also had a closet full of suits he had outgrown since leaving his wife and two kids and moving into his own apartment. I had never worn a suit as expensive as the one he gave me. It was gray flannel and had a designer label inside the jacket. Of course, I needed a beautiful tie to wear with such a handsome suit, and he chose a dark blue silk one with dots from his closet. I'm not sure if the tie was a gift or not, but I never returned it to him and he never asked for it back. When he offered it to me, he said he had not worn it for some time because he had grown tired of wearing it so often. I should have understood then how I fit into his life—as something new and unusual that could lose its luster at any moment. But I didn't. The tie still hangs in my closet, waiting for another opportunity to be worn with the suit.

He had also outgrown a drawer full of dress shirts. These were beautiful pinpoint oxford cotton. There was a blue and white striped one, a solid blue one, and a blue striped one with a white collar. The shirts were tailored along the back and the sides, which is why they were no longer of comfort to him. They fit me perfectly when I tried them on. I didn't get these shirts at the same time that I got the suit and the tie, but they came into my possession soon thereafter. For a while I wore the shirts to a temp job and pointed out the monogrammed cuffs to my co-workers. The initials were not mine, of course, but I found them full of extravagant subtext when I explained that the letters belonged to the name of my boyfriend.

There was a period, too, where I gave him clothes. He loved to wear T-shirts from luxury destinations and I bought him many from the places we visited together or separately. I gave him shirts from Hawaii, Palm Springs, San Francisco, Key West, East Hampton, and Disney World. I could not afford to travel to all these places without his help and my gratitude was always bound up in the design I chose for him. These gifts were not without their inherent problems, however—a few faded or shrunk in the wash and were never seen again after their initial wearing. And one of the sturdier ones would haunt me for over two years—I later learned that the weekend we spent apart and the day I had chosen the shirt for him, he had spent celebrating another, younger, boyfriend's birthday.

Six weeks after I first met him in a bar, he took me to a store and offered to buy me an outfit for my birthday. I had never had anyone take me into a clothing store with this in mind except for my mother, and since he was older and I was younger it felt both paternal and perverted, as if I were a young hustler he had discovered in a bar and wanted to make more presentable. Nonetheless, I found his gesture to be authentic, but much too extravagant for someone I had known for such a little time. I decided to only let him buy me a pair of pants. The ones that I was wearing at the time were faded and shredded at the cuffs and knees and crotch, though only the threads at my ankles were truly discernible to anyone other than the wearer.

The pants that I chose were olive green khakis and I wore them about a year before they faded and shredded themselves, too, from overuse. They did not set him back too many bucks and, in retrospect, I think it was a good investment.

He gave me other gifts on other birthdays, too. One birthday he gave me a sporty and moderately expensive watch. He was not a man full of romantic or intimate notions and for a brief moment I felt as if we had exchanged rings. A watch is not an intimate gift, of course, but I took it to be an intimate gesture because there was nothing else even mimicking it in our relationship. When my next birthday rolled around I had lost the watch and he questioned me about its whereabouts when he noticed I was no longer wearing it. I said it was in need of a new battery and I would have it fixed in a few days. The watch had not stopped and it had not really been lost; it had been stolen by a trick I had picked up one night in a bar and taken back to my apartment. It took me four paychecks to save enough money to buy a duplicate of this moderately expensive watch and by the time I had bought it, it was clear to me that our time together was finite and soon to end.

There was a time, however, when I loved him and I tried to use as many connections as I could to arrange invitations to take him to places where I could show him off as a boyfriend. Several of these places and occasions were black tie events, and the first couple of times we went together, I wore a tuxedo I had owned since college and had bought second-hand when I sang in the glee club. There was a time, too, when he outgrew his own tuxedo and I took to wearing that one while he opted to dress in a more comfortable-fitting all-black suit, shirt, and tie. I never returned the tuxedo to him because I always hoped that there would be another place we could go together, but he did return to me, a year after we had broken up, some clothes that I had left behind at the summer house. He had decided to sell the house because he did not wish to go there alone anymore. In the bag he handed me were jeans I had left behind at that house that no longer fit my waist because I had fallen into a depression of eating and drinking too much. A few of the T-shirts still fit and they felt, when I put them on for the first time after an absence of months, like an old friend who had called on the phone and wanted to make sure I was doing all right.

    Not long ago I lost the baseball cap he had given to me when he went on a trip to Palm Springs. It was a brown khaki color with pale green lettering and a darker green palm tree between the words. The day I lost the cap I was shopping for winter coats. I had put it on when I left the house because it looked like it would rain and had taken it off to look at myself in the mirror when I tried on a coat in a store. When I got home, I realized I had left the cap behind on a display shelf. It saddened me to think that I had lost it in this way, that I had not tossed it out from anger or grief or relief but that it had simply disappeared because of my careless oversight. Sometimes when I wear my new coat I think about the missing hat. It was a good hat. And, at the time I wore it, it fit me well.

A FEW MINUTES WITH LIBERACE

One of the things that irony teaches us is never to be surprised. This thought ran through my mind in Las Vegas as I stood at a souvenir counter in a strip-shopping mall and debated whether or not to buy a Liberace ashtray. I am neither a Liberace fan nor a smoker, but I enjoy collecting local tchotchkes from my vacations. I was looking for something distinctly Vegas to buy. The gift shop is in one of two sites the Liberace Museum occupies in storefront spaces located in a one-level strip-shopping mall. Outside, between the two buildings, rows of metal roofs and hoods of cars wavered in the desert heat of the black tar parking lot.

I'd flown to Vegas to meet my college roommate, John, for a vacation. I had been on business in Chicago; he lived in San Diego. On my arrival I found myself jet lagged, and my skin over sensitive to the sun from pain medication I was taking for a back problem. Our days were spent taking monorails to look at the insides and outsides of the giant casinos such as Luxor, Caesar's Palace, and the Venetian, as if they were architectural wonders full of priceless art. In the evenings we crashed early, exhausted from all that motion and our stomachs bloated from early-bird bargain buffets.

We took a break from Vegas for a two day trip to see the Hoover Dam and the northern rim of the Grand Canyon. On our way back into Vegas we decided to use the rental car to spend a few extra minutes to visit the Liberace Museum, located on the outskirts of the main Vegas area. It seemed like the campy, gay thing to do, after all. This was the first vacation I had planned in some time which had not been planned around a gay-resort destination.

The gay scene in Vegas is about as underground as it can get, unless you factor in the one or two drag revues playing at the casinos which feature female impersonators doing the usual Cher, Bette, and Diana imitations. Our first night in Vegas John and I had made an attempt to locate a gay bar. From one of our guide books, we had read that there were none located where we were staying, at the southern end of the Strip, the generic nickname for the town's main drag, Las Vegas Boulevard, but that there was a cluster of gay bars and businesses nearby, settled close to one another in an area called the Gay Quarter, along Paradise Road, just below Tropicana Avenue. The streets of Vegas are laid out in a pseudo-grid version that look easy to decode on a map, but are actually more difficult once you get out into the distracting lights and signs of the casinos. We decided that by walking a few blocks east we would reach the local gay bookstore and inquire about the nearby bars. One block in Vegas, however, is worth about ten in another city, and leaving the Strip we were soon walking within a dimly lit industrial nightmare: undeveloped land, no traffic, confusing street signs, and not a clue to where we were headed. After we reached the first intersection, about thirty minutes later, we luckily flagged down a taxi driver who dropped us off at the intersection we had set out for (and which would have taken us another hour to reach by foot and bravado). We spotted the gay bookstore and went inside.

The bookstore was relatively empty (maybe two other people besides ourselves and two men behind the sales counter) and sold more erotica items and videos than they did books. One of the two young men behind the counter, the one with the wide smile, long hair, and the earring (in his left ear, not his nostril or eyebrow) pointed out the scenario of bars within the Quarter, an area of one-story street front commercial looking buildings. We tried to inquire what kind of scene was happening at each bar but John and I were dressed in our most "vanilla" outfits (polo shirts and khakis) and our own lack of gay specificity didn't elicit detailed descriptions. (We reeked "tourist" to the "nth degree.")

Outside on the sidewalk, John and I debated which bar to check out first, when a dark-looking, well-built man who had been smoking a cigarette nearby provided us with a better description than the sales clerk had about the two bars across the highway. (One had a better dance scene than the other but it started later.) We jaywalked behind him across the highway and followed him inside the supposedly busier bar without the dancing.

There was not much of a crowd here, however. The requisite slender, young bartender in T-shirt and jeans was working the center of a circular, wooden bar counter. Inside the bar it was darker than the night was outside. There were maybe ten customers and the only difference between this bar and one which you would find in, say, Worcester, Massachusetts, was that along with the cigarette machine, juke box, and scattered gay publications by the door, there were slot machines recessed into the top of the bar counter so that a customer could easily "drink and play."

We bought our new friend a drink. (I thought he was possibly interested in hooking up with John, as is usually the case when the two of us are out together.) But as it happened, our friend, a personal trainer by trade, was more interested in trying to sell us admission cards to one of the larger jazz clubs on the Strip. ("Hey, a lot of gay guys like you go there." Translation: guys who pass for straight—or worse—married guys away from home and out looking for "trouble.") But when it was clear we were not even nibbling at his wares, the trainer left disgusted and we fell into a conversation with another young man, a reedy blond with large, blood-shot blue eyes and a gravelly voice, who talked about how many crack heads there were in this town (and included himself).

It was still early according to "gay time"—barely after 10 p.m.—and John was much more determined than I to party. We had another drink, watched a repairman come in and fix one of the bar counter slot machines, and then asked the bartender to call us a cab to take us back to our hotel. John debated whether to stay behind on his own but decided against it. The wait for the cab was a long one—and our bar hunt was to be the only gay excursion of our trip. That is, until we decided, impulsively, to visit the Liberace Museum.

The Liberace Museum houses the late showman's collections of antique, rare, and gaudy pianos, automobiles, stage costumes, and jewelry. Opened in 1979 by Liberace himself, among the things you are likely to find are Chopin's piano from the early 1800s, a mirrored-tiled Rolls Royce, and the world's largest Austrian Rhinestone, totaling 115,000 karats and weighing over 50 pounds. The Museum is also filled with mannequins wearing the performer's trademark gold lamé dinner jacket, ostrich feather and mink capes, and the notorious red, white, and blue hotpants used in his salute to the 100th anniversary of the Statue of Liberty.

The walk through the rooms and exhibits of the Liberace Museum took less than an hour and was full of eye rolls, smiles, and giggles. It occurred to me by the time we entered the second building of the Museum, that the visitors were easily divided into Us and Them and the Us team was clearly in the minority. Nowhere in the Museum was Liberace's homosexuality revealed. (This was the man who successfully sued a British newspaper for hinting at his homosexuality early in his career and later in life suggested he was dying from a watermelon diet and not AIDS). The closest moment of truth arrives in a video segment broadcast on a television monitor when, amongst guests such as Debbie Reynolds, one of Liberace's young protégés is introduced to the studio audience. (Wink, wink.)

Today, Liberace's closeted but flamboyant homosexuality has become synonymous with his name. Nobody likes a Liberace queen (though they may find him entertaining). But unlike other closeted stars and celebrities whose sexuality have been revealed and dissected after their deaths (James Dean, Rock Hudson, Montgomery Clift, for example), Liberace has not become a gay icon or role model. (Nor was that his intent. He deliberately developed an audience outside of the gay community.) I can't say that I ever met Liberace or saw him perform live in concert. And I never wanted to. If he was ever on a television set that I was watching, I changed the channel quicker than you could say "Lawrence Welk." If the truth be known, as a boy, Liberace appalled me. I spent twelve years studying the piano and did my best to be serious about it. I did not want a flashy costume to get in the way of my performance. Or overpower it. And behind my closed bedroom door, listening to show tunes on a portable stereo player, it seemed somehow all right to emulate Barbra or Liza. But Liberace? *I don't think so.* Liberace was not part of the same sexual consciousness that summoned up images of Steve Reeves in a toga or Marlon Brando in a torn T-shirt.

But Liberace did seep into my consciousness, nonetheless. I knew who he was and I didn't want to be him. I once had the opportunity of meeting Liberace. In the mid-Eighties, the publicity firm where I worked representing a Broadway play was also publicizing Liberace at Radio City Music Hall. But I declined to see both the show and meet the performer. The sad thing about Liberace today is not that he never owned up to his sexuality in public but that this campiness and outrageousness has outstripped any appreciation or respect of whatever genuine talent he might have possessed. Fame, it seems to me, pushed him harder than art did. Or maybe I have misread him entirely. Perhaps he was never a great talent. Perhaps his art was his campiness and his music merely incidental to the image. How easily, for instance, can you identify Liberace playing on the radio?

I'd like to say that the Liberace Museum was merely a frozen moment in time, an homage to a man and his closet, a product of its own era. But the truth is that it is reflective of Vegas today: showy, glitzy, with all meaning and subtext hidden. Sin City is family and tourist oriented now in the same way that Times Square has been Disneyfied. It's also reflective somewhat of the state of a large public unawareness of the history of gay life in the United States. Nowhere to my knowledge is there a museum devoted to an individual's struggle with his gay sexuality nor to our collective gay experience with identity and acceptance. (Even the Andy Warhol Museum in Pittsburgh plays minimal interest to the artist's sexuality.)

I ended up not buying the Liberace ashtray. And I didn't buy a Liberace scarf, a Liberace necktie, or a Liberace T-shirt. What I bought was a chilled bottle of spring water with the Liberace script "L" logo on the label. I was dehydrated. We had been driving for hours that day and the heat outside was over 100 degrees. The water was pleasant, welcome, needed, and replenishing, something the Museum was not. Outside, walking to where we parked the rental car, I spotted a familiar looking store across the highway. I looked around and told my friend John that we were in the exact area of the gay bars we had been looking for a few days before, struggling in the dark to find the Gay Quarter. He did a double take and laughed, recognizing the gay bookstore we had discovered and the ironic moment we had just uncovered: The Liberace Museum is at the heart of gay Vegas.

The empty Liberace bottle stayed in the hotel room for another day or so, my unintentional shrine to the superpopularization of a man who despaired of the public really understanding him. It went in the trash before we checked out. I suppose I could have filled it up with water from the sink and carried it with me. But somehow that didn't seem right. Why adorn the substance when the substance is what is merely desired? I went thirsty for a while. And then somewhere at the airport I drank water from a fountain.

TWILIGHT ON THE ESPLANADE

The days are getting shorter, the weather cooler; already it is mid-September, 2000, the first year of the new millennium or the last of the old one, depending on your point of view. Labor Day has come and gone and this is the first weekend all summer that I have taken my roller blades from their nook in my kitchen and gone skating on the Esplanade, the ribbon of concrete that weaves between grassy knolls and the congested West Side Highway and stretches beside the Hudson River in Manhattan. Last summer, I was there quite a bit. This summer, more things than a lack of good weather have interrupted my outings.

My summer began with a trip to the emergency room. Rundown from a stressful week and putting up an unexpected houseguest, a former college roommate in town from California, Memorial Day weekend arrived with intensifying discomfort in my lower back. I've had growing back problems for about two years now, something I attributed to less time spent at the gym and more time spent at aging, as well as the increased pressures I've often forced onto my lower back from a variety of household projects—cleaning out my storage space, assembling a bookcase, rearranging the tower of fruit crates that create the writing workspace in my apartment. Though I was tired that week, I could not pinpoint a specific source for the sort of sharp, needleprick pain I was feeling. I tried to relieve it with an ice compress but the discomfort was only momentarily dulled, then tried painkillers and analgesics which seemed to help psychologically for a few moments, and then turned to ointments and creams recommended for sore muscles and other aches, hoping they could alleviate the persistent symptoms of something I felt was not entirely due to a back problem. Not even a hot bath and a few drinks offered a lasting respite.

By Saturday, it was impossible for me to sleep, impossible for me to find a position to remain in for more than a few minutes without the pain returning. Lying on my back, face up, staring at my blank ceiling, offered me no comfort. Neither did turning stomach down nor curling into a fetal position. Breathing became both a problem and a luxury. Could this be because I was now forty-four years old and still sleeping on a fold-up, fold-down futon which mimicked neither a sofa nor a bed? Or were my back problems borne out of years of being without a decent mattress in a tiny New York City apartment? Or was something more serious at work in my body? Was I in some kind of deep medical crisis?

Like many Americans I turned to the Internet first for advice. I plugged my symptoms into a search engine and began to worry over kidney stones, liver infections, and an inflamed appendicitis. By Sunday, a rash had erupted around one side of my waist which I attributed to an irritation from the ice packs and ointments. When I found that I had trouble reading and couldn't concentrate, I tried to psychologically imagine the pain away. Then, not wanting to spend the weekend confined to bed, I made it a few blocks down the street to meet a friend to see a movie, thinking that being outside of my apartment might also allow me to be outside of the pain. *No such luck.* In the lobby of the theater, explaining my predicament to my friend, I showed him the rash that was now ringing the left side of my waist. His diagnosis was easy and forthright. *Shingles.* After the movie, with the pain more intense and my mind a jumble of anxieties, instead of walking home, I walked a few extra blocks to the emergency room of the nearest hospital.

I have never invested much faith in doctors. Years ago, an ophthalmologist diagnosed me with cataracts (which another doctor could not find) at a time when many of my friends and co-workers were battling their own inexplicable battles against

HIV and AIDS. As I migrated through jobs and changed the direction of my career, I often changed medical insurance carriers and health plans, the last time selecting a general physician in my new HMO guidebook who was also amenable to gay patients.

My relationship with this physician had consisted of a routine medical exam and the explanation that sometime during my late twenties, while being tested for HIV, it was discovered that I also had a heart murmur, something that several other physicians I had seen before him had also been able to detect. During this exam, the doctor detected that I also had an abnormal EKG (a test that provides information about heart rhythm) and suggested that I make an appointment with a heart clinic to have an echocardiogram done, which I did a few days later. The clinic, located in a room of one of those expansive East Side hospitals, did not provide me with the results of the test or a discussion of their findings. Those were sent directly to my physician's attention. Or so I thought.

In all my years in New York City—more than twenty now—I've considered myself lucky to have never required an overnight stay in a Manhattan hospital. I'd also never had to rely on a city emergency room. Walking uptown to St. Luke's-Roosevelt, the emergency room nearest my apartment, I had visions of being in the midst of dangling, nearly-severed limbs and bullet-wounded bodies spewing blood on the floor—years of images culled from watching too many TV shows. Instead, I found the waiting room remarkably calm and vacant. In less than an hour I had seen a doctor and was given medication to ease the pain and a prescription for a drug to kill the virus which causes shingles. (It is an adult manifestation of the chickenpox virus.)

I was also advised to make a follow-up appointment with my general physician. I might have let that appointment slide by the wayside if I had not already booked a vacation to Las Vegas the following week. I cannot begin to accurately describe the searing pain shingles causes, but an approximation could be finding yourself inside a medieval torture apparatus where long, thin nails hammer your tendons into your bones. I was concerned that once my ER-supplied pain relievers ran out, the discomfort would return while I was out of town. During the follow-up visit with my physician, he suggested I have another general physical examination when I returned from vacation, and then asked, offhandedly as he checked his notes in my medical folder, if I had gone for the echocardiogram at the heart clinic. The shock must have registered in my face. It had been almost two years since I had had those tests done.

I would have cast this off as another cog in the wheel of the great doctor-and-insurance company shell game had it not been that for the fact that when I got home that evening, I discovered my doctor had left me a hasty message on my answering machine. He had had the heart clinic fax him the missing results. My echocardiogram showed that I had more than just a murmur. My heart was also enlarged and thickened. And it was something that needed more testing.

* * *

It is late afternoon when I enter the park at Christopher Street, but the sunlight is still bright and sharp in the sky—only a few clouds scattered against a sheet of blue. The roller blades are snugly packed in my knapsack and I sit on one of the benches and unlace my sneakers. Because of the cooler weather today, I have worn sweatpants and a jeans jacket over my T-shirt, even though others enjoying the Esplanade are not so warmly dressed. I've become more cautious this year than in others; the last thing I want is to catch a cold before winter even arrives.

The skates are tighter this year, too, bought second-hand a few years ago from a friend-of-a-friend who decided to abandon the sport when he realized he could not maintain his balance. I've added an extra pair of socks on top of the ones I normally wear to keep my heels from blistering and I have to adjust the pre-set snaps two notches wider. I've added close to ten extra pounds since last summer and I know from the larger waist sizes that I've been forced to wear that the extra pounds did not fall directly to my feet.

With the sneakers packed up, my sunglasses on, I head downtown along the path that is designated for bikers and skaters. In the past I've always bladed listening to cassette tapes, but today, since I'm worried about being a rusty on the wheels, I have left them at home. Instead, I simply let my surroundings keep me entertained. And there is plenty to look at: On one side, the light dances off the water as kayakers and boats navigate the river; on another, the flowers are still in bloom in the strips which separate the park from the West Side highway. And in front of me there is plenty of eye candy to enjoy: guys in tank tops and shorts, with a few of the hardier souls showing off their chests or six-pack abs.

I suppose if I were to pick a favorite place in Manhattan this would be it. I've made it here a few times this summer, sans roller blades: I walked here once on a date, another time on Gay Pride Sunday, another time to read a book in one of the new landscaped areas north of Christopher Street. To be here at twilight when all else is pulsing around town is to discover an unruffled inner world within the city. These are my favorite moments to be on the Esplanade—the Battery Park buildings jewel-like as the sun stretches down to the water and a feeling of being a part of a big city and apart from it at the same time—a sort of out-of-body experience that I've never been able to duplicate in any yoga or new-age movement class I've taken in the city.

I suppose if I were to deconstruct my preference for the Esplanade it would have as much to do with the water as with the view. Not long ago I read somewhere that the Chinese believed being near a body of moving water was meditative and relaxing, a philosophy I realize I have consciously accepted. The patterns of waves in the overall movement of water entertain the brain in the same way as patterns in fire or a flock of birds overhead in the sky. Many writers have described the effects of water on the human psyche and this is not the place for me to try to recount them. But it is clear that something ingrained within the mind responds to the splash and flow of water. For me, my mind opens up, expands, wanders, wonders. Things always seem to come into perspective out here by the Hudson River. The smell is not entirely of the sea or salt air, but not entirely clogged from the city, either. And at times, with the drumming ribbon of traffic along the highway, it is almost possible to imagine the steady sound of tires against concrete as waves lapping against sand.

As a journalist and an editor I heard a lot of discussion about the merits and minuses of the new construction under the auspices of the Hudson River Park Conservancy, the umbrella organization initiating the changes to the waterfront area, among them the reduction of prostitution and drug trade but also the loss of a safe zone for minority gay youth who are underage and can't congregate at bars. The transformation of the area seems to have accommodated the youth in the same way that the zoning of sex shops by the Giuliani administration did not entirely displace those stores, only made them a little harder to spot. Among the parents pushing strollers and dogs straining at their owners' leashes, the gay youth still come to see and be seen. And I notice a level of safety that exists now that didn't in years past. But the best thing about the new waterfront development is that it has opened up a host of activities for many city dwellers that were luxuries belonging only to suburbia, from the day-glow bowling alleys and dank-smelling equestrian stables at the Chelsea Piers to the put-put-golf course just north of Battery Park.

I skate around the pot holes in front of the large yellow building that blocks off Pier 40, and then out onto Pier 34 toward the ventilation shaft that rises from the Holland Tunnel (and looks as if it should be some kind of important war memorial). Instead of taking a seat on a bench as I might normally do, I head back toward the Esplanade. My goal today is to prove that my heart is no longer damaged goods. I want to physically test my stamina, to do the loop that I used to do last summer—down to the Winter Garden and back to Christopher Street.

Before I reach the awkward ascent into Battery Park, I stop to find my water bottle in my knapsack. I've not really skated very far but I'm dehydrated from carrying the skates while doing errands before reaching the Village. The water is not cold but it is satisfying and replenishing. The best thing so far is that the skating has not winded me; already I am thinking of skating further than I had planned.

* * *

The day my doctor told me my diagnosis, I went to a bar and got drunk, flagged a cab home, and passed out without undressing. I'd developed a growing dependency on alcohol since the end of a four-year relationship that had never become what I had hoped it would be. I'd turned to liquor—white wine, actually—in the same addictive way that I once reached out for cigarettes, anti-depressants, and sleeping pills. I hadn't reached the Ray Milland extreme in *The Lost Weekend*—hiding bottles under the sofa and pawning my wares for money to buy booze—but I had reached the point where I recognized my problem and that perhaps my drinking was creating a few more. One thing I'd learned about myself—even as I continued pouring glass after glass—was that I am prone to obsessive-compulsive behavior. (It's funny how as we get older we are able to look back on the shapes and folds of our lives even if there is little we can do to amend the behavior. I know now that I cannot have a pint of ice cream or a bag of cookies in my apartment, for example, without finishing them all in one sitting.)

I did not confess my growing alcoholism to my doctor when I returned for the general physical after my Vegas vacation. I only mentioned that I was a social drinker. I still felt it was something I could and would conquer on my own, in the same way I had overcome my other addictions. As it happened, I was more worried that day about a mole on my right leg which was changing texture. The doctor ran through his tests—blood was drawn, I stuck my tongue out, he looked in my eyes—and, at the end of this short, expensive session, he gave me the name of a referring dermatologist to have the mole removed and advised that I repeat the echocardiogram in order to measure any changes which might have occurred since the last test. This time, he said, call him and tell him when the test had been done; he would see to it that the results would be read in a more timely fashion. In my mind this was my doctor's subtle attempt to exonerate himself of any legal liability I could devise for his earlier oversight.

When I called the health clinic to make an appointment for another echocardiogram, I was referred to a satellite location instead of being sent directly to the hospital. The satellite clinic turned out to be a cardiologist's office on the Upper East Side. In order to have my medical insurance pay for another echocardiogram test, I also needed a letter from my doctor requesting the additional examination. My doctor's officiousness this time was a surprise, but not as much as the letter's content. When he faxed me a copy of the letter the shock of a concrete diagnosis registered for the first time. There it was in black-and-white type. I was a patient who had "a history of hypertrophic cardiomyopathy."

* * *

Hypertrophic cardiomyopathy, or HCM for short, is a condition in which the muscle of the heart is abnormal in the absence of an apparent cause. There is no particular symptom or complaint, but there may generally be a shortness of breath, chest pain, palpitations, lightheadedness, and blackouts—all the signals, really, of an oncoming heart attack. The major abnormality of the heart in HCM is an excessive thickening of the heart muscle. Heart muscle can thicken as a result of high blood pressure or prolonged athletic training, but in HCM the muscle thickening occurs without an obvious cause. Usually there is a significant increase in the thickness of the muscle of the left ventricle (the large pumping chamber of the heart). The most common area of the increased thickness is on the ventricular septum (the wall of the heart muscle that separates the left and right ventricles) just below the aortic valve. Parts of the heart commonly affected in other conditions (the heart valves and main coronary arteries) are normal in HCM, but cardiology tests are strongly recommended to detect for any obstructions to or irregularities in the heartbeat.

An echocardiogram is a non-invasive sound wave imaging test that allows a physician to observe the heart as it is beating. It allows for the measurement of muscle thickness, degree of obstruction, chamber size, valve movement, and blood flow. In the examination room at the satellite clinic, I removed my shirt and lay down on my left side on an examination table, my left arm hooked behind my head, my right arm falling behind my back. A technician lubricated a spot on my chest with a KY-like gel and placed a hand-held microphone against my skin at the site of my heart. The lights in the room were lowered and the mic returned echo waves of sound which were captured by a computer and converted into pictures. This technology allows the internal structures of the heart to be visualized, permitting an accurate measurement of heart wall thickness.

In this particular room there was a shelf on the wall above the examination table. On it was a monkey-like sculpture that appeared to be made out of polished and painted dark wood. Lying on my side, staring at this monkey-doll, I had the strange sensation of déjà vu—that I had been here before—the room was familiar to me in a way that I could not exactly pinpoint.

There was no immediate diagnosis given to me that day. I saw only a technician that visit whose most telling comment was a suspicious "ooohhh" as he located my heart with his electronic wand. He asked me if I fainted often and what kind medication I took. My answers also seemed to surprise him: I had never fainted before in my life and I wasn't on any sort of medication for my heart.

Outside on the sidewalk in front of the cardiologist's building, standing and squinting at the sun, déjà vu arrived again. I had a mental image of leaving this office years before. Then, somewhere in my past, I had smoked a cigarette and walked away, propelled by the irony that a heart problem could be my fate when I was so worried about becoming HIV-positive. That inner turmoil would make it somewhere around 1985 in my Manhattan chronology. That had been a summer of fear for me, the year I hadn't imagined myself living long enough to develop a heart problem because I was too worried about dying from AIDS.

* * *

The results of the second echocardiogram were the same as the first: I had a significant thickening of the septum. Even though there was no progression of thickening between the two tests, my doctor suggested that I return to the heart clinic to meet with a cardiologist. The cardiologist who had evaluated both echo tests had also advised my physician that I should have another test done—a Holter monitor. This monitor, an octopus-like contraption of electrode pads connected to wires connecting to a recording unit, is worn for twenty-four hours and records the sequence of heartbeats in order to detect any irregular rhythms called arrhythmias.

It was a four week wait before I could get an appointment with the cardiologist and have the Holter monitor test. Enough time for me to forget about the potential trouble of my health. Or so I thought. Because two things happened right away that changed my state of mind. The first thing was I begin to research my heart condition on the Internet. The second was I stopped drinking.

Knowledge is power, or so the dictum goes, but sometimes too much information can also be a horrendous thing. In retrospect, I wish I had tolerated my stupidity and gone about my summer without being so curious. Ignorance is bliss, after all, or so another dictum goes. On the Internet I discovered several new facts about hypertrophic cardiomyopathy, among them that there is no known cause or cure for the disease. No treatment is available that returns the heart to its normal operation. The outlook for patients facing this diagnosis is also inconsistent. There are some patients who remain asymptotic and lead a normal life. Other patients live with the increased risk of a premature and sudden death which can occur with little or no warning.

Sudden death. Now that was an alarming concept to me. And it's incredible how much power a simple combination of words can have over you. I did not feel unhealthy—even while battling shingles—until my doctor handed me an untreatable diagnosis. At first I used it to explain a lot of inexplicable things about myself: the poor circulation in my feet (which was why I always wore socks, even on the hottest days of the summer), my lack of concentration and lightheadedness when I was stressed and overworked, my growing insomnia and inability to focus on long distances. But then I began to convince myself I *was* ill. I had a diagnosis. I had an incurable disease.

As the days ticked by, I grew increasingly anxious about the test. I was aware of the increased force of my heartbeat; at times an extra beat could be felt rising up into the arteries near my collarbone. At night, lying on my left side, the force of my heart was outrageous; there was no way I could find to control its speed or lessen its thuds. Walking down the street I started to become dizzy, my vision blurring. At the gym, I was so worried about fainting that I began to wear a bag around my waist that contained my health insurance cards, apartment keys, and notes to strangers in case I blacked out. Things seemed finite to me; I was living in a tunnel. I began to worry about my unfinished writing projects, about dying alone in my apartment. I made out my will, and, on one sleepless night, I typed up instructions to a friend in case my body was discovered if I succumbed to a premature, sudden death.

And that was not the end of it. In the days leading up to the Holter monitor I began to experience a burning sensation in my left shoulder. Somewhere I had read that that kind of pain was a prelude to a heart attack—an early warning sign. Like the pain from the shingles, this was a pain I could not relieve or will away. Now, in retrospect, I realize after more reading on the Internet that some of these problems might have been due to my withdrawal from alcohol. Drying out from booze can cause muscle cramps as well as other psychological and physiological discomforts. For me, this was a period when my jaw tightened and my tongue ached for the sweet memory of alcohol. For days I couldn't concentrate. This is what the Web sites don't tell you: Drying out is another fight in life.

Yet the simple, honest truth was—or so it seemed to me at the time—I had become afraid of my life. Of living. One weekend alone in my apartment I was convinced that the muscle spasms which had started in my chest were a preface to my sudden death. The cramping was not as painful as it was frightening. Trying not to panic, I packed an overnight bag and walked uptown again to the emergency room. In my mind I rationalized that if I could successfully make to the hospital then I would have another option of either checking in or admitting that there was nothing *really* wrong with me and returning home.

The walk was both lovely and disturbing. It was one of those cool July evenings, not yet fully dark, very little humidity. My walk took me along the strip of Ninth Avenue in the West 40s where I used to live, an area of town that is rapidly gentrifying in the same trendy fashion that Columbus Avenue did two decades before when I first moved to the city. The actors and theatrical professionals, who have moved into the neighborhood housing before rents skyrocketed, seemed to be even younger and more attractive than when I lived there. Gay male couples holding hands in public were now as comfortable in this neighborhood as they are in Chelsea and the Village. I was aware of them all as I walked—aware that I was different from them going about their normal, fabulous lives on a Saturday night—I was worried, alone, and unhealthy. I couldn't even wallow in self-pity by drinking.

When I reached the hospital, I circled the block, thinking all the trouble was merely of my mind's fabrication. For all I knew I could only have heartburn, something that happened whenever I ate rich or spicy foods cooked in oil or butter. But I knew this wasn't heartburn—but I also hadn't completely convinced myself that this *was* a heart attack. Don't you just drop down to the ground in agonizing pain when that happens? Don't you have to have someone call an ambulance to take you to the hospital?

I went inside the corner bodega and bought a bottle of water and sat on the steps of St. Paul's Church, watching two men load boxes into a van. I stayed there till it was dark and the only light around was from the traffic and overhead street lamps, then decided I was okay and walked home. On my walk downtown, I stopped at the video store and rented a movie—*Shakespeare in Love*, even though I had seen it before during its initial theatrical release. Then I walked across the street to the liquor store and bought a bottle of wine. The bottle was finished before the movie ended, the alcohol comforting in the same way as the movie. Both were familiar, lighthearted, and necessary. I fell easily asleep that night, momentarily untroubled by the course of events and my desire to challenge them.

* * *

The skating goes slower when I enter Battery Park. The slick, hexagonal tiles of the sidewalk pose no problem for rollerblading, but there are more people to navigate. A year ago, I would have brought a book or a magazine in my knapsack and stopped at this point and read for a while. But that was before my doctor made me restless. The day he explained my heart condition to me he said, "You have one of those types of hearts you hear about athletes dropping dead from for no apparent reason."

I am not an athlete—far from it. In high school and college I shied from as many athletic activities as I could (even as I lusted after the boys who succeeded at them). I didn't enter a gym until my mid-twenties—and only as a national fad to be pumped up embraced the nation and I felt it might increase my chances to find a steady boyfriend. But even then I seldom had much enthusiasm for it—the working out—I once gave up a membership to the Chelsea Gym because I couldn't relax around all that testosterone and heavy-handed cruising—it didn't seem the right place for me at that time nor the right kind of guy I wanted. It wasn't until my mid-thirties when the one-two punch of stopping smoking and a failed relationship sent me emotionally crashing that I turned to exercise as a therapy against stress, anxiety, and depression. My activity of choice in those years was cycling—not in a gym class but out in the countryside or at parks—and I did it so often I ended up with some shapely gams (as well as some muscular problems around my knees). Which was why I was thankful for the rollerblading boom when it happened—skating allowed me an alternative exercise to biking.

I've often remarked to my friends that I skate like "a little old lady." Speed is not of importance to me; in fact, I find it frightening. Skating is simply a slightly faster, more MTV way of watching the world. And if the truth be told, I enjoy looking around as much I do the physical activity. And I know I'm not the only person with that opinion. Today, one biker, a middle-aged man out with his son, creates a near-accident when he spots an outdoor pool table in Roosevelt Park and abruptly stops and shouts to point this out to his son. All of us nearby respond to the father's cry of "Hey, look!" What I notice is not so much the outdoor pool table but a player enjoying being outdoors. He is shirtless, tanned, and buff, and looks like he could be the perfect pitchman in television land: the guy washing the sports car in the driveway or out throwing a Frisbee to his shaggy dog. If I felt I was in better shape, I would dream about meeting him. Instead, I sigh and skate on.

Ahead the State of Liberty stands out in perfect, sharp detail. Lady Liberty. The beacon of hope. The whole scene of the New York harbor unfolds—the mega yachts harbored while a few sail boats take to the wind, the shoreline of New Jersey on the other side of the Hudson, the birds dipping and swooping in the air. I skate until I reach the plaza of the Winter Garden, to me, one of the most breathtaking spots in the city. It looks as if it really belongs in another city—somewhere in

Europe, I think, a modern day Europe, really, a combination of old world elegance with modern architecture. When I reach an area shaded by two rows of dense, arching trees, I decide it's time to turn around. I've been skating for almost forty-five minutes. My thighs and hamstrings and glutes have begun to ache. Instead of going back along the water, I decide to take a sidewalk in front of a row of shops where there are not as many walkers. But after two blocks I miss the water and it's back into the crowd I go. I skate slowly, letting my eyes get the most exercise.

* * *

It was a miserable morning when I showed up at the clinic to be strapped inside the Holter monitor. The sky was gray, the air thick and steamy; a steady stream of rain pounded into puddles as if the water was boiling. By the time I made it to the reception area I was soaked and cranky—the subway was at its worst: hot, humid, crowded with grouchy commuters making their way to work. I felt small and miserable as the nurses and technicians moved about me, like a dog brought in from a storm but made to stay in a corner because he was smelly and wet.

In an examination room, a nurse shaved away portions of my chest hair with a disposable razor and taped a set of gummy electrode pads in place against selected sites on my chest and rib cage, the wiring from the pads leading into a portable electrocardiogram, a small recording device which I strapped to a belt that looped through the waist of my pants. The rain had made my khakis damp and heavy and the weight of the recorder—about the size of a portable cassette-player—made the pants hang so low I felt as if I were wearing the wrong size of clothing. The purpose of this test was to determine the presence and severity of disturbance in your heart rhythm by wearing the device over a period of twenty-four to forty-eight hours. The monitoring device can correlate heart rhythm disturbances with symptoms you may be having, such as dizziness, palpitations, or fainting spells, all of which are also hand-noted throughout the day in a diary.

After being fitted with the monitor, I had a consultation with the cardiologist that lasted well over an hour. A small, Asian-American woman, she reviewed with me the reason for the test and we discussed the history of my health and heart condition. I attributed the possibility of an abnormal heart from being a premature birth; born two months premature, I had weighed less than four pounds. Other than my recent bout with shingles, I mentioned that I had no health issues other than those brought about by my anxieties over the test. We did not discuss my alcohol consumption—for I had made it through a four-week period of sobriety—but we did discuss my exercise and gym routines. I confessed that I had changed my routine about a year before to include more aerobics than heavy weight-lifting, due to the fact that I was unable to shed some extra pounds and was hoping that this would help. She seemed to be concerned about the amount of exercise I did, and asked that my trips to the gym be suspended until she had finished with her testing.

She then suggested that my heart condition could be genetically-caused. I tried to dismiss this notion by explaining that I come from a strong-hearted family. Even with a family history of diabetes, prostate and colon cancer, both of my parents were still alive in their mid-seventies and my grandmothers had lived to their nineties. I felt the doctor was grasping too hard at this cause as we discussed my brother and sisters. Her questioning made me uncomfortable with the realization that I had always maintained a remote relationship with my siblings.

The rest of session was spent detailing my rising anxieties over the heart tests and my concern that my daily health was at risk. When I explained the burning sensation that had occurred in my shoulder, the cardiologist suggested I meet with the unit's clinical psychologist during my testing process. I agreed—and, at the close of our session, her assistant scheduled an appointment for me to meet the psychologist the following day when I returned the Holter monitor.

It's odd how the mind records things when it's under stress that it might otherwise forget. It's curious, too, what images are retained when the mind is confronted with the body's mortality. The diary I kept that day is full of senseless and useless details of importance to no one but myself. (I ate pasta for lunch. Do you care?) But what floated through my consciousness were some larger issues as well. How do I explain this to my family? Or should I? Have I reached the place where I will die? What could I do to give myself a passion to keep on living and working? Should I think about moving to another city? Could I survive if I were to go on medical disability?

The rest of the day was uneventful; I stayed at home watching the rain, reading, making notes for an article such as this. My one excursion out into the storm—lunch with my friend Jon, a playwright, ended with a climb up the stairs of his building to his fifth floor apartment where, winded, I unbuttoned my shirt and allowed him to take photographs of my wearing the Holter monitor.

The day would have ended like that if I hadn't, upon waking from a nap, remembered something about my youngest sister. The year I moved to Manhattan—more than two decades before—my mother had made a passing remark about my sister going through medical tests. I tried to recollect what there were about—her blood pressure? Her heart? A blood clot? I knew I would have to contact my family to get at this truth. Before I could spend more time fretting about this, I reached for the phone.

I tried calling my sister but the telephone number I had for her had been disconnected—I knew she had moved into a new house in North Carolina but hadn't known she had changed her number. Long distance information had no listing for her. So I called my parents in suburban Atlanta and my father answered the phone. I explained to him why I was concerned about my sister's health and wanted to contact her. He took the news of my heart tests with his usual detachment and said it wasn't necessary to bother my younger sister. He knew about those tests. And what he also gave me were some remarkable details about the state of my own health and history.

* * *

I had not been expected to live, my father told me, the odds were against me. I was too little, too sickly. "You weren't doin' too well," he said, when we talked on the phone. My mother had returned home from the hospital without me to take care of my older brother, then four years-old. After six weeks in the hospital, my mother convinced her doctor to set up an incubator in the house, the first time a hospital had ever allowed the equipment to be set up in a private home. "It was nothing but a box with a lid," my father said to me. "There was just a pan of water, a towel to keep the humidity in, and a 100-watt lightbulb to keep you warm." This was where I lived for the first three months of my life.

As for my younger sister, she was not born premature but during her physical for her college admission, she was discovered to have an abnormal EKG. Additional cardiology tests discovered that she had a small hump on the exterior of her heart, something that posed her no difficulty or obstruction in blood flow and was not a tumor. My mother's father, however, had died of heart attack at age fifty-three. He had been admitted to the hospital at the time because he was diabetic and his blood sugar was high.

What my father didn't mention was my grandfather's extra weight and obsessive drinking problems might have also caused his death. My mother had once confessed that the reason why her teeth were so crooked was because sometime during her teens "her daddy stepped on her retainer and he wasn't about to spend all that money again for another one." Several versions of the story later, I learned that her "daddy had been drinkin' that night."

Like many religious Southern families, our problems were kept unmentioned, hidden in the closet or swept under the carpet. When I came out as gay to my family the fact was not repeated beyond immediate family members for fear of what the neighbors or members of the church might think. My brother's behaviors have also met with a similar secrecy. Once, while out drinking, one of my brother's buddies shot my brother in the leg with his own shotgun and left him on the side of the road to bleed to death because he wasn't ready to return home yet. I only heard about the incident when my sister called and mentioned my brother might want to receive a phone call while he was in the hospital recuperating.

But the fact is I can't really blame my alcoholism on my family or heredity. Some of it is my own fault, after all. And genetic or not, my father has a standard of self-control and discipline that I certainly did not inherit. The unfortunate thing is that I do think some of this behavior has been aggravated by coming out into a generation of gay men who socialized and befriended one another in bars and clubs. I started smoking in gay bars because I was tired of looking bored or frightened that I would have to leave alone. I finally stopped the cigarettes when I realized that few of my friends continued smoking. I turned to anti-depressants to weed myself of nicotine, then spent a few more years trying to weed myself of the need of an artificial substance to make me feel better about myself. I suppose that the drinking now serves both as a reason and a release from self-pity. For the record, I'd like to stop the habit, but then I'd also like something in my life to make it feel a little better as well. It's such a vicious cycle that I often worry where I will go next: Will I turn myself into a chaste Christian praying hourly for God to give me strength to resist the urges that are, well, what make me human?

* * *

Skating back toward Christopher Street my right foot begins to hurt. I know it is because the boot is too tight but I skate on, adapting my pace to the pain, thinking that I will stop and adjust it and drink more water when I reach the point where I entered the park. Ahead, I see another skater—a fortyish woman with a hooded sweatshirt that bobs against her back with the same pulse as her ponytail—swerve when a fast-paced cyclist passes by too close to her. She doesn't lose her balance and fall but she skates out of the lane and stops, turning around to see the path the cyclist is now taking. Our eyes meet as I skate by her and I notice her disgust. I know she must be thinking how his recklessness has impacted her recreation, and it makes me think how even when the weather is glorious we are still at the whims of both the random and deliberate paths we choose throughout the day. The truth is this what-does-destiny-have-in-store-for-me speculation has crossed my mind often in recent weeks. It's no secret that I have constructed my own unstable house of cards in New York. As one of those New Yorkers who live hand-to-mouth from paycheck to paycheck because of high-rents and middle-class lifestyles, an injury or health crisis would probably cause a tremendous change in my life. Without any savings or investments at my disposal (those are luxuries available to Upper East Siders and not an aging, struggling West Side writer), a simple broken bone would probably mean the difference between my staying in New York or leaving it. Without the ability to earn a weekly income, I'd be forced to give up my apartment and seek shelter with either family or friends.

Somehow one thought displaces another and I forget about the nagging pain from the too-tight boot. I skate until I reach the spot where the vendor who sells soft drink parks his cart. Instead of sitting down, removing the skates, and taking the subway home, I decide I'm not ready to give up skating; I've met my goal and now want to best it. I skate around a small construction site and continue my path northward. On my left the sun hangs low in the sky like a fiery basketball on the rebound. Twilight is approaching but not quite here.

* * *

I'd always believed I inherited my anxieties from my mother and her side of the family. My grandmother was a chronic complainer; I remember when I was seven or eight years-old I overheard my father's comments about her—that no matter how good she felt, she never felt good enough, something was always "actin' up" on her. My mother never complained in that sort of fashion, perhaps, because she knew my father's opinion about "that sort of behavior." My mother did, however, worry a lot. She worried about my father's heartburn, my brother's broken back, my sisters going out on dates too soon. The last thing she wanted for me was to see me move to Manhattan, away from the rest of the family, meaning her. She worried about where I would live, what I would eat, how safe I would be walking the streets of a big city.

    I tried to remain pleasant with the nurse when I returned to the hospital the next morning to have the Holter monitor dismantled and removed. It was still raining and the relentless humidity and the inability to shower and shave had left me smelly and disheveled. When I realized that tape from the electrode pads had left a gummy residue on my skin, I decided to return home and clean up before seeing the psychologist. (A feat which required crossing Manhattan island from its extreme east to west sides and vice versa with the help of public transportation, a journey I would not wish on anyone but an enemy during such foul weather conditions.)

    By the time I arrived back at the hospital for my appointment with the psychologist, I felt gloomy and defeated. I've suffered from self-diagnosed depression since the mid-Eighties, the year I willingly left a lucrative career as an entertainment publicist to try to be a professional writer. I never expected it to be a high-income career, but I thought that after more than a decade of part-time work at the craft of writing during evenings, weekends, and holidays that I might have achieved the ability to commit myself full-time to it and not have to rely on an assortment of odd jobs and temporary positions to maintain a decent income to survive in Manhattan. This was one of the things I confessed to the psychologist early in the session, my anxieties over still having to scrape a living together while many of my friends were raising babies and buying vacation homes. A middle-aged man with a scrappy black-and-gray beard, the psychologist quizzed me about my work—asked me my income, what publications I had written for. I mentioned that most of my work dealt either with the subjects of gay men or AIDS and that the personal impact of the epidemic had also created stretches of depression. He countered with the suggestion that perhaps I might give up writing and get a "real job" instead of continuing at it as a part-time freelancer—Wasn't I at the age to begin thinking about things like health benefits and retirement?

His suggestion left a burning resentment in my chest that I was unable to shake for the remainder of the session. This was not why I had come here or what I had expected to hear. I had anticipated some guidance and discussion of the daily workings of my heart which the cardiologist and her staff had not provided me—so far in my appointments and consultations no one mentioned facts such as the appropriate blood cholesterol levels, what was an acceptable daily limit of caffeine, how cold medications might affect my heartbeat, if alcohol or saunas could cause dehydration, what kind of warning signs I might look for, if I should join a support group—information and questions which I had gleaned while surfing the Internet. To his credit, the psychologist did ask if I did any drugs, either recreational or otherwise. When I admitted to drinking a bit too much in the solitude of my apartment, he made it clear that it was not something he wanted to focus on. In fact, he said, the only drug he was really concerned about was cocaine. *Cocaine?* I had only tried cocaine once—about twenty years before. *In the Seventies.* Experimenting my first year in the city. My first year away from the reigns of my family. When I was young.

Toward the end of the session we spent a few minutes learning how to meditate and the psychologist suggested I consider taking yoga classes—perhaps that might help me with my anxieties. The session ended with the doctor discussing his fees and suggesting a follow-up visit while my other heart examinations continued.

Outside, walking to the subway, I barely noticed the rain had stopped; I was too concerned that I had become a puppet of the medical system once again—something had convinced me that there was a problem with my heart even though I continued to function as I always had—even with its natural level of depression. Something else had led me to believe that my growing worries were, well, growing out of control even though they were just normal worries. The more the shock of the session began to wear off, the more I felt psychologically raped and abused. Mentally, I knew I was healthy enough to function on a daily basis. And I wasn't about to stop writing. That was the thing that kept me going. My reason to live. It was my *passion*.

* * *

It was another two weeks before I returned to the clinic for further testing. In that time I had returned to drinking, trying to find a way to break the anxiety of the job, trying to convince myself to continue working on a novel I had started four months before. The truth is I had plenty of desire to write but I was also paralyzed about embarking on a large project, something I might not complete, thinking, what would it matter?—the end was coming soon, wasn't it? In all this time there was no word from the cardiologist—she had told me she would call me with the results of the Holter monitor within a few days of the test. And no word from my physician, either—for some idiotic reason I thought maybe the cardiologist would have relayed the results to him. Once again, medical disinterest created my heightened apprehension; I was wrestling with mortality and nobody was giving me the attention I wanted to have.

I had been sober for twenty-four hours the morning I showed up at the clinic for the next stress test—I thought that was the least I could do to prepare for the event. I was led into a small room where I changed into a hospital gown and then into another where I met the three technicians who would be running the tests. They tried their best to keep me relaxed and focused as more hair was shaved from my chest and I was strapped into another set of electrode pads and wires. One man complimented me on the watch I wore—I learned during the hour of the test that he and his wife sold watches and cameras at a weekend street fair in the Bronx. Another technician passed along to me his wife's public relations business card, suggesting I contact her if I wanted to find more freelance writing outlets. The cardiologist and the third technician—another Asian-American woman whom I had briefly met before this visit—ran me through another echocardiogram. As I lay on the examination table, the lights of the room dimmed, the wand at my chest, the computer capturing the crashing waves of sound—another thought ran through my head that I should at least be thankful that I had maintained a health plan from a former job. How much was this costing? Three technicians, a doctor, a room full of hospital equipment. Everyone here just because of me. Silly ol' sick me.

After the echocardiogram I was led to a motorized treadmill where I started another test by walking slowly. Gradually, the incline was raised, making it more physically difficult to continue my pace. Throughout the test my heartbeat and blood pressure were measured and monitored. This test was to see how far I could push my heart (without passing out). Every three minutes, when the elevation changed, someone in the room yelled out to me to make sure I was okay and capable of continuing. I walked for eighteen minutes, reaching the steepest incline the technicians wanted to test, my heartbeat reaching 180 beats per minute.

From the treadmill I was quickly led back to the examination table where another set of echocardiograms were done to capture the heart beating at this faster pulse, in order to detect any current or potential obstructions in the blood flow. As the cardiologist and the technician examined these photographs, I got dressed again in the changing room.

The whole experience ended while I was tying my shoes. The cardiologist interrupted my dressing to say that I only had a minor obstruction when my heart was beating at such a fast pace. The Holter monitor had revealed that I had a few extra heartbeats, but nothing which posed a serious daily threat. The bloodwork my physician had supplied to her had not indicated any additional areas of concern. Death was not imminent. No surgery was necessary. No medication was prescribed. No other cardiology tests were needed. Only a minor warning was issued. "Don't lift heavy weights at the gym," she said. "The pressure could cause your pulse to be too rapid."

* * *

The skating turns rougher after 14th Street. There are fewer people but the lane narrows near the sanitation warehouse and the surface becomes an unwieldy a mix of sand, gravel, and potholes. I stumble a bit but never completely lose my balance and fall, the blading more cautious steps than slow skating. In some places, only a chain link fence separates me from the West Side highway; in others, a concrete divider barely thigh-high, the cars so close I could lose my balance if I don't concentrate on my own journey.

When I reach the southern entrance to the Chelsea Piers, a man in an orange vest waves me to detour through the internal structure of ramps, warehouse-like buildings, and parking garages—the outside access lane is closed today due to repair work. I skate along a boardwalk into a hallway where the entrance to the brewery and the bowling alley are located and where large black-and-white photographs hang, historical pictures of the giant passenger ships such as the U.S.S. Washington, the Mauretania, the Lusitania, and the Carpathia and the crowds that used to gather here to watch or board them. I keep my pace slow to avoid crashing into pedestrians while I study the photos and read the captions, my mind wandering from history back to the future and how badly my legs and back might ache tomorrow from even this simple exertion.

When the hallway intersects with one of the parking garage exit lanes I decide to skate outside again, thinking that I have traveled far enough north to bypass the road construction. Outside, I learn I have not skated beyond the repair work, and I stop to lean down to adjust the snaps on my left boot a bit wider—the pressure is now unbearable.

Instead of backtracking, I decide that there is enough room to skate close to the garage exits, and I pick up a bit of speed as I continue to leave the area. My position near the wall does not allow me to monitor the traffic exiting the upcoming garage portals, but since the area is closed to traffic, I am not expecting to have to negotiate any cars. Suddenly, as soon as I skate in front of an exit, a Jeep appears: black, dusty, and headed directly into me. When we collide I use the palm of my hands to bounce back away from the body of the Jeep in order to keep my balance and not fall or slip beneath the tires. My strategy works and when I clear my head from the shock of what has happened, I notice my handprints on the dusty black finish of the Jeep.

A woman riding in the passenger side shakes her head at me as if this were all my fault. I mouth an obscenity wide enough for her to detect and skate in front of the Jeep toward the exit lane and the rocky path of the Esplanade which continues a few feet away.

The near miss with the Jeep will be what I remember most about the outing, my afternoon mission on the Esplanade. It will not be that I reached and exceeded my skating goal. It was that I cheated death one more time.

Skating again on the Esplanade, toward the heliport and the Javits Convention Center, I take a quick inventory of myself. The palms of my hands burn from the near accident, my wrists ache slightly from being pushed so quickly backward. Otherwise I am fine, though my heart is racing at a faster pace than it has been at all day. I think about what a friend said to me two summers ago when he almost drowned but didn't, swimming to shore to survive an unexpected undertow. "I guess my time's not up," he said, spitting out a throat full of salt water into the sand.

I guess my time is not up either, I think, feeling the swollen colors of twilight now around me. The air is both warm and cold against the sweat of my back. And something in the universe has made me lucky. At this moment I am happy and sober. This is a something I can write about. This feeling. This is something else I can try to understand.

WHAT DID NOT CHANGE

The view has changed. What was there before is there no longer.

In the hours after the attack on the World Trade Center I heard many reporters and journalists say that life as we knew it would never be the same. But in this same period of time I found myself answering many questions about my life in New York City, questions from my parents, my relatives, my friends out of town, my friends in other parts of the city.

Our connections with one another at these moments were meant to reassure each other that we were still alive and doing well. Nonetheless, I was aware of the ironies contained within my responses. My life had not changed, the basic quality of life as I knew it had not been disrupted. At home and at the office my electricity worked. So did my other utilities: water, gas, phone, even cable TV arrived without any glitches. (HBO and Showtime were still broadcasting movies, QVC was still offering tremendous bargains.) At my job at a company in Times Square, even though I and my co-workers were able to watch the attack on television, we were not sent home early the day of the attack or in the following days of chaos. In fact, we were encouraged to continue working. On Wednesday, September 12, the day after the collapse of the Trade towers, as nearby landmarks such as Grand Central and Penn Station were being evacuated by bomb threats, the chief financial officer where I worked made announcements over the building's fire command system that the safest place for all of us was to remain at our desks, *working*. The irony of this, too, did not escape me, that the ruthlessness and greed of corporate America could not be broken by a mere threat. Later in the day I would hear a story about workers in the south Tower who were sent back to their desks when they attempted to flee because the neighboring Tower was on fire. An announcement, too, had told them they were in no sort of danger.

But did my life change in these moments? Really change? My first thought at this time was an idea that had surfaced in my consciousness in the mid-1980s: I had survived something others had not. In those past days the news was filled with losses from the AIDS epidemic, not just the announcements of rising infection rates and obituaries of single men coded with the wordings of "prolonged illnesses," but the rumors of gay men who had leapt from the balconies of their apartments in order to avoid what they considered a more ignoble kind of death. As I placed phone calls and sent e-mails in the minutes after the terrorist attack—to check in with those I knew—it soon became clear that though I and my friends had survived this attack, we were not to be spared the stories of those who did not. Suddenly the news was filled with stories of workers missing, of firefighters caught in the collapse, of companies wiped out on the upper floors of the buildings. And the rush of grief that I had successfully come to terms with years before came tumbling back into my consciousness. How do you deal with devastation like this when the accumulation of grief is so swift? What had once slowly seeped into my consciousness was now ringing like an unanswered cellphone.

So the question remains: Did New York City change in these days? Yes and no. The streets were empty, many were blockaded, late in the week fighter jets could be heard overhead, trucks full of oxygen tanks or moving equipment would race down the streets with an escort of sirens, yellow "caution" tape circled every public and government building for days. On the block where I live stands a police precinct and I had to get permission to enter my building on the evening of the attack. But at the company where I work my bosses reacted to the tragedy by creating more busy work for me to do. On a usual business day my job as a temporary officer worker seems frivolous to me—I merely type and distribute correspondence and corporate legal documents—and on the day of national mourning I found myself in front of a fax machine waiting for a hundred pages to be successfully transmitted between New York and Boston because Federal Express was not operating. Was this how my life was to change? Since I had been spared a personal grief, was the rising level of my frustration to be the psychological hurdles that I must leap over?

For days each morning I awoke hearing explosions and sirens outside my apartment, a refuge off Ninth Avenue that does not normally harbor those sounds. Even before my body had fully awakened I turned on the TV expecting a worse turn of events. The news would greet me that no one was rescued, that bodies might have been pulverized in the collapse, and that the wind had shifted and the strange bitter smell I now detected in my apartment was the aftermath of a burning building. Was this what the newscaster meant that life as I knew it would never be the same again? That I had now learned that death and terror and fear possessed a different kind of smell? But had my emotional balance really changed or had it just been momentarily disrupted?

And did my life, the core being of my existence, change in these moments? After work one day I met a friend for drinks at a gay bar on the Upper East Side. By then I was aware that the gay community had also suffered losses in this tragedy—a co-pilot of one of the hijacked planes was gay, a gay couple and their adopted child had been on board another. I stood in a room with a drink in one hand fully aware that I was socializing at a moment when in another part of the same town a fireman was confronting a mass of smoldering debris. What kind of person did that make me? Was I in shock or denial or just not willing to yield to the potential fear? Or was I seeking out the company of others as a solace *from* this fear?

The ironies of the times would surface when I ordered another drink. The gay guys who ignored you continued to ignore you; if the world was collapsing, which many thought it was, some gay men would still not acknowledge that you existed within the same room.

But this would be what I could not truly escape—a sense that I was living a life without disruption while others so close by were not as fortunate. Still, my life *was* different than others in the city. Earlier in the day a co-worker proudly arrived at my desk and said she was going to give blood at a Red Cross center on the other side of town and did I want to go with her. My response was a mumble of words and coughs and excuses. Though she was aware that I was gay she was not aware that gay men were still not allowed to donate blood in this country. How do you layer this kind of helplessness into all of the other ones you feel? Do you admit your frustration with anger? Or do you tell her the truth—that even in times of national emergencies when patriotism reaches an all-time flag-waving fever pitch, gay men are considered, well, as something *sub rosa* in this country.

Ironies would continue to fill my hours and thoughts. A friend e-mailed me that a reading of his new musical was being postponed because of the attacks. Within minutes of this postponement another friend had asked me if I wanted to go to a party that would occur on the same date and time of what was not happening. Why was one considered in bad taste and another not? And it soon became clear, too, while wandering around the city, that the media was overplaying the image of a transformed New Yorker into a generous and considerate citizen. True, that was the case in several situations, and there were avenues and avenues of cheering men and women in the city, and countless good deeds went untold. But the local news was filled with reports of hotel owners gauging stranded tourists. Street vendors suddenly appeared hawking World Trade T-shirts and souvenirs to make a buck off of suffering. A taxi driver would still try to sideswipe you while crossing a street. Pedestrians were still paying more attention to their cellphones than they were to each other. And the day after the attack a woman I worked with complained about the inconvenience of having to walk to work because the subway was not running. The thoughts and words of many New Yorkers could still continue to boggle your mind.

Another night, over dinner, a friend confessed to me that this could be the final straw, the thing that could push him to live outside the city. I agreed with him, of course—businesses were sure to suffer now, the thought of working in a high rise in a visible city seemed perilous as the country moved toward a feeling of war even though an ineffectual President could not identify an enemy. Who wants to live in a target zone? I thought. In the moments of attack the last place I wanted to be was in New York. But a few days later when a friend offered an invitation to spend the weekend in Long Island I turned it down. I could not leave the city behind me. I could not watch news of my home from any other place other than my home.

But when the weekend arrived a need for closure surfaced and could not be found. What was found, instead, were hours dazed in front of the television, watching news that seemed to be repeated over and over and over. A trip to the pharmacy for razor blades for myself turned instead into an impulse purchase of toothbrushes and socks for the firemen and rescue workers. A walk through town to visit the impromptu memorials created at fire houses and Union Square ended in a visit to a church and a candlelight vigil. What was clear to me then was that I was not a hero in this story. But neither was I a casualty. I was an ordinary person trying to maintain his normal life in a city that *always* challenges you. Was this what had changed—that normalcy now seemed to be an ideal, a goal, to achieve? That life as we knew it—or perceived it as we *wanted* it to be—would never seem normal again? Or was the true irony of all of this that America finds no normalcy in gay life, that Jerry Falwell can blame us, that the Red Cross can turn us away from it doors, that the military can refuse to let us serve our country. Was the change in my life the recognition of what did not change with a tragic event? That what was before was still there, still a basic part of the view.

DO I KNOW YOU?

Dear Richard and John,
   Thank you so much for sending me the invitation to your Impending Grand Nuptials. I'm very honored and touched to be included as part of your Great Day. And I'm certainly impressed by all the grandeur and the expense of the Big Occasion you are mounting. (The invitation alone could become a museum piece—Heavy-weight paper! Embossed borders! Gilded edges! Translucent Insert!) You must be planning an Elaborate Affair for Hundreds—a four o'clock wedding ceremony on the beach followed by dinner and dancing in town. I'm already dazzled and excited! And I just love that "Festive Attire Requested" bit. No black tie necessary! No suits and neckties that no longer fit me because time and gravity have taken their toll!
   But I must confess right up front that I can't exactly place the moment—or place—where we met and bonded enough that you would be so generous to include me in your Special Celebration of Commitment to One Another. Are you the Rich who works out at my gym or Rick-the-personal trainer who gave me his cellphone number a few weeks ago? There is a Rick-with-a-goatee who lives in the apartment two floors above mine. Is that you? Or are you the Richard who works on the floor beneath me? You're not the Dick with the huge cock and the sling on East Fifty-Third Street, are you? Or Richard the therapist that I met at the Townhouse about two years ago (and who had that fabulous loft)? I'm certain you're not the Ricky I hired as a hustler last fall—he would need a lot of work before he could land into such nuptial bliss as what you are up to—I mean, even those *Queer Eye* boys would be hard pressed

to convince him to dry out and sober up enough to say, "I Do," but, then again, he *was* a beautiful piece of work, with a dick that could get as hard as a good dick can get... And a rich man could certainly entice him into sticking around for the Next Big Thing he could try... Is that you? Are you that Dick? That Ricky? That Richard?

I know there was a friend, Rick, from my ACT UP days, but he is long gone from this planet and that can't be you. And then there was another Richard who was on my phone tree list—that's not you, is it, after all these years? Or are you that older Richard, the Richard I met at the Man's Country baths back in the late Seventies? My God, that would make us both, what?—well, almost ancient and shriveled-up and certainly almost-off the marriage-market list!

So it must be John whom I know—Is this John from the Black Party in 1995? (The guy in chaps I gave such a long, delicious blow job to in the balcony?) Or the Jon who was the volunteer at the March on Washington in 1993? (We shared a bagel together while waiting to head down to the Mall). You're not the JJ from the Gay Pride Parade in Manhattan back in, well, 1986, are you? (Jonathan James Something-Or-Another, as I recall... the guy who was an ex-boyfriend of my ex-boyfriend—the one who was in the hospital at the time and didn't live much longer that summer?) You're not Johnny, the chorus boy, whom I dated briefly when I was just out of college, are you? Or are you the Jonathan I had the three-way with back in the early Nineties? You're not the John who was married to Sharon-Lee, are you?—the guy who swore he was going to get a divorce from his wife and wanted me to fuck him a second (and third) time the night we hooked up. You can't be John from Hewlett Packard—that really well built dude who showed up at my apartment to fix more than just my printer—he told me he was really straight, but didn't mind having sex with a guy and so he did—have sex with a guy—*me*—and more than once, too, as I recall. This isn't you, is it?

So maybe it is Richard I know after all. Are you the Richard on Perry Street with the beautiful nine-inch cock I greedily devoured one night in 2002? The one with the massage table? Or are you the Dick I had a blind date with (about 4,000 blind dates ago)—the guy I met at Starbucks on Eighth Avenue on April 16, 1999 (and who, by the way, looked nothing like the photo he e-mailed me in advance). Are you the Richie from the summer house in 1985 I fooled around with when our boyfriends weren't around? Or the one on Fourteenth Street in 1991 with a gold Labrador and who liked to do watersports in his bathtub? You can't be Richard-the-Republican I slept with at the Warwick—I mean, he would have had to gone through a lot of therapy to come out of the closet, you know—but, then again, that was something like fifteen years ago, so, well, it could be you? Are you that fucked up Dick?

Come to think of it, there was the John I shared a heart-pounding handjob with during a van ride from the Miami airport to Key West in 1983 (when that near-monsoon canceled our flight and we were driven south in the blinding rainstorm courtesy of the airline). Or did I meet you on the rooftop of Kevin's apartment building on the West Side during his Fourth of July party back in—what—1979? The John with the big blue eyes who was a really great kisser? I hope you're not the John I threw up on during the boat ride around Manhattan when my boss was retiring in 1987. (Who knew gin and tonics could be so deadly on an empty stomach and a swaying vessel? But then you were so sweet—we went back to your place and showered and fooled around for like, well, hours and hours and hours and hours.) Is this you again, after all these years?

Whomever you are, how ever I know you, I am so glad you have each found your Significant Other and I am thankful that whatever past I shared with either (or both) of you did not make a strong enough impact for you to abandon your quest to find your True Soul Mate For All Eternity and thus, you found Each Other. I am so looking forward to being present at your Special Recognition of Commitment Between Two Gay Men and listening to you exchange your Vows of Companionship—especially, after all the time and memories that have passed between us (unless you're the Richard from the chat room

I met last week—then we simply have to smile and nod and keep our little secret, huh?—consider it one of those things that bachelors do before they get hitched).

So, *Yes*, absolutely, I've enclosed my RSVP card (prestamped by you, no less, how *truly* generous). And of course, I'll be sending a thoughtful gift along before the Big Date happens—a quick Google search already shows that you are registered at Bloomies, Tiffany's, and Crate & Barrel! But my big, burning Question of the Day—the one I am saving up to ask when we meet again—is not really How did *We* meet? but How did *You* find each other?—How did *The Two of You* meet? How did it happen? Where did it happen? Details, details, details, dearies—I want to know all the facts. (Because, God knows, I've been trying to meet someone just like you for decades! I have been a Husband Hunter from my Gay Day One!)

I'll also be bringing lots of Kleenex with me to the Big Event, expecting to sob my eyes and heart out because of your fortunate happiness and new marital ecstasy. I'll share my tissues with anyone who needs one, you know, and I'll have a few unused condoms in my wallet, too, just in case there is someone who might be interested in seeing what happens. You never know who you might meet next—he could be Mr. Right, after all. Then again, even if he's not—even if he is just Mr. Right Now, I'm not too old yet to overlook a new adventure—and you never know what else you might find along the way... As I always say (and probably said to you), it's good to keep an open mind and be ready for the possibility to change.

All my best and see you soon,
xoxoxo
Jimmy
(aka James, Jameson, Jamey, Jim, JC, or just plain J!)

LOVERS

After two months of dating Scott he told me it had to end. We were spending an afternoon in Central Park, sitting on a sheet I had taken from my apartment and unfolded on the lawn of Sheep Meadow. I was telling Scott how I wanted to see more of him, get to know him better, and that maybe we could make some trips together or take a share in a summer house in the Hamptons or the Pines. Scott answered by saying that things could go no further between us because he was getting back with his ex-lover Donnie. Scott and Donnie had been a couple for three years and ex-lovers three weeks before I met Scott at a bar on the east side of town. "It has nothing to do with you," Scott said after he told me he was breaking things off between us. Of course, it felt like it had everything to do with me. I felt like a failure because I had not convinced Scott that I could be a better lover for him than Donnie was.

It took Scott another three weeks before he actually broke things off between us. "I don't know how I can give this up," he said the afternoon we walked back to my apartment from the park and had discarded our clothes and fallen into bed again. Scott was forty-one years old and going through more crises than just breaking up and getting back with Donnie or staying with me. He had been laid off from his job as a stock analyst for a Wall Street firm, and his idleness, or lack of motivation to find a new job, was what had provoked the trouble with Donnie. Scott was not enjoying his forties; a series of root canals had left him cashless and feeling vulnerable, and the night I had met him he had complained of his brown hair graying too quickly, even though I told him it was one of his more distinctive and handsome features. I was twenty-seven years old that year and tried to prove that, together, Scott and I were ageless in bed. Scott was short and thickly built, looking more like a truck driver than a business executive, and he had a cock like a serpent, long and slender with a slightly wider head. I let him stay deep inside my body for what felt like hours; he loved it when I straddled his furry thighs so he could bury his face against my chest, whispering, "Yes, keep me here, right here, don't let me out." I was of the age that I believed that if I was passionate and involving in bed with Scott, he would be passionate and involving with me out of bed, a mistake I would make many more times with many other men.

Scott did his best to prove that it was not the quality of sex that provoked our demise. In fact, he said it was the reason why he had such trouble letting go and returning to Donnie. I did my best to show my pride was not wounded or to admit that I was again a failure as lover material by recommending Scott to a friend of a friend, a headhunter I had once dated and who specialized in finding displaced executives Wall Street positions.

Scott never thanked me for recommending him to Keith, my headhunter acquaintance, which, in turn, I also got over. Sometime later, maybe about nine or ten months, I ran into Keith in the lobby of an off-Broadway theater with our mutual friend Barry, both of whom knew of my woes with Scott. Keith mentioned that Scott had found a job at one of the city's larger banking corporations and had finally broken up with Donnie. Keith even confessed that he and Scott had gone out on a date but that there hadn't been much chemistry between them. Then Keith told me that Scott had a new boyfriend and they were part of a house Keith was putting together for the summer in East Hampton.

"I suppose you're not interested in doing a share?" Keith asked me and explained he was still trying to find someone for the final share.

"I don't think so," I answered in my most bitter and campy inflection. In the lobby of the theater, I was left with the hope that perhaps my timing or luck or both had just been out of sync with Scott, and had nothing to do with someone not wanting to know more of me outside the bedroom. Before I left to take my seat inside the theater, I asked Keith if he could recommend me as a boyfriend to any other executives who might pass his way. "Someone like Scott," I said, "but without the extra baggage."

* * *

It was a few years later when I met Paul on a phone line. Our conversation was brief, revealing our ages, height, weight, genital size, and sexual preferences in bed in the most minimal of ways. Instinct usually rules in these encounters, and I had a good feeling that I would not have to be the kind of specific sexual acrobat with Paul that other men on the phone lines so often desired. The only unsettling thing that had transpired before Paul gave me the address to his Chelsea apartment was his asking me, "Are you cute?"

I think I'm cute, and I also think I'm cuter than some of the trolls that I've met online who call themselves "hot," "handsome," or "sexy," so I answered Paul's question with my too slick, too practiced response, "You won't be disappointed," which I always hated having to use. Paul took my response in stride—we were, after all, hooking up to have sex, not make a porno flick, and it was a rainy, chilly Tuesday night, a time when even the hottest, most handsome, and desperately horny men seldom set out to travel, preferring instead their tricks come to them.

Paul met me at the door of his apartment, having already scrutinized me through his doorman's video camera. His apartment was tastefully decorated—solid colors, beige furniture, modern art on the walls—and he had lit candles on the coffee table as a centerpiece. He offered me a drink, which I accepted, and we talked while a hidden stereo system hummed out the notes of a jazz pianist.

Paul was close to as he had described himself; his short, blond hair was thin and balding, but since he was clean shaven and wore wire-rimmed eyeglasses, he looked as academic as his perfect pronunciation had indicated. In fact, in our short conversation, he admitted he taught an urban studies class at one of the downtown universities but worked full-time as an architect for a midtown firm.

On the couch, we kissed for a few minutes, and when Paul felt comfortable, he led me into a bedroom where there were more candles lit—on the nightstands, dresser top, and windowsill. Rain pelted at the window and the stereo had drifted into a sequence of softer lullabies. The overly romantic scenario and the alcohol had finally relaxed me—I'm usually suspicious as these encounters begin—and we lay on the bed continuing our kissing, slowly undressing each other in a randomly aggressive and passionate way.

It was when we were undressed and I was lying on top of Paul that I got an eerie sensation that Paul's attention had been pulled out of the room. Looking over my shoulder, I saw the shadow of a man standing at the door. My body tensed from fear, and a startled sweat broke out at my forehead, armpits, and back. I had not known that there was someone else in the apartment—Paul had not indicated that he shared the space and I had not heard anyone come in, and I had not detected Paul speaking to anyone when he had gone out of the living room and gotten us drinks. I rolled off of Paul and swung my feet over the side of the bed and reached for my T-shirt and underwear on the floor, defensive enough to throw a punch if that was what the scenario required. My heart was beating heavily in my ears, but somehow I heard Paul say, "Happy Birthday, darling."

The man in the doorway moved further into the room and Paul reached out to me and said, "Don't go."

"What's going on?" I asked. I was worried that the man might be angered—I still had not seen his face and he stood at the doorway with his hands crossed against his chest.

"Looks like my gift is as surprised as I am," the man said. The tone of his voice, the same calm, practiced sort of speech as Paul's, was layered with a brilliant glee and made me stop getting dressed, though my heart continued crashing inside my chest.

"You don't think I was going to get you a hustler?" Paul said. "You could have done that on your own."

"So instead, you've hustled our new friend, who seems not to know anything about me."

The man was now closer in the room and I could see he was startlingly handsome—dark, slick-backed hair, dark eyes, with a slender European style about him. I immediately understood why Paul took whatever steps he could to please this sort of man, even to the expense of luring a stranger into bed. The man radiated sex, and it seemed to me that he was the kind of man it was not easy to possess because life could offer him potential distractions it would not necessarily offer others.

Paul introduced me to Tino, his lover for two years. Tino was turning forty the following day, or rather, at the stroke of midnight, only a few minutes away. Tino and Paul settled my nerves and Paul fetched more drinks—a bottle of champagne was opened and poured into long, thin glasses. We talked a bit more in the bedroom—mostly my lobbying questions at Tino to dispel my anxieties, until Paul toasted Tino at midnight. Tino responded with a kiss—first for Paul and then with me, and then he drew us easily into a lovely and unexpected threesome.

* * *

That was not my first or last three-way, and I must confess that Paul and Tino paid more attention to me than they did to each other, as if I were the one celebrating a birthday. I've not done enough of these threesome encounters, however, to be an expert on their psychological construction. But it was clear to me even on that night that there was an imbalance in their relationship. It was a few years later when I think I finally understood what Paul had been trying to do that night we hooked up on the phone. By then I was in my forties and in my first relationship with a man to last more than six months, and I was looking for ways I could justify keeping our unbalanced relationship going. Adam was also in his early forties, recently divorced from his wife and out on his own for the first time as a newly minted openly gay man. His years as a stockbroker in suburban Connecticut had given him a conceited arrogance, and he now found everything about gay life as sexually exciting as would a teenager just discovering the power of his dick. Among his newly articulated fantasies was his desire for a "hot three-way," something that though I did not discourage him from finding, I did not want to participate in with him myself. Adam had a stinginess to his personality which I had grown to dislike the more I knew him better—a sort of this-is-what-I-deserve-because-I-have-been-in-the-closet-for-such-a-long-time—that I knew whatever three-way encounter we could have would leave me as the odd partner out. I could clearly imagine him luring another man into bed in the same way Paul had lured me, yet Adam would never have been as accommodating in the way Tino had. Adam, in fact, would have made me watch him make love to someone else, as if it were a way to punish me for the bad behavior of revealing my insecurities over our relationship. I was wildly attracted to Adam, more so than he was to me, which had set up our inequality since our first date. Adam was the sort of man who wanted a boyfriend who wouldn't mind him having other boyfriends, and though I tried my best to be that sort of man, it just wasn't where I was headed at that moment.

Adam had also complicated our relationship by leaving clues of his other sexual involvements—Post-It notes with names and addresses seemed to float out of garbage pails or wave at me from desk drawers to catch my attention; phone messages would begin on his answering machine while we were in bed having sex, "Uh, Adam, this is Joe, we met last week …"

I suppose I should have just abandoned Adam, given him up, but psychologically I couldn't admit to another defeat. I had come this far. I thought if I found a way not to care about Adam's other activities, I could find a way for our relationship to work for me, and I pursued several options—meditation and yoga, long hours at the gym, easing my confusion with a series of strong drinks—none of which worked. I also considered ways in which I might be more sex-positive; I thought about suggesting we go to a sex club together or participate in a threeway, though I could not commit myself to actually discussing these possibilities with Adam. Which was how I found my way into a bar in the East Village one night and where, slightly inebriated and finally relaxed, I met Jesse.

Jesse was in his late twenties and perhaps the tallest of all my lovers, six-feet-four, long-legged, hairless, and lean, with the pale, chiseled physique of a swimmer. He was a corporate lawyer who spoke in such a soft, dull monotone that I would have to blink to maintain my attention. Jesse was much livelier in bed, however, and he made me feel like a young man myself with his slender legs propped up against my shoulders and his ass willing to accept my cock. It was the fifth or sixth time with Jesse when things turned sour—impotence struck me for the first time in bed with a man. I knew I should have been moving into a deeper emotional involvement with Jesse but I couldn't because I still had Adam lodged deeply in my consciousness. I knew I couldn't go any further with Jesse unless I confessed the truth about myself because I had been dishonest with him from the start—never mentioning that there was another man. It was as if Adam were already in bed with us, commenting on Jesse's attributes, ready to take him for himself.

Jesse didn't seem to mind my inability to perform—he was firmly erect, and I could have gone ahead and been the evening's passive partner. But my frustration was caught in my throat and I began a short crying jag that startled both of us. Jesse held me the way a concerned lover would—exactly the kind of lover I always wanted—and I unraveled the whole misery of my affair with Adam, and for the first time I understood what Scott must have been feeling the afternoon he had told me we could go no further.

When I had finished my tale and restored my emotional stability, Jesse said, "I've not been honest myself." It was now my turn to embrace him as he confessed his ongoing relationship with a guy who lived out of town, his former college boyfriend. Together, Jesse said, they were great in bed, but neither of them would commit to giving up their lives and careers away from each other, so they only saw each other once a month on visits. The moment Jesse began talking about his boyfriend, Chip, the better I felt, as if I knew that I no longer had to be a major player for Jesse, or he for me.

Although our sexual chemistry had failed to ignite that night after our confessions, it was not my last encounter with Jesse. I did not give up on Adam right away, either; I found myself in deeper despair before I found my path out. But there was an evening when Adam and I went as boyfriends to a gallery opening in Tribeca, and we ran into Jesse, who was friends with one of the artists in the exhibit. As I introduced one lover to the other, I sensed Adam's interest in Jesse as a potential and younger sexual partner and Jesse's interest in Adam because he had witnessed my tale of woe over this man. I sensed that I could have possibly engineered a three-way that night, but I didn't attempt it. Instead, I walked away from both of them and their growing conversation, hoping they might hit it off together on their own, without me. They didn't, of course, and I was spared the humiliation of watching one's lovers walk off into the sunset together, arm in arm. But it was a defining moment. Watching them from the other side of the gallery with a drink in my hand, I finally understood I was on my way to someone else.

MY HAUNTED HISTORY

On a recent trip to Edinburgh, Scotland, I noticed when I arrived to check into my hotel that there was a pub next door which brashly advertised its gayness with signs and posters of its special nights, events, and half-priced drinks beneath a rainbow flag and a trail of streamers. I had traveled to Edinburgh for two specific reasons: I could remember nothing of the trip my family made to the city in 1966 when I was ten years old and I wanted to see if I could dislodge any memories. And my father had unearthed our Scottish ancestry and I hoped to find a cultural connection. In my hotel room, after unpacking and settling in, I did a quick Internet search to find out more information about the night spot next door. To my surprise I discovered that I had landed in the "Pink Triangle," a neighborhood enclave of gay-owned or gay-targeted businesses. It was as if I had stumbled onto the ghost of my younger self, the one who had traveled in search of gay destinations, when gay life was not so easily visible and gay history was often learned by word of mouth.

When I first landed in Manhattan in 1978 at the age of twenty-two, I knew few facts of gay history. The new friends I met in graduate school and my first jobs in the theater served as my gay educators: Did I know that Marlon Brando and Wally Cox were once roommates? That Blanche's husband was gay? Why Brick was troubled? Or the rumor where Edward Albee had seen a line of graffiti—Who's Afraid of Virginia Woolf?—scrawled on the toilet wall of a gay bar in the West Village? And then gradually other questions and insights arrived: Had I read Oscar Wilde or Walt Whitman? Did I know about Leonardo and Michelangelo? What did I think about Truman Capote? Or Gore Vidal? Or Andy Warhol? Suddenly I was exposed to a legacy of literature that was shaped by sexuality, time, and place.

I recall I had a particular fascination with the history of Greenwich Village, the neighborhood where I had chosen to first live in Manhattan. I wanted to be a writer, specifically a playwright, and I dreamily saw myself as an "artiste" and a "bohemian," not someone determined to find a job and financial stability, and the free spirit of the neighborhood and its community was something I aspired to belong to. I would take long walks in order to understand the paths of the streets, walking east to west, river to river, north to south, 14th Street to Houston, locating the places where James Baldwin had lived or where Edward Albee's play had premiered, where Truman Capote had gotten drunk, or where the Stonewall Inn had been located.

Greenwich Village's transformation into an Oz-like destination for gay men began around the turn of the twentieth century when New York society living in the neighborhood began to seek bigger dwellings uptown, and the area was taken over by artists in search of cheaper housing. By the 1920s the Village was bustling with speakeasies, many of which attracted, according to press reports of the day "dainty elves and stern women." After the end of World War II, urban gay life came under increasing attack and scrutiny and became more hidden; and gay bars became tucked away establishments on the Village's side streets.

In the years following the Stonewall riots Greenwich village came to stand as a sort of mythical symbol of the epicenter of a visible and open gay life, a mecca where sexual energy, cultural expression, and social interaction with other gays were conspicuously integrated. While many neighborhoods throughout the city's history have attracted gays in large numbers—Times Square's sex emporiums for gay men and Sutton Place's residential enclave for wealthy lesbians—the

West Village became the place where a generation of gay men dreamed of living, including myself.

In my early days in New York, I soon learned I was too practical to make it as either an artiste or a bohemian. Economics forced me into the reality of securing a full-time job to afford an apartment and pay off the loans I had taken out for my education. I moved from apartment to apartment to apartment to keep myself afloat, but no matter where I lived in the city, I always identified as a Villager. But my evolution as a gay New Yorker continued. The books I read and the plays I saw when I was in my early twenties, the years of the late Seventies and early Eighties, made a significant impression on my gay consciousness: the importance of coming out; the concept of pride; and the political, social, and religious hurdles associated with those essentials. Of significant importance were the novels by the Violet Quill writers: Andrew Holleran, Felice Picano, Robert Ferro, and Edmund White; the plays by Charles Ludlam and Harvey Fierstein, and anything published in *Christopher Street*, a gay literary magazine of the era.

The arrival of the AIDS epidemic would provide me with a reason to write and allow me to find my voice. But New York, specifically Manhattan and the West Village, shaped my course as a writer. I would always admit to being a New Yorker and a gay writer. My destination and sexuality would define the literature I would write. But it was also apparent that it was impossible for me to ignore my personal history in the characters I would create and write about. I struggled with another label I was unable to shed: being a Southerner.

* * *

Since I was not born and raised in a trailer park or on a plantation, I've always been hesitant to label myself as a "Southern Writer." I grew up in the suburbs of Atlanta during an era where the emphasis was on shopping malls, high school football teams, and drive-thru fast-food restaurants, and I could never define or detail my boyhood experiences as belonging to either the high-fallutin' society or the dirt poor trash. I was a product of suburbia and American pop-culture, and, once I learned the importance of education, I was determined that this would be my path.

I am not ashamed of being a native of the South, nor of being a gay man from this area of the country; my college years in Atlanta remain among my most happy memories as well as my most enlightening. It's a part of who I am and who I became. I dislike making sweeping generalizations about the South, because for every narrow-minded conservative religious bigot toting a Bible, a gun, and a Confederate flag, there is a determined and fierce liberal, or at least a tolerant do-gooder, even if that open-mindedness is crouched in quotation marks. The true difficulty of being gay in the South is that the coming out process never stops. Society, class, religion, politics, economics are always setting up a battlefield. Most gay men of my generation either left the South or settled in Atlanta or New Orleans. My choice to leave for New York was no different from theirs. I left Atlanta to find my self-respect.

As a writer I've always considered myself first and foremost a "Gay Writer Who Writes About Gay Subjects," seldom straying from this purpose except for an occasional literary, medical or journalism assignment. But the older and more reflective I have become, the more I have also become aware that I do possess a distinct Southern heritage. The South, after all, is a portable place, as evocative for its heat and humidity as it eccentric characters and frustrating conservatism. And the older I've become the less reluctant I am to write about the South and its distinctiveness. It is inherent with conflict, the crux of literature, and something I no longer wish to avoid.

A few years ago at an awards ceremony in Manhattan, writer after writer praised Armistead Maupin and the impact *Tales of the City* had on their lives and careers (and deservedly so). I was filled with joy the first time I read that book and it was instrumental in my wanting to become a writer of gay stories. I was twenty-four when I discovered the novel in 1980 and I wanted to see San Francisco myself as a young gay man, just as Maupin's character Michael "Mouse" does. Michael, if you recall, is a transplant from the South, just as Maupin is; he is a native of North Carolina, and I know that what I saw in Michael was a lot of myself—a young man leaving the comforts of his home to discover a world where he feels he belongs. Gay literature is full of this emigrant experience. Other Southern gay writers have also put their own spin on this sub-genre, among them Allan Gurganus, Andrew Holleran, David Sedaris, and Tony Kushner.

My visit to San Francisco would not happen until a few years after I had read Maupin's novel, when my job as the advance publicist for the national tour of a Broadway show landed me for a week's stay in a Union Square hotel. With me I had the torn-out pages of the San Francisco sections of *Gayellow Pages* and the *Spartacus* travel guide, essential tools to navigate gay life in other cities.

It was both a heady and somber experience. By then, AIDS was changing the landscape of gay life in San Francisco and elsewhere. And I was well aware of the importance of gay history, recorded, unrecorded, ever-evolving. I would use these moments again and again in my fiction.

* * *

If destination can inspire literature, can literature inspire destination? My first recollection of New Orleans is how much I hated it. It was 1976 and I was twenty years old, a college junior in Georgia, on a performance tour with fellow members of my university's glee club. It was spring break and our one-week trip carried us to Houston and back to Atlanta, with a side trip to New Orleans. At that moment in my life I was confused about a lot of things about myself: my religion, my sexuality, my studies, my goals. There were about thirty of us on that tour, including two close friends who would later become my roommates when we moved off-campus the following year. I was deeply infatuated with one friend, a young gay man who was the first boy who had made me mentally question my own sexuality. I was deeply committed to the other friend, a young black man from Maryland, who challenged my conservative Southern background. I don't recall many specifics from that tour; in part, because for years I blocked the memory of it, but I do recall we stayed in a hotel on Rampart Street and a group of us walked to the French Quarter that evening, including me and my two close friends. It was humid and we dodged thick raindrops as we made our way to Bourbon Street, the only spot any of us had heard of. I was appalled at the crowd we found: the rowdy, inebriated behavior of tourists, the hucksters trying to lure us into bars. We made our way into one club where a thin girl about our age danced on a stage the size of a milk crate, her breasts bare and wobbling as she stretched her hands toward the ceiling to the beat of loud, recorded music. I was offended to be in the presence of someone displaying nudity, embarrassed as much for the girl on stage and those in our group witnessing it, and confused by the fact that we were all trying to ignore it but aware of it in front of us. Another college friend who was part of our small bug-eyed group in that strip-bar, a talented young woman and singer who would become a well-regarded theater director, made a reference to this trip when we were reunited years later: Wasn't it terrific that we had discovered New Orleans together? she remarked, though I think her sentiment was mostly directed toward our lost youth rather than to our shared experience on Bourbon Street.

My second visit was equally as miserable. I had been living in Manhattan for less than a year, inching my way into accepting my own gay identity. But I had not entirely left my life in Atlanta behind, or, rather, the smaller town of East Marietta north of it, where I had been born and raised. One hanging thread was a hometown sweetheart I had dated off and on since high school. After graduating college she became an airline stewardess and was deeply committed toward getting me to make a commitment to her. When I fled to Manhattan, she followed me with spontaneous visits courtesy of free airfare from her employer. When she accepted a position based in

New Orleans, she moved to Metairie and asked me down for a weekend visit, a free trip as long as I was willing to say that I was her relative. I accepted and flew south, intent on breaking up with her at the moment she expected more from me.

We spent a hot miserable summer afternoon in the French Quarter, walking through the heat, shop to shop, market to market, zombie-like and directionless. I had no desire to revisit Bourbon Street, less desire to slip away to find a gay bar, and my soon-to-be-ex-girlfriend had no passion to show me her new hometown. I refused to sleep with her that weekend, opting to sleep on her couch, and I returned to Manhattan an unhappy man because I felt I was being unjustly cruel breaking up with her at the moment she expected more from me.

Flash forward through many years, many changes, and many losses from the AIDS epidemic to the publication of my first book in 1993, *Dancing on the Moon*, a collection of short stories about the impact of AIDS on the gay community. During a promotional tour, I was paired in a book reading and signing with Barbara Lazear Ascher, the author of *Landscape without Gravity*, a memoir about her brother's battle with AIDS and his death at the young age of thirty-one. Part of Ascher's memoir is her account of traveling to New Orleans where her brother lived, meeting his friends, and coming to terms with her grief. Meeting Barbara and reading her book was a changing point as to how I regarded New Orleans, making me aware that for many gay men of my generation who grew up in the South, New Orleans had had the same magnetic pull as New York City had for me. Reading other books set in New Orleans removed my initial dislike of the Big Easy. Two literary works in particular, *A Confederacy of Dunces* by John Kennedy Toole and *Lives of the Saints* by Nancy Lemann, inspired a desire to revisit it.

But those years living in Manhattan continued to be tough ones for me: low paying jobs, big literary hopes, and the high cost of living left me unable to travel to many of the places I wanted to visit. After receiving a literary fellowship in 2003, I used the funds to travel to New Orleans to research a novel

I was outlining: an attempt to reimagine an Edgar Allen Poe story within a home in the Garden District. I was forty-seven and it had been twenty-four years since my last trip to New Orleans. But this trip would be another changing moment; for the first time I was a willing tourist in the Big Easy. It was September and the weather was extraordinary; I went on ghost, garden, cemetery, voodoo, and vampire tours. I had my cards read in Jackson Square and my fortune told by a psychic. I had beignets at Café Du Monde and a hurricane at Pat O'Brien's. I rode the streetcar along St. Charles, and crossed that invisible gay marker on Bourbon Street at St. Ann's to find my way to Café Lafitte's in Exile. I easily fell in love with New Orleans in the same manner I had so earlier dismissed it. Perhaps most memorable was the room at a bed and breakfast on Dumaine Street where I stayed for more than a week; it would serve as the inspiration for my novel, *The Wolf at the Door*, about the hauntings of gay-owned guest house in the French Quarter. I think Avery, the main character in that novel, comes close to who I am today, a funny, boozy, overworked, aging gay man, with a backstory of emigration from his hometown and an escape from a conservative Southern religious background.

In recent years I have returned annually to New Orleans to attend the Saints and Sinners Literary Festival, grateful that it gives me a reason to go back to the Big Easy. I am no longer compelled to be a tourist, more intent, now, on revisiting my favorite bars, restaurants, and stores. One of the things I love most about New Orleans is that it wears its history visibly in its buildings, shops, and streets. Echoes of Spanish, French, Caribbean, and Southern history and cultures are everywhere in its food and music and art. I like to think that when I am in New Orleans now that I carry my history around as well. But I am no longer haunted by my unhappiness; instead, I find New Orleans makes me feel vibrantly gay and alive.

* * *

A few weeks prior to my trip to Scotland, I returned to an area of Pennsylvania where I had lived more that fifteen years before trying to recover from death of a friend and bring some perspective to my life. Since leaving the area and returning to Manhattan, I had learned through my father that many of our ancestors had lived in the counties on the Pennsylvania/New Jersey border.

One morning I went to pay my respects to my great great grandfather Jacob and his second wife Mary who are buried in the Easton Heights Cemetery in Easton, Pennsylvania. In 1862, Jacob, a farm laborer aged twenty-three, enlisted as a Private Company A of the 11 Regiment, New Jersey Volunteers, 3rd Brigade, 3rd Division, 2nd Army Corps, Army of the Potomac. His younger brother William, aged eighteen, also enlisted in the same company as a Musician (a drummer). Both brothers fought in several key engagements during the Civil War, including the Battle of Gettysburg. At the battle at Boydton Plank Road in 1864, Jacob was wounded with a Minié ball lodged in his chest and was left on the field for dead. He revived and became a prisoner. He was taken first to Petersburg and then later to Richmond where he was paroled. His younger brother William was wounded in the battle before Petersburg, Virginia in 1864 and his leg was amputated. He died shortly thereafter and was buried in an unmarked grave in Washington, DC.

After the Civil War, Jacob returned to the New Jersey area where his family lived. He married in 1865, and worked as a carpenter until 1874 when he bought a milk route and moved to Chestnut Hill. He died in 1908 at the age of sixty-nine. His first wife Mary died in 1869 at the age of twenty-six, two years after the birth of my great grandfather Charles.

It took me several attempts to locate Jacob's grave in Easton. I first tried on a Saturday morning, wandering around Easton Cemetery, searching for the grave until I located a caretaker who told me he was not buried there. (I thought I was at Easton Heights Cemetery. Instead I was at Easton Cemetery. The two cemeteries are side by side on a mountainside, separated only by poor fencing at their boundaries and I had not traveled far enough up the mountainside to reach Easton Heights Cemetery.)

At Easton Heights Cemetery, the caretaker's office was closed, so I wandered around for an hour trying to spot the grave and finally had to leave to make a lunch appointment in New Hope, an hour's drive south of Easton.

I tried again the following morning, arriving at the cemetery early, before 9 a.m. The caretaker's office was closed and the heat and humidity were already high and unpleasant. I wandered through the southern slopes of the cemetery where the oldest graves were located. I knew from online historical records that Jacob's headstone was not large or tall and could only be read by standing above it. I have little experience of wandering through cemeteries and I don't really know if or what the protocol is of where to step or walk. That morning I think I trampled over many, many souls in search of Jacob and I asked all of them for forgiveness in doing so. I gave up my search, however, then asked God for a sign and tried again, and was finally overwhelmed by the heat and gave up once more. As I was leaving the cemetery I noticed that the caretaker's office was open. I knocked and went inside and asked the woman who was in the office if she had a record of where Jacob was buried. She located the grave on a map of the cemetery, ironically along the south slope where I had searched and given up several times, mentioning that he was likely "buried on a hill."

I set out again, this time using the map she gave me as a compass, again asking God for some kind of sign to help me along the way. When I parked my car in that area there was a deer standing partially in the shade of the trees. We exchanged glances and the deer scrambled away and thinking that this might be my sign from God, I wandered into the area the deer had left. It was the row the caretaker had indicated on the map where Jacob was buried but I could still not locate the grave. I wandered up the slope, out of the shade and into the heat, consulted the map again, wandered around in the sunlight until

I thought I would collapse. I could feel my disappointment and frustration making me upset and cranky and I decided to do a row by row walk of the section I was in. The problem with this cemetery was that there was no logic to the burial rows. All of the headstones did not face the same way and there seemed to be smaller rows embedded within the major rows that weren't exactly full rows. As I made my way down the slope I had convinced myself that I would not locate the grave on this trip either, that this was a foolish exercise and I was not about to die of a heat stroke trying to locate my great great grandfather. What was I thinking? As I was walking the next to last row I noticed two small headstones embedded within a larger row that were behind where I was walking. I looked over my shoulder and caught sight of the American flag first and then the name Jacob. There he was!

I took photographs of the grave of Jacob and his second wife (also named Mary), and noticed that next to the flag was a small round sign with the initials G.A.R., placed to signify veterans of the Grand Army of the Republic. I felt satisfaction and pride in both finding the grave and learning that I was not entirely a Southerner.

* * *

While I was in Scotland, I spent several days walking through Edinburgh and touring the castle, the palace, and the supposedly haunted underground vaults along the stretch known as the Royal Mile. I had a brief moment of déjà vu at the gates of Holyrood Palace, the Queen's residence while in Edinburgh, but it was fleeting and indistinct.

One afternoon walking back to my hotel I stumbled by chance onto a graveyard located on Calton Hill. This burial ground was opened in 1718 and sits on a hill above Waterloo Place. I did not expect it to be a memorable place, but inside I discovered a memorial to the Scottish-American soldiers who had fought in the Civil War. It was erected in 1893 and depicts Abraham Lincoln, one hand behind his back, sixteen feet tall in bronze, standing on a pedestal inscribed with the word "Emancipation." At the base of the monument is the depiction in bronze of an emancipated slave, arms raised in the act of placing a wreath at the feet of the martyred sixteenth President of the United States, astride two unfurled flags.

This was the first statue of an American President created outside of the United States. It is the only Civil War memorial outside of the U.S. The memorial was presented to the city of Edinburgh by American citizens in honor of Scottish-American soldiers who fought in the Civil War, many of whom died in poverty and who were the inspiration for the memorial. Among these financial donors was Andrew Carnegie. The inscription reads "To preserve the jewel of liberty in the framework of Freedom" and is a quotation from the writings of Abraham Lincoln. The American sculptor who created the memorial, George E. Bissell, had served in the Union Army.

My Scottish ancestry traces back to my great great great great great grandfather, who was born in 1720 in Virginia. He was granted land in Virginia from Thomas, Lord Fairfax, Baron of Cameron in Scotland, and he was a private in the 11th Virginia Regiment during the Revolutionary War. He is believed to have died in the surrender of Charleston in 1780, one of the last battles of the Revolutionary War.

His great grandson, and my great great grandfather, was the father of seven children and enlisted as a private in the 14th Virginia Cavalry, Company E in the Confederate States Army during the Civil War. He was assigned to taking care of the horses. This Regiment was very active throughout the war. There were many skirmishes, but two engagements stand out from the rest, and they were the Battle of Gettysburg, July 1-3 1863, and what was to be known as "The Final Cavalry Charge at Appomattox," April 9, 1865, prior to Lee's surrender of the Army of Northern Virginia.

My great great grandfather was captured at Berryville, West Virginia, on September 9, 1864, and taken as a prisoner of war to Camp Chase, Ohio, until his release on April 11, 1865.

Following the war he returned to Virginia and donated land for the establishment of a Baptist church. He died in 1917.

In learning more about my family history, I have discovered that I had relatives who fought on both sides of the Civil War, including two great great grandfathers who fought at the Battle of Gettysburg, one Confederate, the other Union. Both survived. While this memorial in Scotland is to the soldiers who fought for the Union in the War and my Scottish heritage links me to my Confederate relative, I have also learned that there is now an effort led by a Scottish minister to collect additional names to add to the monument, including those who fought for the Confederacy.

I count these many events and discoveries as defining moments of the man I am today. Southerner. Northerner. New Yorker. Gay. American. Writer.

A BOOKSTORE TOURIST

This October I took a cruise to the Mediterranean, visiting Venice, Dubrovnik, Santorini, Corfu, and Ephesus (in Turkey). The weather was gorgeous, as was the scenery, and the overall experience was interesting and relaxing (and which was what I needed). The highlight of my trip, however, was my final day in Paris because of a stopover flight—a bright, sunny Sunday afternoon crowded with Parisians strolling arm and arm through the streets. I walked through the Marais till I found Rue Ste Croix de la Bretonnerie, where I was relieved to discover that Les Mots à la Bouche, the gay bookstore was open. I was tired from the flights and my stamina isn't what it used to be, and I wedged my way through the aisles looking at titles, searching for books that might be familiar to me in their English editions. And there, face out on the shelves with the other works, was *Les Fantômes*, the French translation of my AIDS stories by Anne-Laure Hubert that the French publisher Cylibris had published in late 2005. I'd seen the edition before; I have several copies and have given many as gifts to friends. But I had never seen the book in a bookstore.

It's hard to explain this sort of thrill to someone who hasn't had the experience of seeing their writing displayed in a bookstore. It's immensely gratifying and awesome and exhilarating, probably like what an architect might feel standing in front of his completed building, particularly if you have spent years and years, as I do, writing a book, struggling with the plots and characters and themes and then trying to find a publisher who was willing to release it out into the world. I remember the first time I saw a book of mine in a bookstore—

it was the winter of 1993, late February, and I was temping at a job on Park Avenue in Manhattan. My first collection of short stories had been accepted more than two years before by Viking, but because of a recession and a company freeze on signing contracts with new authors, the book was not slated for publication until that spring. The store was a small Barnes and Noble outlet, situated on a corner of one of the high-rising glass skyscrapers on Park Avenue near Grand Central Station. I hadn't expected to find my book so soon in a store. I was on a lunch break, escaping my desk where I had eaten a sandwich because I was too poor to afford the neighborhood restaurants. It was a winter I could barely even afford to take the subway. I had stepped out of the cold into the bookstore, thinking I might look at a magazine or find a title I might later be able to get from the public library, before I headed back to my dismal job, where, at the time, I was typing up the license plates of cars and trucks that had been abandoned and were sitting in a lot in Queens. And there, in the store on a shelf with the rest of the fiction, were five copies of *Dancing on the Moon*. The first sight of them remains one of the happiest moments of my life, particularly when I correlate it with the unfortunate experiences and deaths from AIDS of the friends who inspired those stories.

That spring and the following one were full of similar thrills. My book found its way into the windows of Brentano's on Fifth Avenue and B. Dalton's in the West Village on Eighth Street. I did readings and signings for the first time—including at Lambda Rising in Washington, D.C and Glad Day in Boston, among other stores. I'm not a widely bought or distributed author and the press runs of my books haven't been the kind to impress any kind of bestseller list, but I've now seen my books in an airport bookshop (in New Orleans), in foreign bookstores (also at Word is Out, the gay bookstore in the Bloomsbury district of London, where I was on the shelves with many of my friends' books), and part of a suggested reading list posted at a university bookstore. And even now, fifteen or so years later, I still get a thrill discovering something I have written in a store, even if it is a used copy of my novel, *Where the Rainbow Ends*, in the second-hand bookstore in my hometown, north of Atlanta.

Hopefully as you get older and wiser, you discover things about yourself that keep you happy. I have been fortunate to have taken some amazing trips during the last two decades—many due to the generosity of friends—and I've learned that I find great joy in being a bookstore tourist. Some people go to museums or sporting events or concerts or restaurants when they travel. I love to hunt for books—and, for the record, not for just my own. I search out local ghost story anthologies, local gay history books, local literary journals and magazines, unusual translations, and all sorts of novels and fiction by both mainstream publishers and small presses. Of all the bookstores I've been to, some other memorable experiences stand out—a déjà vu experience at the Haunted Bookshop in Cambridge (realizing I had already been there decades before with a friend who was now deceased), a boulevard in Pisa, Italy, lined with bookstores, store after store after store, with bins of books outside in the bright sun, the same with Galway, Ireland and the Shinjuku district of Tokyo. I remember the first time I walked into City Lights bookstore in San Francisco and didn't want to leave because the friend I was with wanted to go elsewhere. I can still spend hours wandering along Charing Cross while many of my other friends are out at the theater. And I've often thought I might one day retire to Napa, California—on my last visit there a few years ago I counted more than four bookstores within blocks of each other. I'm not ready for that yet, though. (I still have a few more years left...) And first I'd like to find that town in Wales where there's nothing but bookstores.

A GATHERING STORM

While assembling material for this collection, I was searching through my old computer disks for an essay that I was certain I had written in October 1998 in the days following the beating of Matthew Shepard, a gay college student at the University of Wyoming who was beaten, tortured, tied to a fence and left to die near Laramie, Wyoming. I had participated in the October 19, 1998 rally against hate crimes and the impromptu demonstration down Fifth Avenue in Manhattan and I was sure that I had written about the experience.

What I stumbled across, instead, was the manuscript of a novel I had begun in the aftermath of Matthew Shepard's death. Writing the book had been both a rewarding and painful experience, but I had chosen to forget about my novel because of the personal disappointment I had attached to it.

Like many gay Americans I was moved by the tragic fate of Matthew Shepard, and in the days following the crime I struggled to pull together portraits of the victim and the assailants from the emerging news. One reason why I decided to write *A Gathering Storm*, a novel about a hate crime against a gay man, was because I felt what was missing from the news were the details and stories of the individuals involved—the crime was analyzed and politicized but oddly not humanized. We did not know who these young men were, what they were thinking, what were they doing, why had they been where they were when things went wrong. We only had their generic representations in the media. The national focus on the issue of hate crimes seemed to overwhelm the personal stories.

I finished writing the *A Gathering Storm* in early 2001 and I submitted the manuscript to my editor at the publishing company that had published my first novel and had an option of first refusal on my next one. My contract called for a six-week response, but because I was an unagented writer the manuscript languished at the publishing company, never generating any attention or a formal rejection until my editor casually informed me that he was leaving the press to begin another career.

In spite of this I secured the services of a literary agent to represent the novel, who shopped the manuscript around without much success, and, in my estimation, without much enthusiasm on his part, so I began shopping it around myself to additional publishers and editors. After I found a British publisher who was interested in the novel, the agent declined to act on my behalf, and interest faded away when the British publisher—who saw *A Gathering Storm* as a commercial thriller and not a literary novel—was concerned that I did not have another thriller ready to go as a follow-up.

By then Matthew Shepard had been the subject of too many movies, plays, books, and dramatizations. One editor at a mainstream house declined the manuscript stating "the Shepard murder was discussed and dramatized and debated in the media so much that this novel may have a hard time finding an audience." *A Gathering Storm* was both too similar and too different. My novel was fiction that read like fact. I had consciously changed many details, including moving the location to a college town in the South. During the aftermath of the Shepard murder, the town of Laramie, Wyoming, where the beating and murder occurred, fell under tremendous scrutiny. News reports and other works based on this crime focused sharply on the town. It was my intent to step aside from this location and show that this type of crime could happen anywhere. In choosing to locate this story in the South, I was also able to draw from many of my own experiences and memories and to write it as a story I felt I could tell.

During the course of writing the novel I had also rewritten many details about the Shepard crime and the characters involved with it, weaving in details from other hate crimes against gay men. More importantly, however, I was peering inside the emotional lives of the characters who were living inside my mind, not just presenting the facts. Fiction can oftentimes carry more emotional weight than a news story or a nonfiction account and it was my intent with this work to present a more human face to this tragedy than what was emerging through other works, both in terms of understanding the deep suffering of the victims as well as looking into the psychological motivations and backgrounds of those behind the crimes.

And I had made a conscious decision to write this novel in a different style from the long, complex sentence structure I had favored in my first novel, *Where the Rainbow Ends*. *A Gathering Storm* is a deconstruction of a crime and this time my prose was purposely short and choppy, like a screenplay. I wanted the visuals to rise immediately off the page and to do so I had, in fact, studied many screenplays and true crime narrative accounts and the way they presented both dialogue and action. And since I was deconstructing the crime, I also wanted to deconstruct the narrative structure of the novel, presenting it as linear, circular, *and* fragmented.

Sometime in 2003 I formally severed ties with the literary agent and abandoned the manuscript to pursue other projects. I never expected the novel to be published and had been so upset by the experience of both writing the book and not finding a publisher for it that I had stored all the notes and drafts of the novel into a box and hid the box at the bottom of a closet in my apartment, out of sight and incapable of wounding me any further. But there it was, *A Gathering Storm*, always at the top of a list of my completed work that I keep on a bulletin board above the desk where I write, ignored and overlooked until I *saw* it there again while I was looking for my Shepard essay. Even as I copied the manuscript files of the novel from the floppy disk to my laptop to archive it, I did not anticipate publishing the work because I felt it was surely outdated, even though other authors had revisited the Matthew Shepard crime and had published recent books about it.

What I discovered when I sat down to reread *A Gathering Storm* was a densely absorbing work full of purpose, a novel that I cannot believe I walked away from and I cannot believe I did not find a publisher for. My faith in it had been shattered by the kind but continued rejection of it. One editor who turned down the manuscript remarked on its "enormous integrity" and found it "refreshing to read a manuscript that is informed by such passion." Another called it "a shocking yet timely story that truly gets to the heart of gay hate in America." Still, no one offered to publish it.

I see now that this novel is a bridge to other themes in my later writings, particularly the gay-themed ghost stories that I would publish later in the decade. But I also see it indicative of the evolution of the gay novel during the first decade of the twenty-first century—how it fell victim to mainstream publishers only wanting commercial blockbusters and how smaller publishers decided to mimic this desire—and how during these years gay authors such as myself, because of our gay themes and narratives and characters and the choices of our fictions—had to find other publishers and other ways and outlets to continue to be published and to find readers. I began Chelsea Station Editions to publish work that was overlooked and ignored by other publishers, worthy gay-themed literature that needed to find its way into print, and I am grateful for the advances in technology, economics, and business and trade practices that have allowed me to do so. I have never been a writer who has chased financial or critical success, only a place to publish what I have wanted to write and what I felt needed to be written and shared. I never expected to be a publisher or a bookseller. But I am extremely proud to say that I have created the perfect home for *A Gathering Storm*.

HEARTS

It took Adam six weeks to tell me he did not love me. We were parked in his car outside my building and I was upset that he was leaving town without me, or, rather, that he did not want to leave town with me but with someone else. He did not tell me that there was someone else, but it was not difficult for me to figure out the story. The night we had met he told me he had recently separated from his wife, and I knew that even if Adam could love me he did not want to do so, or certainly was not ready to see if he could. He was a like a sixteen-year-old girl who had just discovered she was popular and pretty, even though he was the graying fortysomething father of two teenagers himself. I knew better than to expect something from him when we started dating, though I stuck around much longer than I should have, waiting to see if he wanted to give something deeper a try.

Scott waited until we were breaking up to tell me he didn't love me. He used the phrase like a weapon, as if the lovers he had found in his past had proven something about him that I had come to believe that he was incapable of himself. Scott taught me how stingy and vulnerable men can be when it comes to expressing love, yet how easy and undemanding they remain when they wish to receive it.

After six months of dating Geoff, he could still not say the words I wanted to hear, even though I sensed he wanted to give the two of us a more serious try. Instead, he used the moment I realized that I could say those words to him by suggesting we both start dating other men while continuing to see each other. In my recollection, this was a cruel thing for him to do to prevent any further intimate feelings from developing between us, particularly since I had recently been through the deaths of several friends and my emotional pitch was higher than normal with him. Time has forgiven him more than my memory has because I still believe he made a big mistake by holding himself back.

Ray would not say the words to me either when I felt I was ready to speak them myself to him. We slept together every night in each other's arms. He let me stay deep inside his body as if that was the perfect place to be. Ray was not perfect, however; he was an arrogant, opinionated man whom all of my friends disliked. He was as far from good-looking and good-hearted as it was possible for me to choose for a lover, but he had an inexplicable sexual hold on me that turned him into an addiction. Ray also traveled with the baggage of a previous lover, something I didn't know when we met and someone he was not yet willing to give up when I learned the facts. I was young enough to give Ray an ultimatum on how to stay with me, but old enough to understand it was not necessary to want to keep him around.

Which leads me to the man I met when I was twenty-five one night at the St. Mark's Baths, whose name now escapes me though the shape of his body is still fresh in my memory. He was an older, toughly built man with olive skin and coarse, black hair, and when we had finished having sex, he suggested we lie in each other's arms and listen to sounds around us. It occurred to me then that I wanted to see this man again, not for sex but to find out who he was and why he desired to be so in tune with the world around him. I wanted to know what made him move through his day, what his likes and dislikes were, and how I myself might fit into the puzzle of his life. This was the moment that I came to define myself as a true gay man—realizing my romantic and emotional desires for a guy were as important and necessary as my sexual and animalistic ones.

It took Jack more than a year to say those words to me and they arrived in a rather backhanded manner. We were lying in bed together at a summer house he had rented in East Hampton. We were both drinking wine, something Jack waited until late at night to do to help him fall asleep. After the first glass his words would get slurry but the truth would spill out of him. I found out a lot about him and how he felt about me in this way, particularly why he thought that I was such an imperfect match for him, and why he was unwilling to let me go. The words arrived that night not in a statement but as a question. "Do you love me?" he asked me sometime after his second glass of wine and before he was ready for sex. "Of course," I answered and wondered if he would remember my answer the next day and not just what we did with each other in bed. Jack was the one who taught me to keep my heart away from my dick, or, rather, that it was trouble to believe they could be aroused by the same thing.

Kevin was the first man to say the words to me, even though he said it as he was dying and I was caring for him and not while we were dating, as if it were more of a "thank you" and not a how-will-I-ever-survive-without-you kind of sentiment. After Kevin died something changed in me; I didn't care as much about where I found love as I felt about wanting to feel it again.

Joel said the words to me four years after we slept together. It came during a phone call when we were separated by three-thousand miles—he was living in California and I was still on the east coast. I had known Joel for almost ten years when we first slept together and I was the first man he had sex with. When I visited him, Joel was engaged to marry a woman and he was headed on a track that I felt was the wrong one for him, though that was not the reason why I reached out to him that night at his apartment. I wanted to have sex with him before his life became lost to me, before he took the route down a path I knew I could not follow for myself. It took me many more years after his phone call to realize that I should have chosen the path beside him at that moment of his confession; hindsight has now turned him into the one heart I should have never let get away.

THE HOUSE OF TEN THOUSAND TEMPERATURES

When I wake the room is cold. I am buried beneath layers of blankets and quilts atop a four poster canopy bed. I am in the bedroom which was formerly used by my two younger sisters. It's the Sunday before Christmas and I am fifty-four years old. My own bedroom has long disappeared from my parents' house—sometime in the my late twenties as I was putting down roots in Manhattan my mother took possession of that room, repainting it a shade of baby blue and turning it into a workroom where she created her floral portraits—drying, preserving, and painting bouquets of pressed flowers—a craft which she passed along to my sister Debbie. When my mother first told me on the phone that she had cleared out my old bedroom, I panicked. Hidden on the top shelf of my closet were magazines I had bought in my college days in Atlanta—copies of *GQ*, *After Dark*, and *Esquire*, where I had admired the men in the clothes more than the clothes on the men. But I had also secretly hidden on that shelf the nervously purchased copies of *Playguy* and *Blueboy*, adult magazines that featured photographs of fully-nude men. When my mother didn't mention the magazines I had left behind I calmed myself into believing that I had tossed them out when I left home years before, along with the mail order dildo and the penis pump I had also hidden in my boyhood bedroom. Instead, my mother told me, "You were right about this room, Jimmy. It gets so hot in here in the afternoons."

"The sun bouncing off the roof of the kitchen," I said over the phone, remembering the afternoons of practicing clarinet in my bedroom when I would be drenched in sweat by the end of the chromatic scale. "The heat creeps right into the room."

"Your daddy made me rearrange things to clear the way for the vents, but that still didn't work," she said. "So I made him go out and buy me a fan."

Now, years later, next door in my sisters' former bedroom, as I slide out beneath the blankets and my feet touch the floor, I reach out and place my hands in front of the portable ceramic heater that sits on the floor beside the bed. A few years ago when I was home for the holidays and sleeping in this bedroom, I mentioned how cold the room was and that I could barely see because all the light bulbs in the overhead ceiling lamp fixture had ceased to work. My parents were getting older, both were in their seventies then, and I could detect that the house and property were falling into disrepair—the toilet upstairs refused to flush, the windows sashes, repainted several times, would not budge open, the leaves on the front lawn were no longer raked. My parents seldom strayed from their own small paths these days. The last time they had been in my sisters' bedroom was probably to store the items which had belonged to both of my now deceased grandmothers.

As I pull on a sweater and step into my shoes, the bedroom door squeaks open as if it is starring in a horror film. The wood of the carpeted stairs creak beneath my steps as I walk downstairs. It is cool in the small hallway near the front door of the house, probably because of a long, thin crack in the wood of the door and the gray slate tiles of the floor, but the living room where my mother has assembled the Christmas tree is blazing with heat. I step inside the room to warm my fingertips and toes. This room, which lies beneath my parents' bedroom upstairs, is on the same thermostat setting. I see the lumpy log of a blanket with an end of spikey reddish brown hair stretched out on the beige leather sofa and realize that it is my teenaged nephew Westley bundled to stay warm. My youngest sister Robin and her family must have arrived sometime last night from North Carolina. I walk through the dining room and into the kitchen where it is a few degrees cooler and set about making coffee.

With a mug warming my hands, I sit in an armchair in the sun room, a large, two-story high room full of windows and skylights situated on the site where our outside patio once was. My father had this room built after all his children left the house. It is paneled with dark wood and decorated with *tchotchkes* my mother gathered from my parents' international travels—ceramic tiles of European villages, salt-and-pepper shakers in the shapes of animals and windmills and brightly dressed dancing peasants, collections of angels and lighthouses assembled on small display stands. From this room you can see inside into the kitchen and outside into back yard. Outside, the room is framed by a wooden deck, where once stood the clothes line and a swing set. Beyond the deck is a small forest of trees that separate our house from our neighbors. Inside the room it is cooler than the kitchen, lightly warmed by the morning sun, and full of chairs and couches and tables. I watch the floating parade of birds that arrive with little thump-thump-thumps where a small feeder has been suctioned to the glass pane of one window. It's a fascinating turnover, as one small bird is suddenly replaced by another and another and another. Beside me on an end table is a guide book to identify the birds, but I have yet to resort to that, enthralled, instead, by discovering the circular path the birds make from feeder to tree to branch to feeder.

My mother appears in the kitchen dressed in her pale blue nightgown and robe and announces she's cold. She goes to the thermostat in the kitchen which regulates that room, the sun room, and the large first floor bedroom where my sister Robin and her husband are sleeping and which was formerly our garage, and she makes the temperature several degrees warmer. A minute later my father is in the kitchen and, having determined on his own that the rooms are not warm enough for any of us to inhabit, adjusts the thermostats again. And so begins another day in the home I have come to refer fondly as

THE HOUSE OF TEN THOUSAND TEMPERATURES

"the house of ten thousand temperatures," where every room in this house will go through a variety of temperatures—both high and low—before the day is over.

* * *

Every year my family comes together to my parents' house in north Georgia to celebrate the holidays the weekend before Christmas. I fly in from New York. My brother Charlie drives down from his home near the north Alabama border. My youngest sister Robin, her husband, and two children arrive from North Carolina. And my sister Debbie, who lives nearby, handles most of the cooking—arriving with a buffet of turkey, ham, sweet potato casserole, cranberry salad, and gallons of sweet tea along with her husband, her daughter Christy, and Christy's two young children.

There is a smaller family gathering at Thanksgiving at my parents' house, but I opt out of joining this one for the opportunity to travel. I've spent Thanksgiving solo and with friends in Amsterdam, Rome, Barcelona, London, and exploring the Mayan ruins near Belize, among other places. I see these trips as educational, inspirational, and a chance for tranquility, one of the few periods of the year when my day job as a corporate paralegal does not follow me on vacation.

By contrast, my trips to Atlanta at Christmastime arrive during a busy time at work. It's usually a short trip for me, always framed by some office event that must be attended to before I leave or when I return, and I am often fretting about the state of the weather and potential airport closures preventing my return to Manhattan.

My travel and work concerns, however, are largely inconsequential in this house, though they do give me a way to voice my presence. My family has never understood my life in New York, never understood why I left Atlanta for the North, why I wanted to work in the theater or what I did when I did or why I gave it up when I decided it was time to move on to something else. They never understood why I was always struggling to earn an income and for years I kept my reasons private, hearing only their disappointment when I said I could not afford to come home for the holidays. I think they largely thought of me as self-absorbed, selfish, and conceited, when what I really felt was different from them in many ways. When I finally came out to my family as gay they understood little about that struggle and wanted to know even less about it. There are no discussions of gay politics in my home, no mention of gay rights or gay pride, no support of gay marriage. There was no interest in knowing of any of my dates or boyfriends or relationships with other men. I stopped sharing my desire to be a writer when I witnessed first their silent reception to my work and then their disappointment over my choice of subjects, so a quiet loneliness always haunts me during my trips to see my family because I feel stifled and inconsequential. My mother once said to me about the fact that I was gay, "We didn't want to tell anyone else in the neighborhood or at church. We wanted to keep it private, only in the family."

After I finish my morning coffee and a muffin, I shave and shower in the upstairs bathroom, joining my father downstairs in his den while we read the morning newspaper. This room has wood paneled walls and is so overheated I keep a glass of ice water near my chair to keep from feeling dehydrated. Hanging on the walls of this room are photos of airplanes my father helped design as an engineer. Years ago my mother studied oil painting, and her bright colored canvases of rural landscapes are also on the walls, alongside photographs and souvenirs brought back from my parents' travels to Hawaii, Alaska, Europe, and the Middle East.

But the centerpiece of this room is the television. My father likes to keep the local news on for most of the day, but he is also a fan of the political opinion shows that Fox news broadcasts. I have more than once left the room when he has settled into watching one of these shows, and it took him a few years to understand that my passive-aggressive behavior was prompted because I did not agree with the commentators. We're not a

THE HOUSE OF TEN THOUSAND TEMPERATURES

family of political debaters and once I moved North I learned my opinions were a minority in the South. By nature I am not a confrontational man and my preference now is to keep my opinions as concealed as the other details of my life are expected to be. I've learned after many family visits to steer the conversation to neutral topics and to seek out harmless programs on the TV that will not reveal anything about myself that my family might find ungentlemanly. I only want to enjoy their company, not engage in an annual, ongoing battle or disagreement or disapproval. As my father is reading the Sunday comics I reach for the remote and change the channel. When my brother arrives a few minutes later we are watching a show about a man who eats bizarre foods in foreign places.

* * *

Growing up, my favorite dessert was my mother's pineapple upside down cake, baked so that the butter melted into the brown sugar and cinnamon to form small nuggets of candy. My family has never been one of healthy eaters, and on my own as an adult I have not been an adventurous cook. The only recipe I ever requested from my mom was the one for her string bean casserole made with cream of mushroom soup. Even the times when I cooked for friends, dates or boyfriends, my culinary skills were limited to simple dishes and today I prefer to survive on take-out meals rather than to cook in my small Manhattan apartment. My sisters, however, cook many of the dishes our mom used to make: fried meats, soupy casseroles, and heavy desserts.

Throughout the house my sister Debbie has deposited her holiday baked goods prior to our family gathering: platters of oatmeal and chocolate chip cookies, a bowl of sugar cookies, a frosted pound cake, and a large round tin of party mix, a recipe that she inherited from our childhood from the back of a cereal box and perfected by experimentation. It is gooey treat of cereal, pretzels, and nuts covered with a sauce made of peanut butter, butter, and Worcester sauce, so addictive you can't eat only one handful and guaranteed to fill your stomach and raise your blood pressure.

Last night, feeling old, vulnerable, and directionless in this house, I reached for the party mix and ate too much of it. It's no wonder that this morning I feel bloated and headachy from all of the sodium. Traveling always makes me constipated and for years I've suffered from a variety of digestive issues: acid reflux, painful air pockets traveling through my intestines, and hemorrhoids that burn and bleed, all of which I know that others in my family have suffered with.

When a tiny Chihuahua taps its way into the den and stares at me as if I am an alien from outer space, I know my sister Robin is up. Boomer, the Chihuahua, is Robin's shadow, rarely straying out of her orbit. I can hear Robin, just steps away in the kitchen, rustling through the cabinets and the refrigerator for something to serve breakfast to her children and husband. Soon, the sizzle and smell of sausage patties is wafting into the den. Parched, dehydrated, and sweating in the heat of the room, I reach for my glass of iced water.

* * *

To an outsider it would appear we are a well-read family. Books and newspapers and magazines are scattered throughout the house. We've lived in the house since 1963, when we moved here from a smaller house about a mile away. I was beginning third grade then and many of the books still in our parents' house date from my school years; there are science fiction novels by Ray Bradbury and Isaac Asimov, books by William Faulkner, Thomas Wolfe, and Rudyard Kipling that were on my library readings lists, adventure books like *Kon Tiki* and *The Last of the Mohicans*, books on UFO sightings and real life encounters with ghosts, biographies of Cole Porter, Judy Garland, and Zelda and Scott Fitzgerald. There are hardcover issues of *American Heritage* and stacks of *National Geographic*. My father joined a book club at some point after our move to the house and large, decorative hardcover editions of classics such as *Treasure Island*, *Dracula*, and *Oliver Twist* fill other shelves, many in slipcovers and with interior illustrations.

But most of the reading material now scattered throughout the house belongs to my father. After his retirement, my father began tracing our family history and in the process became an expert in genealogy. Our family is as much Northern as it is Southern, straddling the Mason-Dixon line with roots in West Virginia and Pennsylvania, before migrations to North Carolina and Florida. After learning that our Scottish ancestors fought in the American Revolution, my father joined the local chapter of the Sons of the American Revolution and began helping others search for their ancestral heritage. Stacks and stacks of folders and papers throughout the house are the products of my father's research. My father, who was stationed in Germany in the immediate years after World War II, marches in veterans' parades, attends dedication ceremonies at cemeteries and civic centers, and delivers speeches on our ancestors to elementary schools and women's groups, often dressed in Revolutionary War attire or wearing a kilt displaying the plaid of our ancestors.

My father traced our family lineage back fifteen generations to Scotland and France, writing up facts and synopses of our history that he uncovered in church registries, census data, and real estate documents. Of distinction are my paternal grandmother, born hearing impaired and educated at the West Virginia School for the Deaf, relatives who fought for both the Union and Confederate forces in the Civil War, an Indian princess of the Delaware Lenni-Lenape tribe, and the mayor of a village in Alsace in the 1600s, but nowhere is there anyone identified as homosexual. It's hard for me to believe that I sprang out of nowhere, that my desires were not shared by someone else in our long lineage, that who I am and my homosexuality is not, in part, biologically determined and shared by other, even distant, family members. The only reference I can recall to another gay person in the family was a subtle, indirect one my father made one year when he was gathering research on our family from the son of a distant cousin in New Jersey. "He's a bachelor like you," my father said, without any further details provided.

* * *

At the time my mother took possession of my boyhood bedroom, my father began using my older brother's bedroom as an office. Inside it now are bookcases filled with books and folders, a large desk, and a hand-built computer that my father proudly assembled from various components. This second-floor bedroom has a window facing the street and is directly above the always overheated family den. I have few memories of this room, in part, because it was my brother's and I was in seldom invited inside it. When I arrived home this year, two days before our family gathering on Sunday, my father asked if I would remove the boxes that I had stored in my brother's bedroom closet because he wanted to use the space to install another bookcase.

His request surprised me. It had been more than thirty years since I had last lived in this house and I didn't recall putting anything in my brother's room and I was sure my father was mistaken. When I asked what were in the boxes, he answered, "Some of your stuff."

The contents of the boxes haunted me until Saturday morning when I entered my brother's former bedroom. The room was so crowded with piles of books and folders there was little room to stand. I know I have inherited my father's inability to discard anything on paper; my apartment in Manhattan is as crowded as this room. I have piles and piles of manuscripts started and never completed, boxes full of notes and research and cassette tapes and disks where I stored more material. A few years ago I helped my father move some items out of the basement of this house because he wanted to have it waterproofed. Everything in the basement was moved to the new garage that my father had built at the end of the driveway, a garage that does not house any of the cars he owns but is used, instead, for the storage of the lawnmower and gardening tools, planting pots and trays, folding tables and deck chairs, and other outdoor clutter acquired over time. One of the items I carried from the basement to the garage were old issues from the 1960s of *Popular Mechanic* and *Woodworker* magazine. Resident in the basement of our house for as long as I can remember is a table saw and my father's hobbies and projects have included making wooden toys and folk instruments. (I still possess the dulcimer he made for me in the 1970s.) When I asked my dad why he was keeping these magazines he had not looked at in years, no, *decades*, I detected his frown as he answered "Why would I throw them out?"

So it was with irony and curiosity that I approached the boxes in my brother's closet, a near impossible task that involved contorting my body to lift and move them to a place where they would not topple over any other items. I maneuvered the five boxes out into the cold upstairs hallway where no heat vents are located, sitting on the top stair to look through the contents and wearing a second sweater because of the cold. Most of the boxes were filled with my college textbooks and the graduate school catalogs I poured through as I was deciding to make my move out of this house. I bagged up the books that I could throw out and boxed the books that I would take to the used bookstore that operated out of a former gas station on the "four-lane highway" as we had always called the main road that ran from downtown Marietta to Roswell. I was able to winnow the five boxes down to one, deciding to keep some college course notes and some childhood memorabilia that had found their way into the boxes, such as the pennants and postcards I had collected from our family's many road trips along the eastern corridor. I found a new space for the solo box in the closet of my former bedroom, in exactly the same spot I once kept my favorite magazines, hoping that the unlabeled box would go unnoticed in the house for a little while longer.

I used my father's tiny electric shredder and set to work shredding my SAT and GRE scores, my elementary report cards, and old letters from high school friends that we mailed to each other our first years in college. I was amazed that I could handle erasing my younger life without regret or nostalgia, though I found it harder to accept that my parents would not cast any sentimentality of their own toward their child's early belongings. Years before in Manhattan, when I moved in with a boyfriend who thought he wanted to be in a relationship, I had cast out boxes of my books and household items onto the sidewalks of New York, painfully watching from my fifth story apartment window as passersby sorted through my former possessions, some which had traveled with me from Atlanta to New York. I still carry a loss for some of those possessions, in part, out of the anger I still harbor against the former boyfriend.

Somewhere near the end of my shredding my father's machine jammed and short-circuited with a tiny, exasperating *zap!* I finished the last items by tearing them up by hand, bagging up the trash, and delivering all of it to the garbage cans outside on the driveway by the garage.

Back in the house I realized my back hurt and I was emotionally exhausted, having traveled through too many memories in such a short time. I told my father I would replace the short-circuited shredder before I left for New York and went to my sister's bedroom to take a nap.

* * *

My sister Debbie arrives at the house at noon on Sunday. It is warm in the kitchen where she and her husband Brian are setting up hot plates and arranging the food she has been preparing all week. The imperfect temperature annoys her and she goes to the thermostat and shuts the heat off completely. I've learned to steer a clear berth while she and the others are working in the kitchen. Years before, when I worried that I didn't offer enough help in the preparations, my mother told me that my parents helped my sister with all the expenses of our family gathering and I realized it wasn't expected of me.

My sister also likes to take command of the house, something she was not entirely successful at when we were all children and she was the lost middle child. I probably made her teenage years more miserable than they should have been; she followed behind a brother with a perfect A grade record and who was his high school class valedictorian. My sister Debbie is a loud, bossy, strident woman, and I don't say that in any sort of a demeaning way. In fact, I believe she is the single person who has held us together as a family. Without her, I think I might have strayed much further than I already have. She has also had her own misfortunes too. Her son, Justin, was as headstrong, determined, stubborn, and combative as she is, and many details I knew about him were relayed to me second-hand through my parents because even in our family, some things are not even discussed between us. Two years before, Justin died at the age of twenty-six of an accidental combination of alcohol and drugs after attending a rock concert. I know my sister must think daily about her son, about all the "what ifs" she could have faced to have made things turn out different.

That "what ifs" are a game I play a lot when I am back in Georgia, driving through neighborhood streets that are familiar to me even as they continue to become overdeveloped with tiny mansions, strip-malls, and multi-lane roads. Long ago I lost my boyish figure, my weight ballooning up because of medication and booze, and though I have many gay friends in Manhattan, I've stepped out of the dating and hookup games. At home in Georgia I think about the life I might have had if I wasn't gay, or the life I might have had if I had kept my sexuality closeted, or if I had taken the insurance job instead of deciding to go to graduate school or if I had decided to marry my high school girlfriend, or if I had decided to tell my college friend that I loved him.

I don't think I became the man I imagined I would become, certainly my life is no longer gay in the way that it used to be. Being gay in my fifties doesn't have the purport that it did when I was in my twenties. My biggest vice, other than imbibing too frequently, is surfing to adult gay sites on the Web. Yet I don't dwell on my regrets, don't fret about decisions I made a certain crossroads, but like every other human on the planet, I still wonder why things happened the way they did and what things might have happened if things were different.

*   *   *

The house now swells with more family. Jennifer and Westley, my niece and nephew, are up and chatting away. Debbie's daughter, Christy, has arrived with her two children: Reese, a large ten-year-old boy who wants to be a football player, and Claire, his six-year-old sister who is the beauty of the family and who is terrorizing Boomer with a dancing, stuffed Santa Claus toy. Brian, Debbie's husband, is a strong, calming center to all this activity, keeping both the cooking and conversation flowing amongst all of us. In the den, someone has flipped the TV channel to a program where bidders are searching for undiscovered treasures in storage units, and my brother and I quiz my mother about potential valuable items in our house. I've often wished we possessed some unknown priceless item or heirloom that could keep us all living in luxury, but anything of value would have to be split four ways with my siblings. I suspect that my sisters might have their eyes on my mother's good china, a set which she purchased the year in the mid-Sixties when we lived abroad in England and hasn't been used in decades, and if I had room for it, I would want my grandmother's Edison phonograph with records thicker than the plates of my mother's coveted china. But the only thing I would battle all of them over is my copy of the first issue of the comic book *Teen Titans*, probably more sentimental than financial value, and lost somewhere in the clutter of this house.

By two we are all gathered in the kitchen. We form a prayer circle and my father recites a blessing that he has used for every meal I have ever spent with him. We parade in front of the buffet of food, filling up our paper plates with the holiday meal, sitting at tables in the sun room, where we gather to eat and talk.

Outside, the procession of the birds to the window feeder continues. I take a seat at the small card table where Brian sits with his grandchildren Reese and Claire. In between bites of turkey and cranberry salad, I ask my six-year-old great niece about her boyfriends, a subject she likes discussing and laughing about.

Soon, however, the inevitable happens. Politics make not one appearance, but many. Complaints ripple around the table about Obamacare. My mother mentions her fear of Hilary Clinton, and then the subject of gun control is the topic of conversation. My father is opposed to any restrictions on the "right to bear arms." He explains that our government was framed so that the people could be able to take action against the government, when and if it becomes necessary.

Drowsy from the trytophans of the turkey, I mistakenly make my way into the conversation against my better judgment, asking my father, lightly, if he is a supporter of the right to bear arms, what guns does he possess? As far as I know, outside of his military service, my father has probably never fired a gun.

Suddenly, my dad points to a pistol mounted near the ceiling of the sun room. I suppose it has always been there, lost among the brickbrak of my mother's souvenirs that cover this room. He mentions that it is a pistol used in the Revolutionary war, and in the den, mounted above the bookcase, are two rifles used in the Civil War. My father also mentions a type of musket he marches with when wearing his Revolutionary War garb.

Astonished, I ask, "But do you have any bullets for them?"

"That's not the point," he answers. "Obama wants to take them away. We couldn't have any of those if he had his way."

* * *

Dessert is over and the young children are restless. Claire and Reese are in the living room where their presents have been placed beneath a tree, lifting each up suspiciously to their ears and trying to determine what might be inside by shaking the box. We all gather in this room to watch them open their gifts. Years before, my sister complained about the expense of giving gifts to everyone at Christmas when we were assembled, and rightly so as we were growing into a larger and extended family. For a few years we tried pulling names out of a hat to give only one gift each to a family member, till one year someone was forgotten and we abandoned that practice to hand out holiday cards instead. Every year I insert into each card a lottery ticket that I have purchased the day before at the local gas station, one of the Georgia instant winner scratch off games. It's a big hit when everyone opens their card, scratches for a prize, and declares their winnings or moans their lack of any. I see this as my subtle inside joke, a way of bringing in a little sin during the celebration of a religious holiday.

This year the kids have received candy and clothes and toys and gift cards. Wrapping paper is strewn around the floor and Boomer is inspecting everything larger than himself with suspicious sniffs and eyes.

We disperse now into various rooms about the house or outside for smoke breaks. All of my siblings and their spouses smoke; both of my parents smoked when they were young but easily gave it up when they began to raise a family. My mother refused to allow anyone to smoke inside the house and after too many years of cigarette butts smashed into the driveway, a clay pot with sand now stands near the back door and is used to extinguish all cigarettes.

Stopping smoking was one of the hardest things I've changed about myself, in part, because I did it while I was fighting a depression over other changes that were happening in my life. Now the vice I keep hidden from my family is the liquor and wine bottles I smuggle into the house to drink at night in the upstairs bedroom to help me fall asleep. I don't recall my parents ever drinking anything alcoholic when I was young, even on special occasions, though my father now indulges in a beer before bedtime because he has heard of its beneficial effects, though I doubt he would feel that way about the amount of alcohol I consume before sleep.

THE HOUSE OF TEN THOUSAND TEMPERATURES

Without a vice to slip into while everyone is around, I sit in a recliner and take a nap while pretending to watch an episode of a program on Animal Planet. Later when I awake, I am sweating around the collar of my shirt. My stomach feels as if I have swallowed a sponge. And someone has turned the heat up again. I go to the living room where the thermostat has always been located and find that the needle refuses to budge. When I snap off the plastic lid, I see that the battery inside has corroded from age. It is then that I remember that my father had all of the dynamics of this house renovated some years ago, about the time my mom began complaining about the heat in my former upstairs bedroom, and that there is no longer one thermostat for this house, but *many*.

I find my brother and father talking about investments at the table in the sun room. My brother has recently sold some of the undeveloped property in North Georgia that he owns with a friend from high school, an investment that is now paying off for him. Charlie has now decided to become a day trader, investing in penny stocks, though one of the obstacles he faces is not having Internet service or cellphone coverage at his isolated mountaintop home. Charlie shares my burly physique, though his full beard makes him distinctly more of a country boy than a city one. My sister Debbie loves to affectionately describe Charlie as a man living after his time. Charlie owns a large swath of property in north Georgia in an area adored by hunters. He lives in a house created out of the metal storage cab of transport truck embellished with hand-built rooms. The year I saw it I thought it was surprisingly roomy but potentially very cold to live in during the winter months. This house was built after the log cabin my brother was building burned down, the aftereffect of his falling asleep while smoking. Charlie has worked as a tree pruner, a window installer, and raised goats with a now ex-girlfriend. One year my mother proudly told me she had bought him a cow. Now my brother grows vegetables and flowers which he sells at a nearby outdoor market in the warmer months, along with the large jars of raw honey that he collects from the bee hives he maintains on his land. This time of year he sometimes sells wreaths made of pine tree branches and naturally grown and hand-made holiday items.

I have often wanted to write about my brother, though I have avoided it out of fear of depicting him incorrectly, or worse, cartoonish. It's easy to say that his temperature—or his temperament—is different from the rest of us and it has taken us all many years to understand this. Though it is also clearly possible to see our family's characteristics and peculiarities resonating strongly within my brother.

When I interrupt and ask my brother how he plans to be a day trader without an Internet connection, he tells me he logs on at the local library. Then he segues into a complaint about not having a neighbor living close enough to him to piggy-back on their Internet service.

* * *

My sister Robin is the first to leave, rounding up her teenagers and her husband Terry. A winter storm is headed toward the Mid-Atlantic States and it is a six-hour drive to my sister's house in North Carolina. I always wish I could spend more time with Robin. She is quiet, like myself, but also reminds me most of our mother. Growing up, I wonder if I gave her as much time and attention as I should have. We suffered through my teaching her piano and how to drive a car, things I don't think I was very good teacher at, but I've often wondered how different her memories and experiences of our family life are from mine. She settled into a career as a catalog production stylist which makes all of us proud, and her son and daughter are certainly more respectful of their relatives than I ever was at their ages. When I see her with her family I wonder about what kind of children I might have raised. What kind of father would I have been?

My sister Debbie and her family are the next to leave, giving leftovers to my brother and parents for future meals. We wave goodbye from the driveway, the winter air feeling moist and invigorating after the close warmness of the house.

THE HOUSE OF TEN THOUSAND TEMPERATURES

Next, Charlie is out the door, wanting to reach to his mountaintop destination before it is dark.

I often thought about how easy it is for them to come and go, driving in for a brief visit and leaving, while my visits during the holiday season must be more planned and that I stay for days in the house we grew up, every year floundering as my adult sensibilities crash against my younger self.

* * *

It has been a long day and I've eaten too much. I am restless, bored, and exhausted. Alone in the house with my parents I know from experience that it will be impossible for me to settle down to read a book or watch a movie without interruption. My mother usually knows when I am preoccupied and insistent on finding me wherever I am hiding and asking me if I am still hungry. Even making a brief phone call to a friend has the potential for interruption, but I decide to walk upstairs and try to reach my friend Andrew on my cellphone, but I only get his voice mail and I leave a message telling him I wish he still lived in Atlanta, so I could go visit him and escape the house.

Downstairs as I walk through the den I catch the weather report on the news, warnings about the storm that sent my sister home early and which is likely to ground life to a halt in several states, before finding my parents seated in the sun room, which is now blazing with lights because the sun is setting. Though I am far from hungry, out of boredom I reach for a handful of my sister's party mix. As I am chewing and swallowing it occurs to me that there is nowhere for this food to go in my body. I've reached my max, but because it is impossible not to eat more party mix, I take another handful.

My father asks me when my flight is tomorrow, and I tell him late afternoon, but if I get to the airport early I might be able to get on an earlier flight.

I explain that every year I am usually able to change flights, though recently the airlines have been cutting back on the number of flights and overbooking the scheduled ones, and

I mention that there were two passengers with the same seat ticket on my flight to Atlanta.

My mother says, "Well, maybe you'll get lucky and you'll find a pretty girl to sit on your lap."

It's an odd comment and my reaction is not one of disgust, mostly surprise, and I shake it off with a laugh. Whatever discomfort I show is not because of any of her insensitivity to having a gay son, but of the party mix and other digestibles churning through my intestines. My need to get to the bathroom is sudden and swift and I abruptly leave my parents in the sun room.

I am on the toilet in the upstairs bathroom when I hear my mother calling my name from the foot of the stairs. Everything I have held inside the last few days is coming out of me and dropping into the toilet. I take a breath and yell to my mom that I am in the bathroom and will be downstairs in a minute.

I am surprised when I hear my mother's voice outside the bathroom door. "I'm sorry, Jimmy," she is saying. "I apologize for saying the wrong thing. You don't hate me, do you?"

It takes me a second to realize what she is talking about, the insinuation that I would like a pretty girl sitting on my lap. I have no idea what my parents must have said to each other after I abruptly left them downstairs, but I realize now that I must have left them with the wrong impression.

"Of course, I don't hate you," I answer and wonder if she thinks that I had fled to the bathroom to sulk or cry. Why would she even think that I would hate her? I might be quiet, passive-aggressive, and secretive, but I am clearly not the kind of grown man who would hate his mother and it depresses me to think that she might have thought that *this* was the kind of man I had become. I take another breath and say, lightly, "I'm on the toilet. I'll be downstairs in a minute."

My bowels constrict because I want to hurry the effort along, so I strain and push and then decide to clean myself up.

A few minutes later downstairs in the kitchen I find my mom and kiss her on the cheek and tell her I love her. Out of the corner of my eye I see my father adjusting the thermostat.

*   *   *

The following morning I have breakfast with my parents and drive to the used bookstore to drop off my unwanted college text books, and am surprised to learn that the store doesn't want them so I toss the books into the dumpster behind the store. I make a stop at a strip-mall where there is an office supply store and buy my dad a replacement shredder and return home.

An hour later I am on the highway on the way to the airport, headed back to Manhattan, wondering if I will be able to catch an early flight. My rental car retains the chill of abandonment as I said goodbyes to my parents. I lean down and study the unfamiliar knobs on the dashboard, cranking the heat up as soon I discover how it can be done.

FIFTEEN MINUTES MORE

MEMO TO: The Screenwriter and Director

RE: The Movie Version

Here are a few suggested scenes that you might wish to incorporate when you make the movie version.

I was twenty-four years old when I met Ethel Merman. She was seventy-two. It was the winter of 1980. I was an apprentice publicist in a small public relations firm in Manhattan that was representing the grand opening of a disco roller rink on the west side of Manhattan. Ms. Merman was a good friend of the two women who owned and ran the PR firm. For the photo op everyone was to wear roller skates, including me and Miss Merman. (Please note that this was before the advent of roller blades, so every boot was a four-wheeler). I was to stand behind Miss Merman and keep her propped up as she did a small kick step for the photographers. I had had an alcoholic drink before I did this. Maybe two. I kept slipping and losing my balance. Ms. Merman, however, was a pro and loudly let me know that I wasn't doing a very good job. She let out an expletive that I will not repeat here and found someone else to hold her up. It was a humbling experience. To this day I am always trying to improve my roller skating skills. Suggested background music for this scene: Any track from the Ethel Merman disco album that she was promoting. (1979, Arista Records)

July 4th weekend, probably that same year. After attending a rooftop party on the Upper West Side, my friend Barry and I drive his car, an old Honda Civic, toward Rhode Island to visit his family. It is dark, except for the light coming from the roads and cars. Somewhere on I-95 in Connecticut we have a blowout. On the side of the road we open the trunk and discover there is no spare tire. (Please note that this was also long before cellphones were available to the general consumer.) Barry and I, in our best summer party outfits, walk along the highway to the nearest exit where we find a service station just closing up shop. The two attendants, about our age, mimic us as they turn us away. Barry and I decide to walk in the other direction, ignoring those fools so they will not kill us. We walk through a bad section of a town. It is dark and spooky. And now close to midnight. Just as we are about to give up hope and begin to truly fear for our lives in this bleak and dismal section of town, we spot a tire store on the horizon. It is brightly lit. And open. A half-hour later, with a new tire, we are back on the road. Suggested phrase for one of us to hum at the scariest moment: The theme song from the movie *Jaws*.

Flash forward several years. I am no longer a publicist. (Thank *God!*) I am working as a temp for a corporate office located in Princeton. I am to be at this position for two weeks. I have nothing to do. The phones do not ring. There is nothing to type. (Unlike an earlier job where I typed rows of license plates of cars which were abandoned property—a *thrilling* job.) I am bored to tears. I do not get along with the man I am working for. He is suspicious of me because I am not female and blonde and big-busted. My belief is that he will never use my temp agency again for sending them a male secretary. One morning he asks me to get him a cup of coffee. I tell him I do not do coffee service but if there is anything he would like for me to type or file I would be glad to do so. I lose the job earlier than expected. I am not invited back to work the second week. A note on casting: the boss should be played by someone short and mean-tempered, think Danny DeVito *without* the sense of humor.

Washington D.C. April 25, 1993. My friend John has recruited us as volunteers for The March on Washington. There are close to a million people participating in this march for gay rights. John and I are given orange T-shirts with the word "MARSHALL" printed on them in bold black capital letters. Our first assignment is to direct every single person emerging from a subway stop to different places on the Washington Mall. We do this for an hour until we are dizzy and another organizer gives us a new assignment. Our new assignment is to organize the order of the procession of the contingents of states in the parade. We walk over to the lawn near the Washington Memorial where thousands of people are assembling. Behind signs marked "New Jersey" and "Illinois" gay men and lesbians wait to march through the streets of the nation's capital proclaiming their pride and necessity for equal rights for all. At one point, I make the entire state of Michigan shift from one side of the hill to another. Several hundred people change their direction when I open my mouth and yell, "Michigan, this way!" This is true power, the ability to move people, to make people physically move. I am empowered! I am proud! I even consider buying a rainbow flag that day!

My brother is ten years old. I am six. We live with our parents in a small house in Los Angeles (Van Nuys, circa early 1960s). We wake up early on Christmas morning. It is still dark out but we are too excited to sleep. We go into the living room where the Christmas tree is set up and we find our presents and the gifts Santa Claus has left for us. We take them back to our bedroom. We open all of our presents. A few hours later our father discovers us assembling my brother's new racing car set. Our father is not happy. His face shows shock, sadness, and a flash of fury. We, however, love our new toys! Our faces are full of love and glee!

Same age. Same house. I am an indestructible first-grader. One day at home I decide that I will turn our nondescript backyard into a playground. I shimmy up the unused pole set in concrete that any ordinary household would use as one end of a clothesline but which my mother refuses to create because she has a new electric dryer. I decide to practice my gymnastic twirl on the side spoke of the pole. I do not remember if the spoke broke or if I did an unsuccessful twirl. But I do remember I hit the ground and broke my left arm. This will be the first incident that affirms a life of unathletic behavior.

Another accident. My brother and I are in the front yard of our house in Marietta, Georgia, a suburb of Atlanta, where we now live. He is twelve and I am seven. My brother has decided he wants to be a juggler. He is using concrete croquette balls. He offers to teach me how to juggle and tosses me the ball. I miss the catch and it strikes my lip, chipping one of my front teeth. This chipped tooth is replaced a few days later with a silver cap. It will be another eight years before I get an enamel cap. I will spend many formative years not smiling.

I am twelve and in the eighth grade. It is an awkward year for me. All of my classmates speak in a sexual subtext I do not understand. Their hormones are raging out of control and mine are not. Every morning I wake up and look under my arm to see if any hair is growing there. My armpit is hairless. One day in class a girl mimics the way I am sitting at my desk while the teacher is out of the room. She crosses her legs, girly style, and swings the top one back and forth. Soon I find that I am holding my books wrong too (in the clutch of my arm, not at my side like a guy is supposed to do). My biggest faux pas turns out to be wearing white socks with my loafers. Soon I am so mortified by my own behavior that I begin wearing dark blue socks with my sneakers. I spend the rest of my life worrying about whether I am doing things the right or wrong way.

I am thirty-eight years old and learning how to roller blade. I have purchased a cheap pair of skates from a discount store on Canal Street in Lower Manhattan. They make a strange noise when I wear them, like there is sand caught in the ball bearings. My boyfriend and I skate from his apartment on the Upper East Side to see a concert in Union Square. (Betty Buckley, former star of *Eight is Enough* and now a Broadway diva, is performing for free.) After the concert, we skate back along First Avenue. At the steep downward hill at East 58th

Street I lose control. I do not know how to brake and skate at the same time. I crash into a brick wall to stop myself from crashing into a lane of traffic headed toward the 59th Street bridge. My tooth is not chipped and my arm is not broken. Luckily, all that is wounded this time is my pride.

Please note that there are several themes running through these suggested scenes. Among them are "skating," "celebrities," "pride," and "jobs." At another temp job, working for a publishing company located in a building on Broadway, I am the assistant to a team of advertising salespeople. It is a lackluster job that makes me miserable. One morning, en route to the mail room with a stack of envelopes in my arms (carried the proper, butch way), I am waiting in front of the elevator. The light indicates that the elevator doors are about to open. Instead of courteously waiting to the side, as I normally do, I wait at the center of the doors, not expecting anyone to arrive to work at this late hour. As the doors open, I collide with a man who is exiting. He smiles at me and says hello just as I say, "Excuse me." The man is John F. Kennedy, Jr. I do not remember if the packages made it to the mailroom but I remember thinking we might be best friends now.

I realize that I have dropped names at the beginning and the end of this memorandum. Please let me reiterate here that I am not a star fucker, a celebrity worshipper, or a celebrity myself. (In the terms of a friend and fellow writer, I am merely "baby famous"—because living and working in Manhattan for more than four decades has put me in contact with many famous people.) If I consciously wanted to drop names and celebrity situations I have been in I could say that I've ridden in a limo with John Travolta, had lunch at Sardi's with Eve Arden, visited Alec Baldwin in his backstage dressing room, and had Liza Minnelli flick the ashes of her cigarette against my wrist. None of these, however, would make terrific scenes in this movie. They would only prove my character to be hysterical, moody, bored, insipid, and awe-struck. These moments *could* make for a nice montage or offer a skilled and talented director a chance to give his industry friends a few cameos to boost the appeal of the script. I would be willing to elaborate on any of the above, as well as suggest songs for the soundtrack.

I have also left out the day I stood in line behind the Academy Award-winning actress Julia Roberts at the take-out burrito place on 23rd Street and Eighth Avenue. (Okay, it didn't happen to me, it happened to a friend of mine, but I did see her once walking on Ninth Avenue.) I feel certain that if we could work in a role for Julia Roberts into this script it would also make the project more timely and bankable. Nobody will turn down a Julia Roberts vehicle, even if it stars another famous actress *pretending* to be Julia Roberts.

I would suggest that no scenes be included which depict me typing or working at a computer in my apartment. Not that I don't think I am unphotogenic in my pajamas, but a movie about my life should show some true action and drama.

And books. The books cannot be overlooked. I should always be depicted as carrying books, reading books, shelving books, looking at books. Perhaps a scene at a bookstore, or a library, or a book fair, I am sure there is a way you can instill drama into a life with books.

And while there are many moments from my life that a good screenwriter and director will be able to shape into serious moments of dramatic acting, I would like to stress that I want to be depicted as a man who is grateful to be alive and happy to have the life he has been given. Imagine a character at a fork in the road and he chooses the correct path. Here is one particular example. It is August 2015 and I am fifty-nine years old and working on the final version of this lengthy collection of intimate writings. I have to stop and start working on it many times, primarily because I have a day job with too many responsibilities where I have to show up five days a week in order to earn enough money to pay my rent and run a small publishing company. On top of this I have scheduled an appointment with my cardiologist, in order to get a prescription renewed. Every appointment I have ever had with a cardiologist takes hours and hours away from my life, because I must go through a series of tests and procedures only to be told that I have an incurable heart disease and will likely die very soon. A few years before I had a muscle spasm in my left shoulder that mimicked a heart attack and I was sent through more tests, including having an angiogram in a hospital (which confirmed it was only a muscle spasm) and several consultations with another cardiologist who wanted to implant a defibrillator in my chest in case I had a real heart attack (and which I refused to have done). The August morning of my appointment I walk forty-five minutes across town in the blistering Manhattan heat, stopping at a bodega to buy bottled water. When I reach the doctor's office I am drenched in sweat and struggling to catch my breath. When I see my cardiologist I tell her that I feel fine, other than a strain in my neck, which I can attribute to the way I sit in my apartment in my pajamas and work at my laptop on this lengthy collection of intimate writings. The cardiologist sends me through a battery of tests before she will renew my prescription. At the end of a few hours, she sits in a chair and with a serious expression asks me about my medication. I tell her about the aggressive therapy I have been doing to relieve the arthritis in my legs. She frowns and looks more concerned. I think she is preparing me for the worst. She says, "I don't know how to tell you this," and then pauses dramatically. In her pause I imagine being rushed to the hospital in an ambulance and tossed on top of an operating table. Instead, she sighs and says, "Whatever you are doing is working. There's nothing wrong. Your heart is normal." I spend a few minutes asking questions and find that there has been no further thickening of my heart muscle. My doctor does not tell me that I am cured and I do not say that I believe in miracles. Instead, she writes me a new prescription and tells me she wants to see me in a year. I feel certain that a good screenwriter will be able to craft some pithy dialogue for this scene in the movie of my life and that a good director will be able to capture the vibrant summer day as I leave the doctor's office and make my way through the city to the office where I work. But I know it will take an extraordinary actor to capture the kind of joy that I feel at this moment, that after years of being told that I am likely to die at any moment, that instead, I can go out and live another year. Even though I gave up dreams of being an actor years ago, I would like to be offered the opportunity to audition for this role. After all, I've been rehearsing for it for a long time. And I've got the perfect way to drop my jaw before I break out into a smile.

ACKNOWLEDGMENTS

Without an ongoing association with other authors, editors, and publishers, most of the writing in this collection would not exist, and I am indebted to their advice, assignments, and acceptance of these works.

"A Bookstore Tourist" was first published in 2008 on the author's blog, *Where You'll Find Me*.

"A Few Minutes with Liberace" was written in 2000.

"A Gathering Storm" was first published in 2014 as the introduction to the author's novel of the same name.

"A Personal History of the Epidemic" was first published in 1998 in *Body Positive*, and in 1999 in *Dallas Voice, Impact, The Bottom Line*, and *Lambda Book Report*.

"Actors" was written in 2001.

"Art History 101" was first published in 1996 in *Architrave*.

"Behind the Screen" was written in 1992.

"Between The Lines" was first published in 1993 in *Backspace*, in 1995 in *NEBO Literary Journal*, and in 1996 in *Apocalypse*.

"Buddies" was first published in 2003 in the anthology *Sex Buddies* and was included in the author's collection, *Desire, Lust, Passion, Sex* (Green Candy Press 2004, Chelsea Station Editions 2013).

"Caution" was first published in 1990 in *In Touch for Men*.

"Dates" was written in 1989.

"Desperado" was first published in 1994 as "Up from the Ashes" in *The Philadelphia Inquirer Magazine*, and in

1995 as "Desperado" in the *Cleveland Plain Dealer Sunday Magazine*.

"Dicks" was written in 2001.

"Do I Know You?" was first published in 2004 in the anthology *I Do/I Don't*, and was included in the author's collection *Still Dancing: New and Selected Stories* (Lethe Press 2009, Chelsea Station Editions 2011). It was reprinted in May, 2014 in *Chelsea Station*.

"Excerpts from a Stonewall Diary" was written during Pride Week, June, 1994.

"Fifteen Minutes More" was written in 2015.

"Finding New Hope" was first published in 1992 in *Christopher Street*.

"Friends" was first published in 1991 in *Au Courant*.

"Funny Guy" was first published in 1994 in *Body Positive*.

"Glasses" was written in 2001.

"Haircuts" was first published in 1990 in *In Touch for Men*.

"Hearts" was written in 2001.

"Hometown Sweethearts" was written in 2001.

"How Does My Garden Grow?" was written in 1990.

"Invitation to Dance" was first published in 1987 in the *New York Native*.

"Isn't It Romantic?" was first published in 1990 in *In Touch for Men*.

"It" was written in 1994 for World AIDS Day.

"July" was written in 1984.

"Just Looking" was first published in 1990 in *In Touch for Men*.

"Lessons" was first published in 1998 in the anthology *Men Seeking Men*, in 2000 in the anthology *Overload*, and was included in the author's collection *Desire, Lust, Passion, Sex* (Green Candy Press 2004, Chelsea Station Editions 2013).

"Lovers" was first published as "Three Lovers" in 2005 in *Velvet Mafia* and in 2009 in the anthology *I Like It Like That*.

"Magic Carpet Ride" was written in 1998 following the author's book tour for *Where the Rainbow Ends*.

"My Haunted History" was written in 2014. Portions were previously published in *Chelsea Station* and on Facebook.

"Old Things" was first published in 1993 as "Keepers" in *The Philadelphia Inquirer Magazine* and a revised version was published in 1994 as the introduction to the paperback edition of the author's collection *Dancing on the Moon: Short Stories about AIDS* (Penguin 1994, Chelsea Station Editions 2011).

"On a Day I Am Not Myself" was written in 2001.

"One Way or Another" was written in 1990.

"Passing Grades" was first published in 1987 in *The New York Native*. It is the author's first published work.

"Remnants" was written in 2001.

"Rock Hudson's Vacation" was first published in 2014 in *Assaracus 14, Joy Exhaustible*.

"Something From The Rain" was written in 1990. It was revised and first published in *Backspace*, 1994.

"Stages" was first published in June, 2014 in *Chelsea Station*.

"Still Dancing" was first published in 2001 in the anthology *Rebel Yell*, and was included in the author's collection, *Still Dancing: New and Selected Stories* (Lethe Press 2009, Chelsea Station Editions 2011).

"Strength" was first published in 1995 in *Lisp*.

"That Summer" was first published in 1993 in *Backspace*, in 1994 in *David's Place Journal*, in 1996 in *The Slate*, and was published in 1994 as "Undercurrents" in *The Philadelphia Inquirer Magazine*, and in 1995 as "Memories of a Lost Summer," in the *Ft. Lauderdale Sun Sentinel Sunshine Magazine*.

"The Child in Me" was first published in 1990 in *In Touch for Men*.

"The House of Ten Thousand Temperatures" was written in 2014.

"The Last Minute Friend" was written in 1984. A revised version was first published in 1988 in *Playguy*.

"The Pot" was written in 1998.

"The Right Man" was first published in 1990 in *In Touch for Men*, and in 1999 in the anthology *Boy Meets Boy*.

"Threads" was first published in 1992 in *Art & Understanding*. It was reprinted in March, 2015 in *Chelsea Station*.

"Treats" was written in 2001.

"Twilight on the Esplanade" was written in 2000.

"What Comes Around" was first published in 2012 in the author's novel of the same name and was reprinted in *Best Gay Stories*.

"What Did Not Change" was first published in 2001 as "Some Things Didn't Change" in the *Philadelphia Gay News*, and as "What Did Not Change" in *Frontiers*.

"What She Gave Me" was first published in 2000 in the anthology *Mamma's Boy* and in 2002 as "And My Heart Goes On" in the anthology *Rebel Yell 2*.

"Where You'll Find Me" was written in 1993.

"Why I Live Where I Do" was first published in 1990 in *In Touch for Men*.

"Writers" was written in 2001.

JAMESON CURRIER

Jameson Currier is the author of seven novels: *Where the Rainbow Ends*; *The Wolf at the Door*; *The Third Buddha*; *What Comes Around*; *The Forever Marathon, A Gathering Storm,* and *Based on a True Story*; four collections of short fiction: *Dancing on the Moon*; *Desire, Lust, Passion, Sex*; *Still Dancing: New and Selected Stories*; and *The Haunted Heart and Other Tales*; and a memoir: *Until My Heart Stops*. His short fiction has appeared in many literary magazines and Web sites, including *OutsiderInk, Velvet Mafia, Blithe House Quarterly, Absinthe Literary Review, Confrontation, Rainbow Curve, Christopher Street, Genre, Harrington Gay Men's Fiction Quarterly,* and the anthologies *Men on Men 5, Best American Gay Fiction 3, Certain Voices, Boyfriends from Hell, Men Seeking Men, Mammoth Book of New Gay Erotica, Best Gay Erotica, Best American Erotica, Best Gay Romance, Best Gay Stories, Circa 2000, Rebel Yell, I Do/I Don't, Where the Boys Are, Nine Hundred & Sixty-Nine, Wilde Stories, Unspeakable Horror, Art from Art,* and *Making Literature Matter*. His AIDS-themed short stories have also been translated into French by Anne-Laure Hubert and published as *Les Fantômes,* and he is the author of the documentary film, *Living Proof: HIV and the Pursuit of Happiness.* His reviews, essays, interviews, and articles on AIDS and gay culture have been published in many national and local publications, including *The Washington Post, The Los Angeles Times, Newsday, The Dallas Morning News, The St. Louis Post-Dispatch, The Minneapolis Star-Tribune, The Philadelphia Inquirer Magazine, Lambda*

Book Report, The Harvard Gay and Lesbian Review, Dallas Voice, The Washington Blade, Southern Voice, Metrosource, Bay Area Reporter, Frontiers, Ten Percent, The New York Native, The New York Blade, Out, and *Body Positive.* In 2010 he founded Chelsea Station Editions, an independent press devoted to gay literature, and the following year launched the literary magazine *Chelsea Station*, which has published the works of more than two hundred writers. In 2013, he edited two original anthologies: *With: New Gay Fiction* and *Between: New Gay Poetry.* The press also serves as the home for Mr. Currier's own writings which now span a career of more than four decades. Books published by the press have been honored by the Lambda Literary Foundation, the American Library Association GLBTRT Roundtable, the Saints and Sinners Literary Festival, the Gaylactic Spectrum Awards Foundation, and the Rainbow Book Awards. Mr. Currier is a member of the Board of Directors of the Arch and Bruce Brown Foundation, a recipient of a fellowship from New York Foundation for the Arts, and has been a judge for many literary competitions. He currently resides in New York.

The cover art for this edition is a collage created in 2015 by Patrick Bremer from a photograph of Jameson Currier taken in 1992 by David Logan Morrow for the first edition of the author's debut work, *Dancing on the Moon: Short Stories About AIDS*. The collage incorporates source material drawn from the covers of the ten works of fiction written by the author and published by Chelsea Station Editions.

More of Patrick Bremer's art may be viewed at: http://www.patrickbremer.co.uk/.

www.ingramcontent.com/pod-product-compliance
Lightning Source LLC
Chambersburg PA
CBHW031611160426
43196CB00006B/90